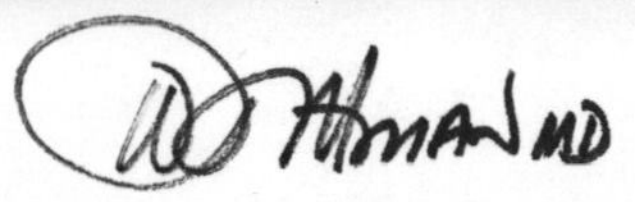

RADIOGRAPHIC ANATOMY OF THE CORONARY ARTERIES
An Atlas

by

Benigno Soto, M.D.
Associate Professor of Radiology
Department of Radiology, Cardiovascular Division
University of Alabama in Birmingham

Richard O. Russell, Jr., M.D.
Professor of Medicine
Department of Medicine
University of Alabama in Birmingham

Roger E. Moraski, M.D.
Assistant Professor of Medicine
Department of Medicine
University of Alabama in Birmingham

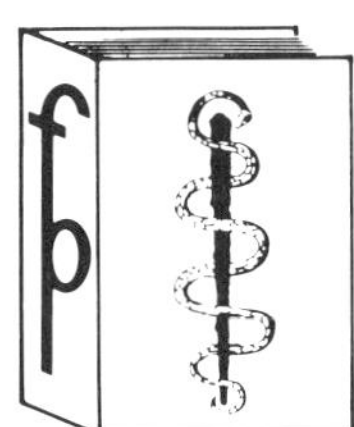

FUTURA PUBLISHING COMPANY, INC.
Mount Kisco, New York
1976

to Teresa
      and to Erick, Pablo and Andres

to Phyllis
      and to Scott, Katherine, Meredith and Stephen

to Patricia
      and to Roger, Jr.

ACKNOWLEDGMENTS

The idea for this book originated with Dr. Alberto Barcia whose demand for excellence in radiography hopefully we have maintained. Dr. Thomas N. James, Dr. Charles E. Rackley, Dr. T. Joseph Reeves and Dr. David M. Witten provided strong and enthusiastic encouragement. We wish to express our gratitude to Dr. William P. Hood, who as Director of the Cardiac Catheterization Laboratory provided help and cooperation. We are grateful to Mr. James Craig who patiently and meticulously performed the photography and to Mr. Luis Zanzi who prepared the diagrams elucidating the radiographic findings. We acknowledge the splendid help and cooperation of many radiography and cardiology technologists. We further acknowledge the excellent secretarial work of Miss Pam Pierce and Mrs. Doris Webster. To Futura Publishing Company, Mr. Steven Korn and Mr. Jacques Strauss, we express our appreciation for the opportunity of publishing this book.

PREFACE

In the past the diagnosis of coronary artery disease was established by a history of angina pectoris or a myocardial infarction. Electrocardiographic recordings during chest discomfort and the response to exercise have provided clinical evidence for myocardial ischemia. Evaluation of coronary artery anatomy became available with the development of coronary cineangiography by Sones. A significant advance in coronary artery surgery was the aortocoronary saphenous vein bypass operation introduced by Favaloro which further emphasized the necessity for precise diagnosis and delineation of coronary anatomy. Several clinical studies have now shown that the extent of anatomical involvement of the coronary arteries is a reliable prognostic index for the individual patient with coronary heart disease.

With the tremendous increase in the number of patients undergoing coronary arteriography and coronary artery surgery, Drs. Soto, Russell, and Moraski provide a timely and useful atlas on coronary arteriography. Salient features of the text are the organization, manner of presentation, quality of coronary arteriograms and the instructive schematic diagrams. The circle loop method for orientation to coronary anatomy, the variations in normal anatomy, commonly encountered coronary lesions, and additional studies on left ventricular aneurysms as well as coronary artery vein grafts provide the reader with a meaningful review of coronary artery anatomy in health and disease.

This text should be particularly useful to clinicians ranging from medical students to house officers and internists to cardiologists. Not only will physicians involved in performing coronary arteriography benefit from the excellent illustrations, but any physician whose patient may undergo this procedure can appreciate the technical aspects of the catheterization and interpretation of the films. An attractive feature of this atlas is the high quality of the large film coronary arteriograms which were obtained along with conventional coronary cineangiograms. The matching schematic diagrams provide further delineation of the coronary artery lesions. The observations on left ventricular aneurysms and postoperative vein bypass angiograms broaden the clinical spectrum for the reader.

The quality of the coronary arteriograms and the useful matching schematic diagrams will significantly contribute to clinical understanding of coronary arteriography, and Drs. Soto, Russell, and Moraski are to be commended for their contributions.

Charles E. Rackley, M.D.

CONTENTS

PART I

ORIENTATION AND NORMAL CORONARY ANATOMY

Chapter 1

Coronary Arteriography: Introduction, Methods and Interpretation

Coronary arteriography may be recommended as an integral part of cardiovascular consultation in many clinical circumstances. Most commonly it is performed in conjunction with quantitative or qualitative left ventricular angiography (very often biplane) and right heart catheterization. In combination, these procedures are highly useful for evaluation of overall cardiac function in patients with angina pectoris, in those with known or suspected ischemic heart disease, in patients with perplexing chest pain syndromes, in patients with primary myocardial disease and in those with valvular heart disease who may require surgical intervention.

Thus, in patients with cardiac disease of diverse etiology, a working knowledge of arteriographic coronary anatomy is highly useful to the practicing physician and student of cardiac disease. To that end, this atlas of arteriographic coronary anatomy demonstrating findings from large film angiograms was prepared with the hope that it will prove useful to all physicians and students of medicine who treat patients with diseases of the heart. Specifically it was designed for physicians and students of medicine who do not perform coronary arteriography, but who may review the films of their patients and who recognize the need for a better understanding of this important aspect of anatomy and medicine.

Clarity and precision in the definition of the pathologic anatomy of the coronary arteries is the cornerstone for the evaluation and investigation of ischemic heart disease.[1] On this data is built the structure for understanding the disease and its impact on the patient's prognosis. The coronary cineangiograms and the large roll film arteriograms complement each other and provide improved visualization and understanding of the coronary anatomy and the collateral circulation. The cineangiograms depict the circulation in motion and the large films provide greater detail of the anatomy. It is the large roll film angiograms that have provided the material for this book. We hope this atlas will complement the monograph by Dr. Thomas N. James — a work which helped to undergird and open the present clinical approach to coronary artery disease.[2]

The approach, methods and interpretations presented in this chapter, and indeed this atlas, are those utilized at the University of Alabama in Birmingham. If coronary arteriography is indicated, the catheterization and angiographic procedure and its potential risks are explained to the patient and his family as an integral part of the cardiac consultation. Written consent is obtained and the deliberations with the patient and family are recorded in the hospital chart.

On the evening prior to arteriography, both the right and left groin are shaved. If a right heart catheterization is planned, the right or left antecubital fossa is also shaved. Catheterization of the right heart may be performed via the femoral vein. On the day of arteriography, the patient is kept in the fasting state for at least four hours and is premedicated prior to being sent to the catheterization laboratory. Mild sedation is obtained with medication such as diazepam or promethazine. Atropine, 0.6-1.0 milligram is given either orally or intramuscularly. If sinus bradycardia occurs during the procedure, supplemental atropine may be given intravenously in doses of 0.4-0.8 milligram.

The right heart is catheterized prior to coronary arteriography or left ventricular angiography. Local anesthesia is adequately obtained over brachial or femoral vessels. Following passage of the right heart catheter into the pulmonary artery, the cardiac output, pulmonary artery and pulmonary capillary, or "wedge," pressures are measured. The cardiac output is determined by either the Fick method or the thermodilution technique. The hemoglobin oxygen saturation in the pulmonary artery is measured by oximetry. The right heart catheter is then withdrawn from the pulmonary artery into either the superior or inferior vena cava depending upon the approach, i.e., from the brachial or femoral vein. During this "pullback," pressure is continuously recorded in the pulmonary artery, right ventricle and right atrium.

The femoral artery is entered by the percutaneous Seldinger technique. At a site just cephalad to the groin skin crease, a Cournand needle is passed toward the femoral arterial pulsation at a 30°-60° angle to the skin. At this location the common femoral artery will usually not have bifurcated. The needle is passed either to its hub or until it touches bone. With this technique the needle may penetrate the posterior wall of the artery. A small drop of blood may appear through the lumen of the obturator as the artery is entered. The obturator is then removed and the needle carefully and slowly withdrawn. It is advisable to support one's hands on the patient to avoid dislodging the needle when arterial blood suddenly arches out the needle, signaling its entry into the arterial lumen. A Teflon® coated flexible guide wire is inserted into the needle and advanced to the descending aorta. Frequently, a j-tipped flexible guide wire is necessary to traverse an atherosclerotic iliofemoral junction and/or abdominal aorta. Great care must be utilized not to shear the guide wire of its Teflon® coating; passage of the guide wire must be accomplished smoothly and gently.

After the flexible guide wire has been advanced into the thoracic descending aorta, a bolus of intravenous heparin is administered to decrease the risk of clot formation; 2500 units of heparin has been found to be sufficient for this purpose. Less heparin (1500-2000 units) is given to females, especially the elderly, to hypertensive patients and to patients with an increase in pulse pressure, as in aortic insufficiency, as the higher dose in these patients seems to predispose to more bleeding after the procedure. In our experience this lesser amount has been sufficient to retard clot formation. Protamine is rarely required.

With the Cournand needle in place a small skin incision is made at the site of entry into the skin using a Number 15 scalpel blade. A tract is created by dissecting along the needle with straight forceps. The needle is then removed, the guide wire is wiped free of blood with a wet sponge, and a tapered tip introducer is passed into the artery with a rotating (back and forth) motion. The introducer should be held close to the skin. The introducer is then removed and a flexible guide wire is again wiped along its entire external length with a moist gauze to remove blood and tiny clots. These manuevers must be performed carefully to avoid inadvertent removal of the guide wire from the femoral artery.

The appropriate preshaped left coronary arteriography catheter is then introduced over the guide wire. The preshaped catheters are available in a variety of "loop" sizes: three and one-half, four, five and six. The three and one-half size is appropriate for small aortic arches, and size six for markedly dilated and/or "uncoiled" aortas. The appropriate size may frequently be predicted from the chest x-ray or by preliminary fluoroscopy.

As the catheter is advanced the tip of the guide wire is maintained in the descending thoracic aorta by retracting it gradually. Once the guide wire is removed, the catheter is aspirated and the blood along with the debris the catheter may have collected in its passage through the skin and subcutaneous tissue is discarded. The catheter is again aspirated and gently flushed in the descending aorta. An undamped arterial pressure wave-form must be obtained with high frequency response characteristics after the catheter has been attached to the injecting syringe and pressure connecting tube. As the catheter is advanced into the ascending aorta, all extra bends in the catheter are removed by appropriate rotation so that the catheter assumes its widest appearance ("open loop") as the tip approaches the coronary artery. Entry into the coronary artery (both left and right) is made under fluoroscopic visualization with constant aortic pressure and electrocardiographic monitoring. Filming is made during deep inspiration. Unless there is damping of pressure (at which time the catheter is instantly withdrawn), the catheter may remain in the coronary ostium until arteriograms in all desired projections are obtained. The left coronary catheter is then withdrawn to the descending aorta. The catheter is aspirated and the aspirate discarded. After the catheter is flushed the Teflon® coated flexible guide wire is reinserted and the catheter is removed. Again the guide wire is wiped clean of blood with a moist gauze.

The appropriate right coronary catheter is then passed over the guide wire and the latter removed when the tip of the catheter is in position in the descending aorta. Again a two syringe discard and flush technique is used discarding the first aspirate. An undamped arterial pressure wave-form is required before proceeding. The right coronary catheter is advanced to the ascending aorta and the tip positioned at the superior vena cava-right atrial junction with its tip pointing leftward ("zero position"). Using a clockwise rotation (considering the inferior surface of the diaphragm as the face of the clock) the catheter is advanced slowly. It is important to remove the torque placed in the catheter by clockwise rotation using intermittent, miniscule, counterclockwise rotations as the clockwise sweep into the right coronary artery is performed. Alternately, the catheter may be advanced to the aortic valve; then with its tip pointed leftward the clockwise sweep is performed as the catheter is slowly retracted up to the level of the coronary ostium. Again torque must be removed as described above. If arterial pressure does not damp or fall the catheter may be left in the ostium of the right coronary artery during the filming sequence. If the pressure drops as the tip of the catheter enters the right coronary artery the catheter must be removed from the ostium and placed again in the "zero position." The patient is then rotated into the desired position and the maneuver of entry is repeated for each oblique or lateral view. The angiographer must be prepared to film immediately, as the pressure may drop again. In this circumstance, the catheter must be removed immediately following the injection. A pressure drop with the catheter tip in the coronary artery is potentially hazardous.

Finally, left ventricular angiography is performed with a pigtail catheter. In our opinion, it is important to first obtain the coronary arteriograms as information on coronary anatomy and pathology is presently unobtainable by other means. If left ventricular angiography is performed initially, hemodynamic deterioration might possibly prevent continuing with coronary arteriography. While it is exceedingly important to know left ventricular size and function, left ventricular performance may be evaluated by other methods should the procedure need to be permaturely terminated following coronary arteriography.

While the pigtail catheter is often easily passed in retrograde fashion across the aortic valve, it is our preference to have the flexible guide wire present in the catheter as there is less bending of the catheter and less catheter whip as it enters the left ventricle. The presence of the flexible guide wire in the catheter also facilitates optimal positioning of the pigtail catheter for left ventricular angiography. If the catheter is properly positioned in the left ventricle, angiography can be frequently accomplished without extrasystoles.

There are three options for entry into the left ventricle using the guide wire. First, it may be positioned with the tip of the guide wire at the tip of the catheter's pigtail. Second, the catheter's pigtail may be left flexible if the guide wire is positioned proximal to the curve of the pigtail. Third, the guide wire may be extruded a variable distance out of the catheter. If entry into the left ventricle is delayed it is necessary to withdraw the catheter into the descending aorta approximately every two minutes in order to vigorously aspirate and flush it. This procedure is necessary to prevent clot formation which may result from stasis of blood in the pigtail.

Following proper placement of the coronary catheter into the coronary ostium, cineangiograms and large roll film angiograms are obtained in multiple views. The cine coronary angiograms are obtained using 250 milliamperes with 3-5 milliseconds of exposure time and 70-90 kilovolts. The frame speed utilized is 60 per second over 3-4 seconds. The film used is Kodak Double-X Negative (5222)® and is processed in a Fisher automatic processer® at 78° at a rate of 15 feet per minute; this gives a fog of 0.31. The large roll film angiograms are obtained using 1000 milliamperes with 6 to 12 milliseconds of exposure time and 60-90 kilovolts. The focal spot is 1.2 mm. The films are taken at 3 to 6 frames per second for 3 seconds. The film used is Cronex-6 (Dupont)®; lightning plus screens are used and the grid is linear with a ratio of 12.

The cineangiograms of the left coronary artery are made in two to four projections: 50°-60° and 20°-30° right anterior oblique; 60°-70° left anterior oblique and at 90°, which is the lateral projection. Cineangiograms of the right coronary artery are made at 60°-70° left anterior oblique, 20°-30° right anterior oblique, and at 90°, (lateral projection). Filming is of sufficient duration to visualize collateral vessels, cardiac veins and late filling of arteries distal to obstructions or stenoses.

Following cineangiography of each coronary artery the catheterization table is moved into position over the large film changer. With the lateral tube large roll film angiograms of the left coronary artery are made in the lateral position, 20°-30° right posterior oblique (visualized as 60°-70° left anterior oblique) and 60°-70° left posterior oblique (visualized as 20°-30° right anterior oblique) projections. The patient is positioned by two radiology technologists under the supervision of the radiologist.

The contrast medium used for coronary arteriography is Renografin 76®, a combination of meglumine and sodium diatrizoates. It contains 37% of iodine and 0.19 milliequivalents per milliliter of sodium. This contrast agent has been demonstrated to be quite safe.[3,4]

While the entire anatomy of the coronary arterial tree is studied and recorded, lesions that are present in larger vessels and that have importance to the cardiovascular surgeon are graded. Particular attention should be drawn to the left main coronary artery, the left anterior descending artery with its large first septal and its larger diagonal branches, the left circumflex artery and its obtuse marginal and other marginal branches, the ramus intermedius (the occasional third branch of the left main coronary artery between the left anterior descending and left circumflex branches), the right coronary artery and its posterior descending branch. Also identified are the sinus node artery, the conus artery and the atrioventricular node artery.

The location of each stenosis is recorded. For example, a lesion in the left anterior descending artery may occur before or after the first septal perforating branch and/or the first diagonal branch. In the left circumflex artery a lesion before or at the origin of the obtuse marginal branch is particularly significant, whereas a lesion beyond this region may have less surgical significance. Although responsible for angina pectoris a lesion beyond the obtuse marginal might not be surgically accessible for saphenous vein bypass grafting. Similarly a lesion before the bifurcation of the right coronary artery into the posterior descending and distal right coronary arteries is of more significance surgically than stenosis in the distal right coronary artery. Thus the lesions are categorized by location as occurring in the proximal one-third, the middle one-third, and the distal one-third of the left anterior descending coronary artery. Lesions in the proximal one-third of this artery are further characterized as being either proximal or distal to the first diagonal branch and to the first septal perforating branch. In the left circumflex artery lesions proximal to the obtuse marginal are considered in the proximal portion and those beyond the obtuse marginal as in the distal portion. In patients whose left circumflex artery has several marginal branches the lesions are located in relation to those branches and the obtuse marginal branch is identified. The right coronary artery is subdivided as follows: The proximal portion of the right coronary artery extends to the origin of the posterior descending branch. This portion may be divided conceptually into proximal, middle and distal segments or thirds. The distal right coronary artery is that portion of the right coronary artery beyond the origin of the posterior descending branch.

The severity of lesions is determined in multiple projections by estimating the percentage narrowing of the normal arterial diameter.

CORONARY ARTERIOGRAPHIC REPORT

Left main coronary artery (LMCA) — normal without obstruction.

Left anterior descending (LAD) — greater than 90% stenosis in the proximal one-third before the first septal and diagonal branches with a size B distal vessel filling by septal collaterals from the posterior descending coronary artery.

Left circumflex artery (CX) — 50-70% stenosis in the proximal portion before the first marginal branch; the 1st marginal branch has a 100% occlusion near its origin; it fills by intercoronary collateral from a diagonal branch of the LAD and is a size C vessel distally.

Right coronary artery (RCA) — dominant; 50-70% lesion in the proximal one-third before the right marginal branch. The remaining vessel is normal. The sinus node artery, the atrioventricular node artery and the artery to the pulmonary conus are present and normal.

Each lesion is graded as either 0-50%, 50-70%, 70-90%, greater than 90% or 100% obstruction of the artery. Although this method is semi-quantitative, after extensive use of this system the authors usually agree on the severity of the diameter narrowing when each reviews the arteriogram independently.

The relative size of the vessel beyond the stenosis is also evaluated. This is of importance in predicting the surgeon's chances of constructing a satisfactory saphenous vein anastomosis. The arterial lumen distal to the stenosis is graded as either A, B, or C. An "A" vessel is one with a normal lumen, or a lumen approximately equal in size to the undiseased segment of the vessel proximal to the stenosis or obstruction. If a vessel lumen distal to a lesion is reduced in size but thought to be adequate for receiving a graft then it is graded a "B" vessel. A "C" vessel is one with a small lumen into which a satisfactory graft probably could not be placed.

The collateral communications between major vessels are also noted.[5] Examples of intercoronary anastomoses include the septal branches between the left anterior descending and posterior descending coronary arteries and communications between the marginal branches of the left circumflex and right coronary arteries.

The intracoronary anastomoses connect a proximal and distal portion of a vessel that has been "divided" by an occlusion. The sinus node artery and Kugel's artery may also provide major pathways of collateral blood flow. Examples of these collateral networks are shown throughout this text.

An example of a typical report of a patient's coronary arteriogram is shown on page 7. It is obvious that a standard method of describing the coronary anatomy is invaluable for those participating in the care of patients with coronary artery disease.

References

1.   Gensini, G.G.: *Coronary Arteriography.* Futura Publishing Company, Inc., Mount Kisco, New York, 1975.

2.   James, T.N.: *Anatomy of the Coronary Arteries.* Paul B. Hoeber, Inc., New York, 1961.

3.   Paulin, S. and Adams, D.: Increased ventricular fibrillation during coronary arteriography with a new contrast medium preparation. *Radiology,* **101**:45-50, 1971.

4.   Banks, D.C., Raftery, E.B., and Oram, S.: Evaluation of contrast media used in man for coronary arteriography. *British Heart Journal,* **32**:317-319, 1970.

5.   Jochem, W., Soto, B., Karp, R.B., Russell, R.O. Jr., Holt, J.H., and Barcia, A.: Radiographic anatomy of the coronary collateral circulation. *American Journal of Roentgenology, Radium Therapy and Nuclear Medicine,* **116**:50-61, 1972.

Chapter 2

The Sinuses of Valsalva and the Origin of the Coronary Arteries

The ascending aorta is a tubular structure with a proximal dilatation called the "bulb." The bulb is formed by the sinuses of Valsalva and is separated from the tubular segment by the relatively narrow supravalvular aortic ring (Figure 2.1). The coronary arteries originate from the aorta at the level of the sinuses of Valsalva.

There are three sinuses of Valsalva (Figure 2.2). The right coronary sinus (R) contains the ostium of the right coronary artery and the left coronary sinus (L) contains the ostium of the left coronary artery. The sinus of Valsalva without a coronary artery ostium is designated the non-coronary sinus (NC).

The right coronary sinus is anterior and in an intermediate position between the non-coronary and left coronary sinuses of Valsalva. Figure 2.3 is an angiogram of the aortic bulb in the antero-posterior and lateral projections demonstrating the relationship of the right coronary sinus (R) to the other two sinuses. In the antero-posterior projection the right coronary sinus does not form the lateral borders of the bulb; in the lateral projection the right coronary sinus forms the anterior border of the bulb.

The left coronary sinus is posterior and to the left as demonstrated by the angiogram in Figure 2.3. The left coronary sinus (L) forms the left border of the bulb in the antero-posterior projection and the posterior border of the bulb above the non-coronary sinus (NC) in the lateral projection.

Figure 2.4 demonstrates an angiogram of an unusual aortic bulb. The aortic valve orifice faces to the left and the left coronary artery has an almost vertical orientation from its origin in the left coronary sinus.

In the majority of cases, the coronary arteries originate in their respective sinuses of Valsalva just below the supravalvular ring.[1] In Figures 2.2 and 2.4 the ostia of the coronary arteries are seen originating in the central portion of the sinuses of Valsalva. Occasionally, however, a coronary ostium may be found immediately above the supravalvular ring. Figure 2.5 illustrates the left coronary artery originating just above the supravalvular ring.

The left coronary artery usually arises from a single ostium. Occasionally the left anterior descending coronary artery and the left circumflex artery originate separately, each with its own orifice in the left coronary sinus. The orifice of the right coronary artery is double in number in 50% of patients.[2] In these instances the second ostium in the right coronary sinus of Valsalva is that of the conus artery.

With the oblique positions used during coronary arteriography changes should be noted in the orientation of the sinuses of Valsalva. In the left anterior oblique projection (when the obliquity is close to the lateral projection), the right coronary sinus forms the anterior border of the bulb (Figures 2.1, 2.3, 2.4). The left coronary sinus is posterior and forms the posterior border of the bulb. This projection is useful for catheterization of the right and left coronary arteries. In the right anterior oblique projection (Figure 2.6) the right coronary and left coronary sinuses of Valsalva overlap and this projection is less suitable for catheterization of the right or left coronary arteries.

Based on the knowledge of the anatomy and relationships between the sinuses of Valsalva, several practical points may be emphasized regarding coronary arteriography: 1) The tip of the catheter must be directed anteriorly when attempting to catheterize the right coronary orifice; 2) The tip of the catheter must be oriented posteriorly and to the left when attempting to catheterize the left coronary artery; 3) When the orifice of a coronary artery is located above the supravalvular ring cannulation of that artery may be quite difficult. When the ostia are located in the central portion of the coronary sinus, catheterization is most easily accomplished (Figure 2.4).

References

1.   Paulin, S.: Coronary angiography. A technical, anatomic and clinical study. *Acta Radiologica Supplementum*, 233, 1964.
2.   James, T.N.: *Anatomy of the Coronary Arteries*, Paul B. Hoeber, Inc., New York, 1961.

Figure 2.1:   Lateral view of the ascending aorta demonstrating the bulb (B) and tubular segment (T), divided by the supra-valvular aortic ring (arrows).

Figure 2.2:   Diagrammatic representation of an opened aortic bulb. The sinuses of Valsalva are labeled as right (R), left (L), and non-coronary (NC). The upper limit of the bulb is the supravalvular aortic ring; the inferior portion of the bulb consists of the aortic valve cusps. The coronary ostia are located below the supravalvular ring.

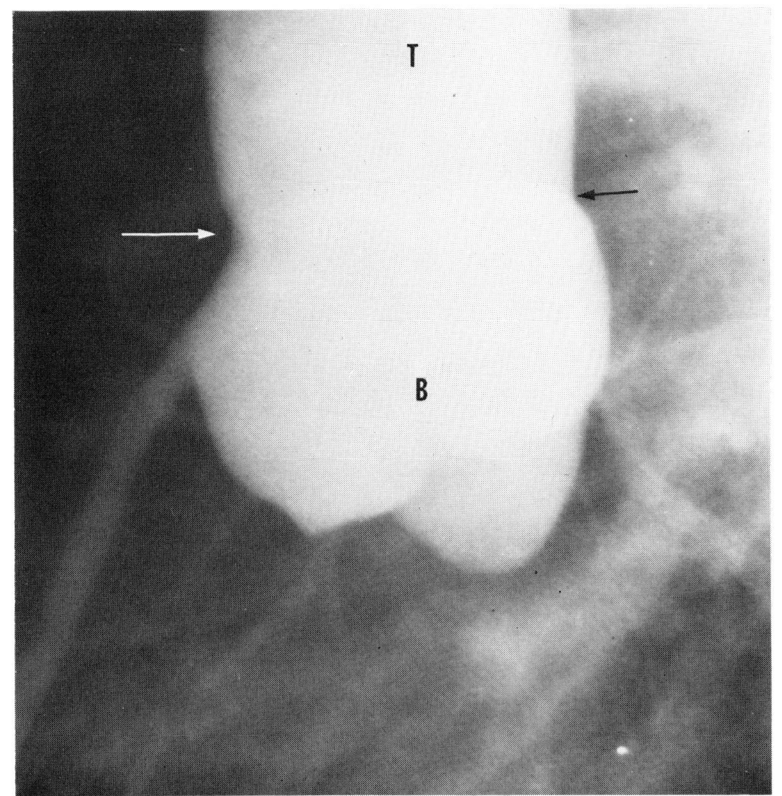

FIGURE 2.1

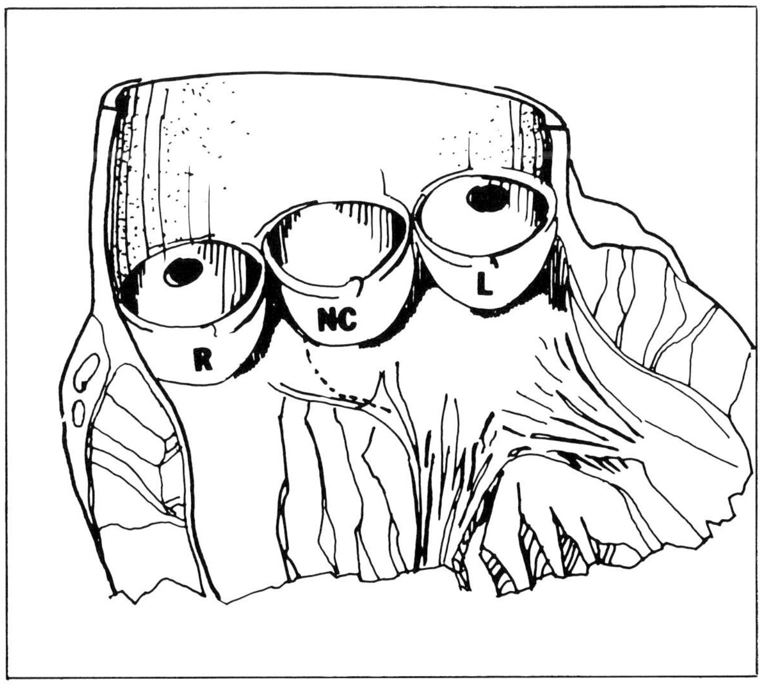

**FIGURE 2.2

Figure 2.3:   Aortic angiogram during diastole demonstrating the relationships of the sinuses of Valsalva. The antero-posterior projection (**A**) is above and lateral projection below (**B**). The right coronary sinus (R) is located anteriorly and medially. The left coronary sinus (L) is located on the left and posteriorly. The lower-most sinus is the non-coronary sinus (NC).

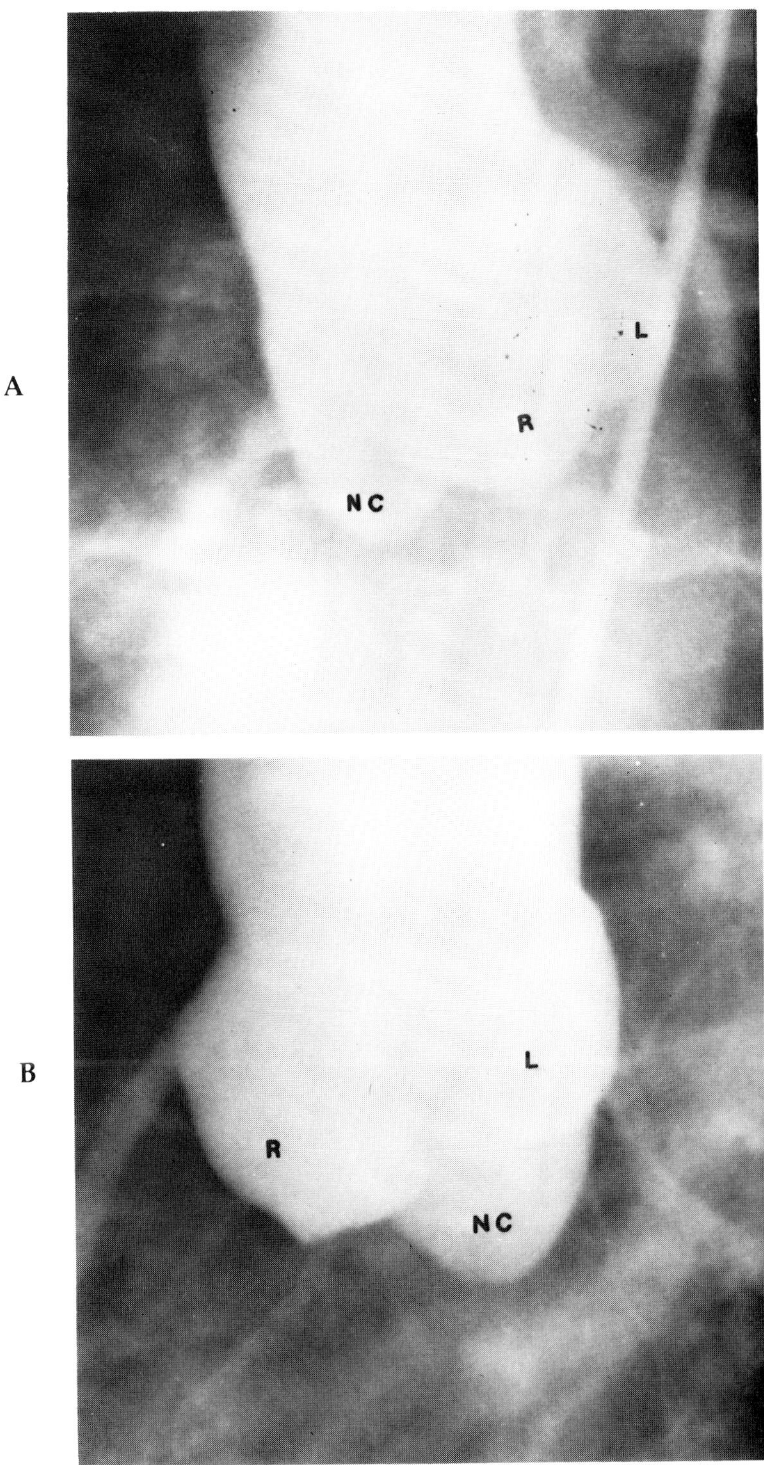

FIGURE 2.3

Figure 2.4: Aortic bulb with an unusual orientation; **A** (antero-posterior projection) and **B** (lateral projection) filmed during diastole; **C** (antero-posterior projection) and **D** (lateral projection) filmed during systole. The orientation of the aortic orifice is to the left and the left coronary artery has an almost vertical take-off. Note that the coronary orifices are located in the central portion of the sinuses.

R = right coronary sinus. L = left coronary sinus. NC = non-coronary sinus.

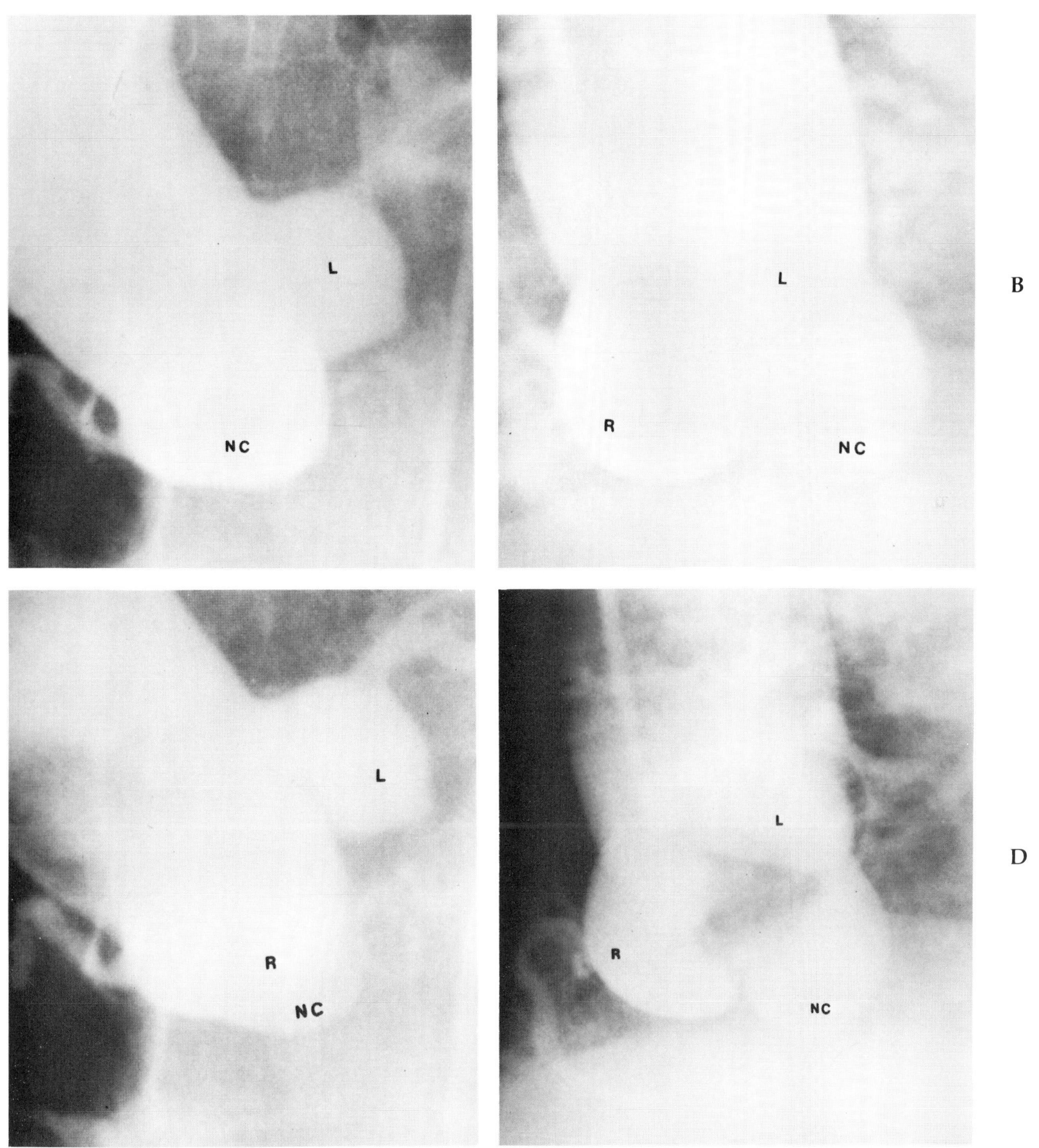

FIGURE 2.4

Figure 2.5:   Aortogram in lateral projection: diastole (**A**) and systole (**B**). The supravalvular ring is well demarcated. The left coronary ostium is located immediately above the aortic ring.

Figure 2.6:   Aortogram in right anterior oblique projection.

A. The right (R) and left (L) coronary sinuses are anterior; the right coronary sinus is higher than the left. The non-coronary (NC) lies posteriorly and inferiorly. The over-lapping of the right and left coronary sinuses in this projection makes their identification difficult. Thus, this is not an ideal projection for catheterizing the right or left coronary arteries.

B. Diagrammatic representation of **A**.

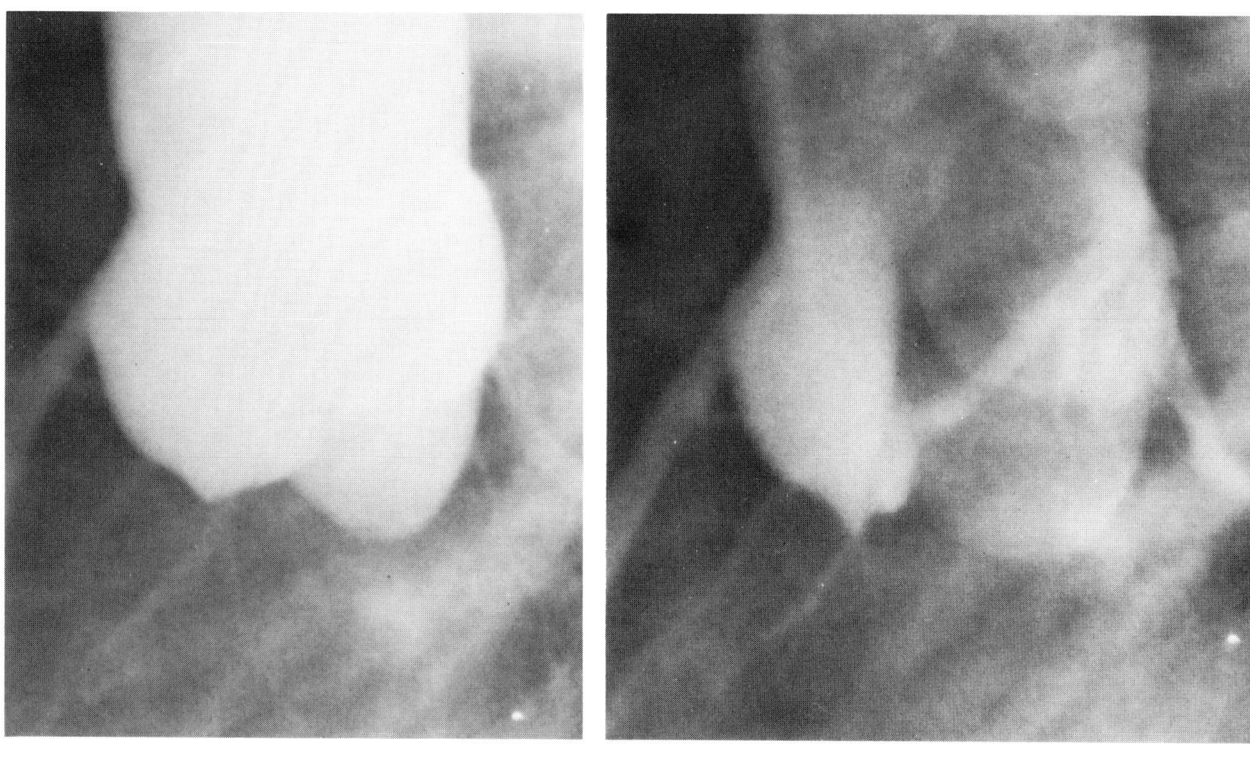

A   **FIGURE 2.5**   B

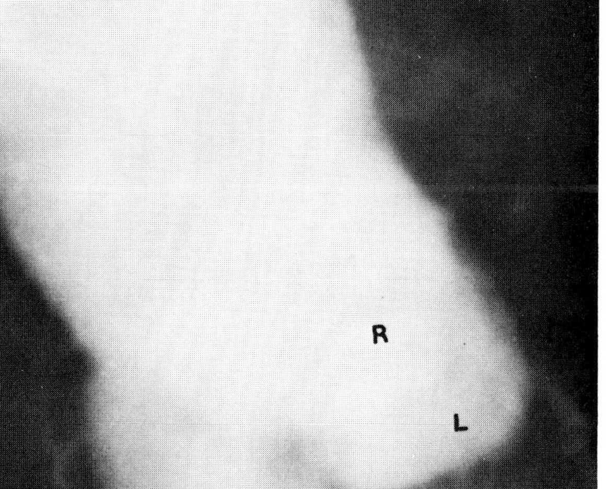

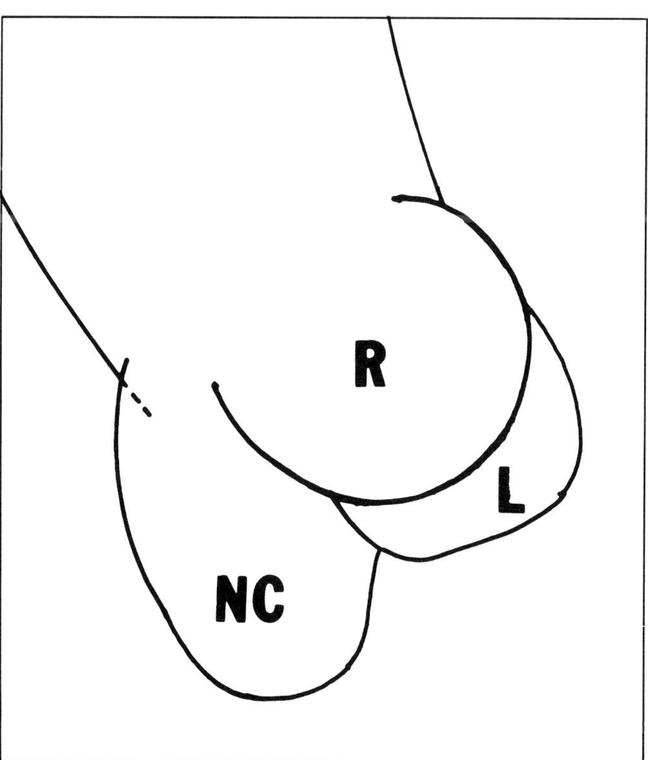

A   **FIGURE 2.6**   B

Radiographic Orientation: The Circle-Loop Concept

The coronary arterial tree lies about the heart in such fashion as to form a circle and a loop which can be appreciated radiographically.[1] The circle is formed by the proximal and distal right coronary arteries and the left circumflex artery as they course in the right and left atrioventricular sulci from their origins in the sinuses of Valsalva toward the crux of the heart posteriorly. The loop is formed by the left anterior descending and the posterior descending coronary arteries as they course in the anterior and inferior interventricular sulci from the aortic bulb toward the apex of the heart. The orientation of the circle and the loop is shown in Figure 3.1. The circle and loop are joined at two points: 1) the anterior junction is located at the origin of the left anterior descending coronary artery and 2) the inferior junction is located at the origin of the posterior descending artery at the crux of the heart. The crux of the heart is located posteriorly at the junction of the atrioventricular groove and the interatrial and interventricular sulci.

As demonstrated in Figure 3.1, the loop is foreshortened by rotation into the left anterior oblique (LAO) projection (right posterior oblique, RPO) and the circle is seen in profile. Figure 3.2 demonstrates the left anterior oblique projection as usually seen during coronary arteriography. Since this is the optimum projection for the circle, the proximal portion of the right coronary artery and the circumflex artery are well visualized.

In the right anterior oblique (RAO) projection (left posterior oblique, LPO) the loop is seen in profile. Thus in Figure 3.3 the left anterior descending and posterior descending arteries are well visualized.

From Figures 3.1 and 3.4 it is appreciated that the circle and loop are seen in a true oblique or intermediate projection when viewed in the lateral projection.

It is necessary to use the three projections described for complete and proper assessment of the coronary arterial tree. Since the left anterior oblique view projects the circle in profile this is the best projection for maximal visualization of the proximal portion of the right coronary artery and the left circumflex artery. The right anterior oblique projects the loop in profile and this is the optimal projection for visualization of the left anterior descending and posterior descending coronary arteries.

Figure 3.5 diagrammatically illustrates the ascending aorta and the bulb, the heart and the coronary arteries. The circle and loop can be easily appreciated.

If an obstruction is demonstrated in a vessel, collateral filling of that vessel can be easily recognized if the location of that vessel is predicted by use of the circle and loop concept. Examples of this will be shown throughout the text.

Figures 3.6 and 3.7 illustrate the anterior and inferior surfaces of the heart respectively. The anatomical relationship between the coronary arteries and the structures of the heart are demonstrated.

In a heart with a right dominant circulation, the right coronary artery reaches the crux and supplies the posterior descending coronary artery. If the posterior descending coronary artery is supplied by the left circumflex coronary artery, the coronary artery circulation is left dominant.

References

1.   Daves, M.L.: Cardiac roentgenology: The loop and circle approach. *Radiology,* **95**:157-160, 1970.

Figure 3.1:   Diagrammatic representation of the coronary arterial tree as a circle and loop. The right anterior oblique (RAO) projection will project the loop in profile and the left anterior oblique (LAO) projection will project the circle in profile. The lateral projection is a true oblique of the coronary arterial tree.

RPO = right posterior oblique.
LPO = left posterior oblique.

(From Daves, M.L.: Cardiac roentgenology. The loop and circle approach. *Radiology,* **95**:157-160, 1970. Published with permission.)

Figure 3.2:   Diagrammatic representations of the coronary arterial tree and the circle and loop in the left anterior oblique (LAO) projection. The right coronary artery (RC) and the circumflex artery (Cx) are well demonstrated. The proximal portion of the left anterior descending artery (LAD) and the posterior descending branch (PD) of the right coronary artery course toward the observer in the LAO projection.

LC = left main coronary artery. SN = sinus node artery. A = atrial branch of left circumflex coronary artery. LM = left marginal branch of left circumflex coronary artery. D = diagonal branch of left anterior descending coronary artery. S = septal branch of left anterior descending coronary artery. RM = right marginal branch of right coronary artery. AVN = atrioventricular node branch of right coronary artery.

(From Barcia, A., Fuertes, A., Karp, R.B., and Soto, B.: Coronary angiography techniques and new areas of investigation. Reproduced with permission from *Horizons in Cardiology 1972: Proceedings of the Third Annual Texas Heart Institute Symposium,* R.J. Hall, ed., p. 26.)

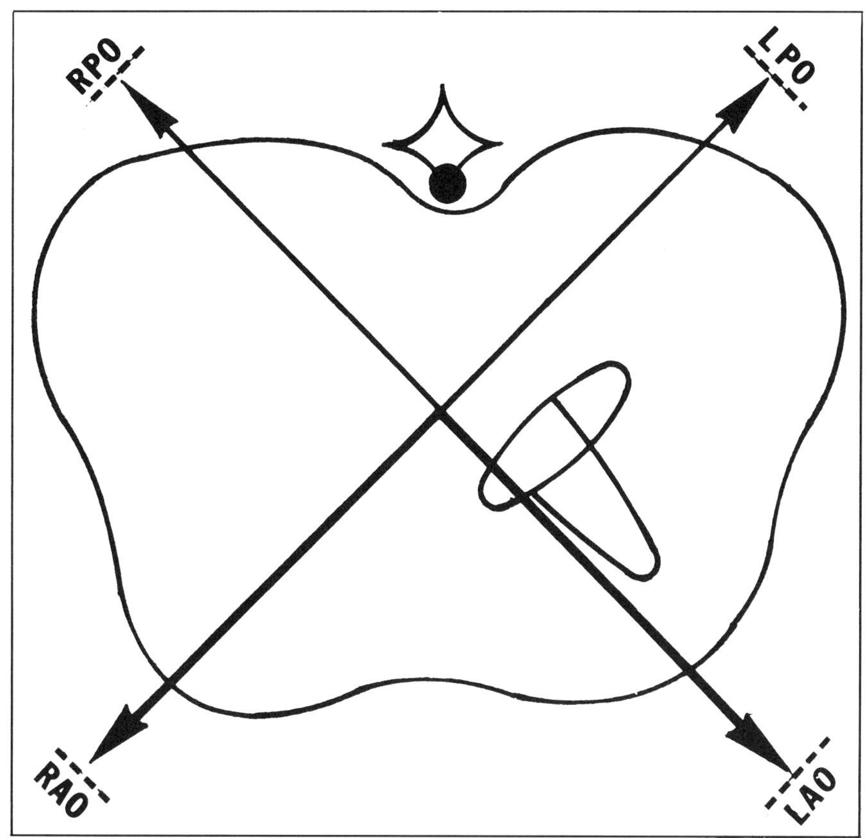

FIGURE 3.1

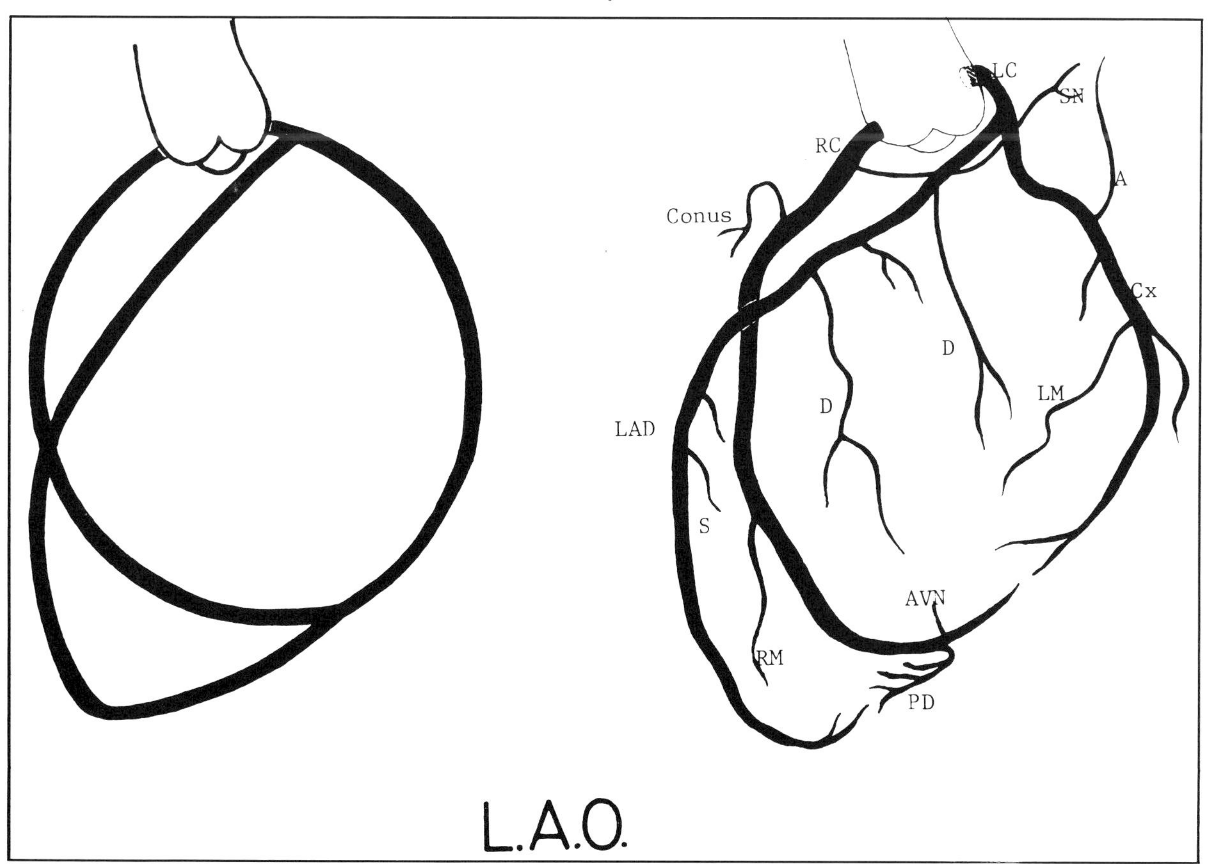

FIGURE   3.2

Figure 3.3:   Coronary arterial tree in the right anterior oblique (RAO) projection. The left anterior descending (LAD) artery and the posterior descending (PD) artery are well visualized as the loop is in profile in this projection. Abbreviations are similar to those in Figure 3.2.

S = septal branches of left anterior descending and of posterior descending coronary arteries. These septal branches are readily identified in RAO projection.

(From Barcia, A., Fuertes, A., Karp, R.B., and Soto, B.: Coronary angiography techniques and new areas of investigation. Reproduced with permission from *Horizons in Cardiology 1972: Proceedings of the Third Annual Texas Heart Institute Symposium*, R.J. Hall, ed., p. 26.)

Figure 3.4:   Coronary arterial tree in the lateral projection. Since the circle and loop are in an intermediate projection, this is an optimal projection for evaluating the entire coronary tree. Abbreviations are similar to those in Figure 3.2.

(From Barcia, A., Fuertes, A., Karp, R.B., and Soto, B.: Coronary angiography techniques and new areas of investigation. Reproduced with permission from *Horizons in Cardiology 1972: Proceedings of the Third Annual Texas Heart Institute Symposium*, R.J. Hall, ed., p. 26.)

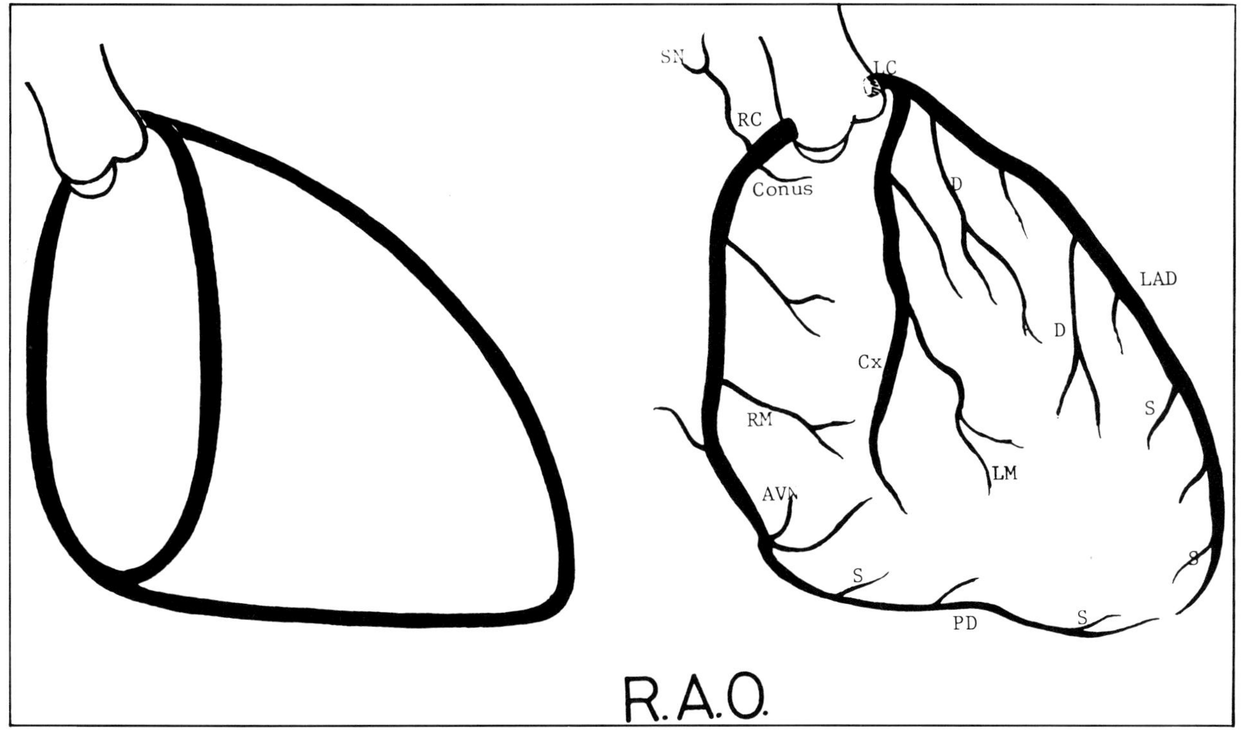

FIGURE 3.3

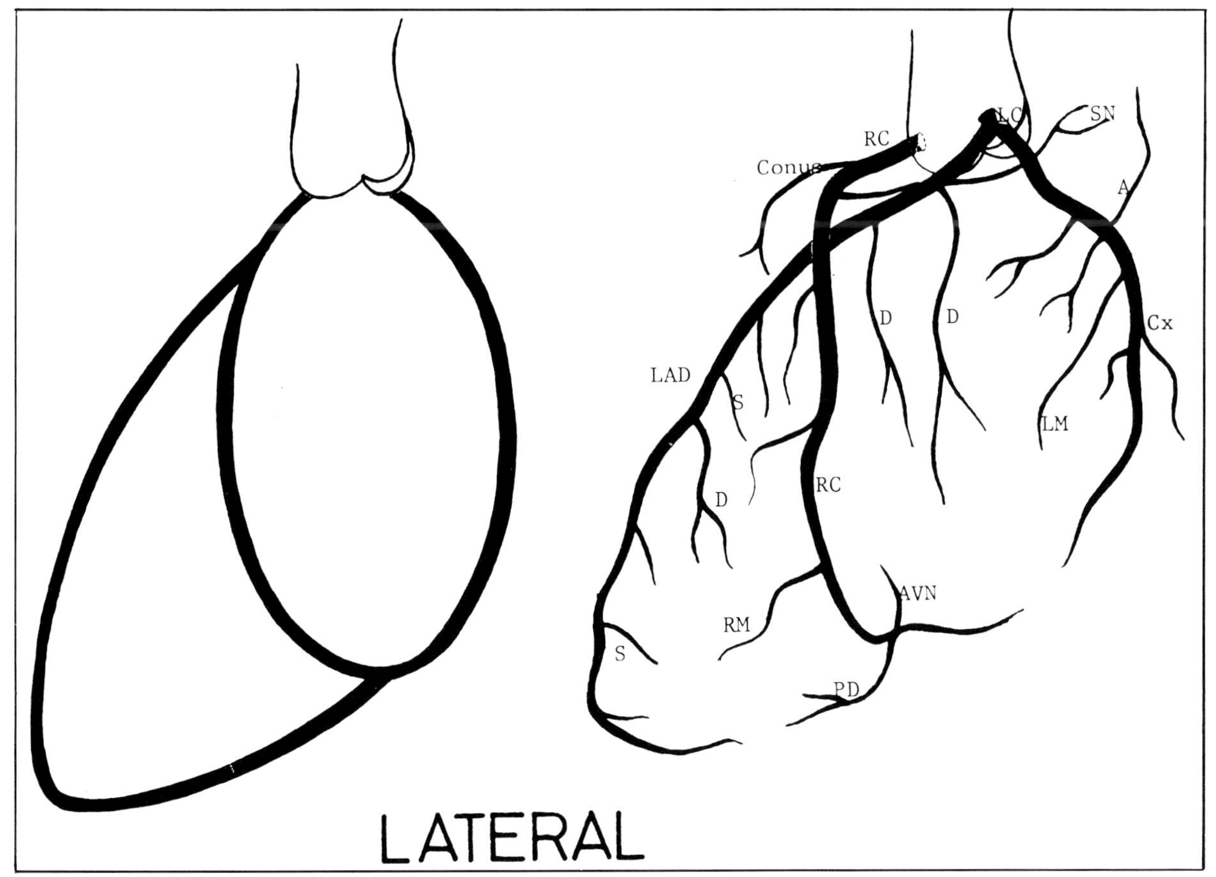

FIGURE 3.4

Figure 3.5:   Diagrammatic representation of the heart and the coronary arteries. **A**. Right dominant system; **B**. Left dominant system. The right coronary artery and circumflex artery are located in the atrioventricular sulcus forming a circle. The left anterior descending and the posterior descending arteries are located in the anterior and inferior interventricular sulci, respectively, forming a loop. Abbreviations are similar to those in Figure 3.2.

C = conus artery.

(From Fuertes-García, A., Soto, B., Montero, J.C., and Barcia, A.: Coronariografia selectiva: Tecnica y resultados, Figures 5 A and 5 B. *Revista Española de Cardiologia*, **26**:481-494, 1973. Published with permission.)

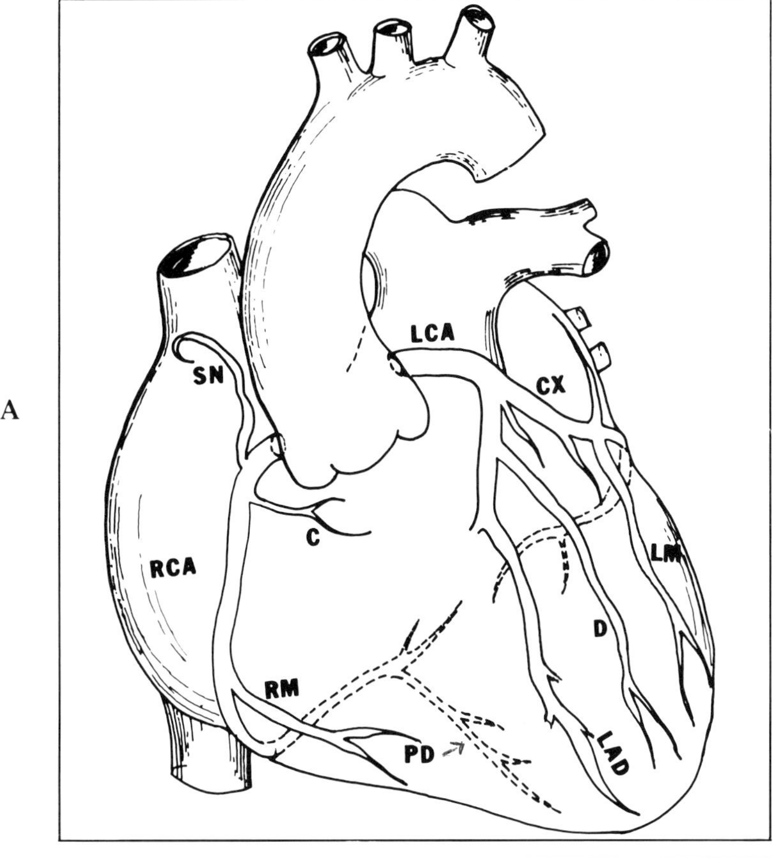

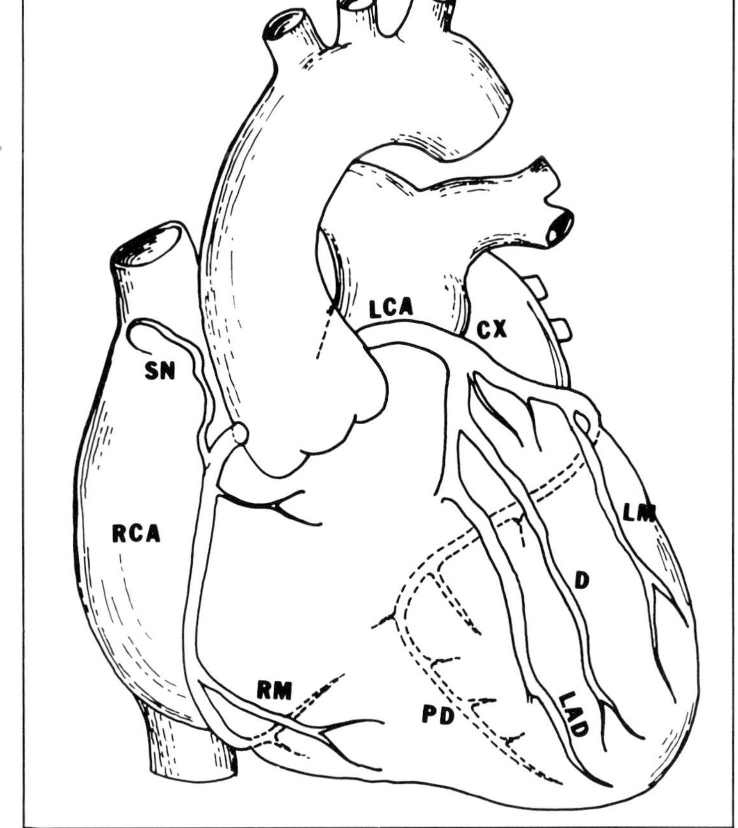

FIGURE 3.5

Figure 3.6:   View of the anterior surface of the heart externally. The origin of the left (LM) and right coronary (RCA) arteries are seen at the base of the ascending aorta (AO). The left and right coronary arteries course to the left and right of the pulmonary artery (PA), respectively. Shortly after its origin the left main (LM) coronary artery branches into the left anterior descending (LAD) and left circumflex (CX) arteries. The right coronary artery (RCA) courses in the right atrioventricular groove toward the inferior surface of the heart.

SVC = superior vena cava; PV = pulmonary veins; LM (branches of CX) = left marginal artery; RM = right marginal artery; SN = sinus node artery; D = diagonal branch of left anterior descending artery; LA = left atrium; RA = right atrium; LV = left ventricle; RV = right ventricle.

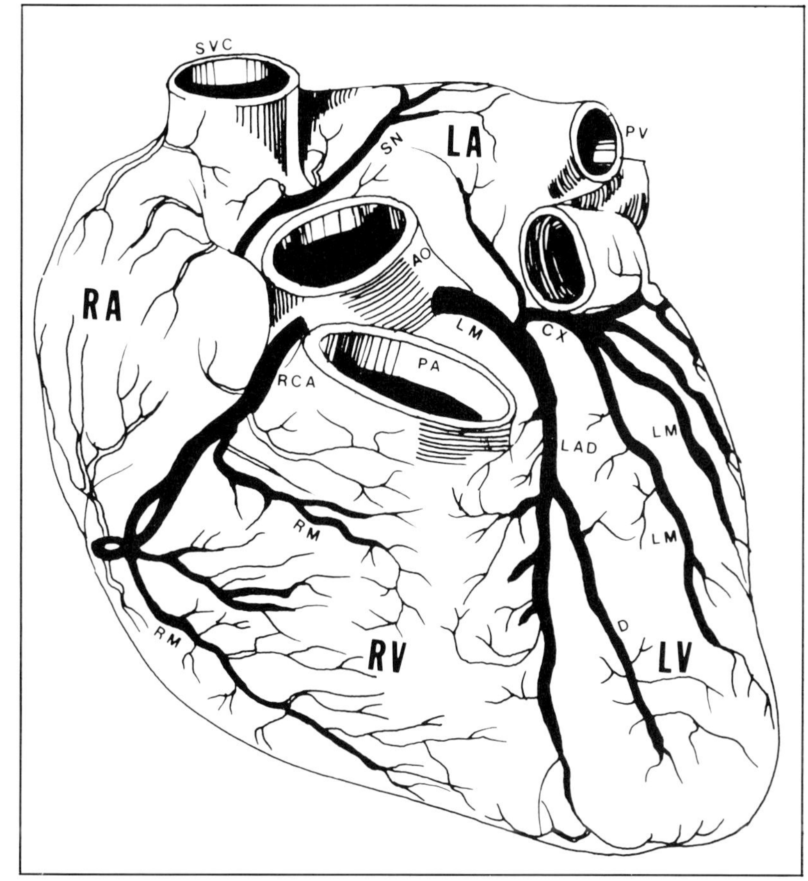

FIGURE 3.6

Figure 3.7: View of the inferior surface of the heart externally. The right coronary artery (RCA) is seen wrapping around the heart in the right atrioventricular groove anterior to the inferior vena cava (IVC). At the crux of the heart the right coronary artery divides into the posterior descending artery (PD) and the distal right coronary artery (DRCA). The distal segment of two left marginal (LM) arteries are seen at the left border of the heart.

SVC = superior vena cava; PV = pulmonary vein; SN = sinus node artery; RM = right marginal artery; LA = left atrium; RA = right atrium; LV = left ventricle; RV = right ventricle.

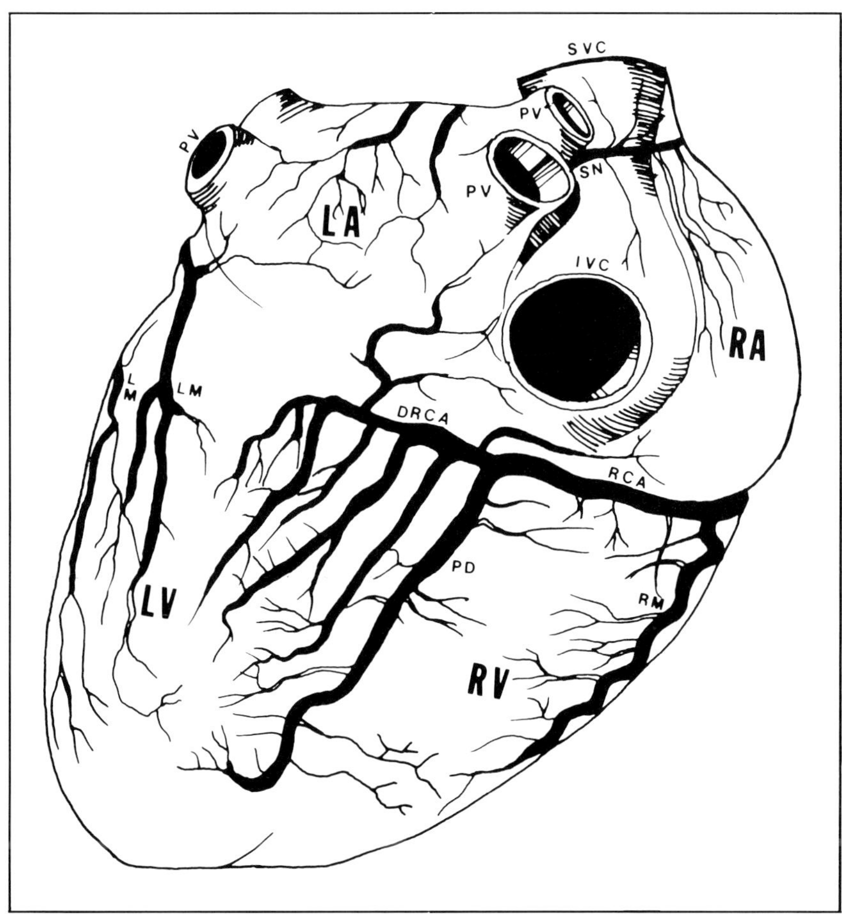

FIGURE 3.7

PART II

NORMAL CORONARY ANATOMY

Chapter 4

The Normal Left Coronary Artery

The Left Main Coronary Artery

The left main coronary artery originates from the left coronary sinus of Valsalva and is a short vessel which varies from 0-40 mm. in length.[1,2] Shortly after its origin, it courses between the pulmonary artery and the left atrial appendage in an inferior and leftward direction. Rarely, two left coronary ostia are present without a left main coronary artery.

The radiographic visualization of the left main coronary artery is of utmost importance. In the left anterior oblique projection, the left main coronary artery is seen originating posteriorly from the aortic bulb (Figure 4.1). In this projection its course is seen only partially. The distal segment of this artery and its bifurcation are better seen in the right anterior oblique projection (Figure 4.2). In the lateral projection (Figures 4.3-4.5) the left main coronary artery is foreshortened and may be completely obscured by its branches. This is especially so in patients with horizontal hearts (Figures 4.5, 4.6). Thus, it is advisable to examine the left main coronary artery in both the right and left anterior oblique projections. Occasionally neither the left nor right anterior oblique views will be adequate. In such instances additional views have been demonstrated to be very useful.[3,4]

The left main coronary artery terminates at the left atrioventricular groove by dividing into the left anterior descending coronary artery and the left circumflex artery.

The Left Anterior Descending Coronary Artery

Originating as a continuation of the left main coronary artery, the left anterior descending coronary artery courses over the anterior surface of the heart in the anterior interventricular sulcus. It usually runs down the entire length of this sulcus, frequently around the apex of the heart, and extends for a variable distance into the inferior interventricular sulcus (Figures 4.7-4.10). Occasionally the left anterior descending is seen as a short vessel which does not reach the apex of the heart (Figures 4.11, 4.12).

The left anterior descending artery is usually of larger diameter than the left circumflex artery, except when the left coronary system is dominant (Figures 4.9, 4.13).

Occasional variations in the course of the left anterior descending artery are seen angiographically and a few of these are demonstrated in Figures 4.14-4.16.

The left anterior descending coronary artery gives rise to two types of branches: 1) the septal arteries and 2) the diagonal arteries. The septal arteries are small in diameter, arise almost perpendicular to the left anterior descending artery and run deeply into the interventricular septum. The first septal artery arises from the proximal one-third of the left anterior descending artery and is the largest of these vessels (Figures 4.5, 4.7). The first septal is the most frequently involved of the septal arteries with atherosclerotic narrowing.[5]

The diagonal arteries usually two or three in number, are larger than the septal arteries and run over the epicardial surface of the free wall of the left ventricle (Figures 4.4-4.7, 4.9). Occasionally, it is possible to visualize diagonal branches to the right ventricle (Figures 4.12, 4.17). These branches may be well developed collateral channels when there is occlusion of the left anterior descending coronary artery.

When one recalls the circle-loop concept, the left anterior descending coronary artery is best visualized in the right anterior oblique projection (Figures 4.2, 4.7, 4.8, 4.13 A). In this projection it is a large prominent artery running in the anterior interventricular sulcus. The diagonal vessels and the perpendicular septal branches are easily appreciated. In the left anterior oblique projection, the left anterior descending artery is somewhat foreshortened and the septal arteries run almost parallel with it (Figures 4.1, 4.10). In the lateral projection (Figures 4.3-4.5, 4.9) the left anterior descending artery is located at the anterior border of the cardiac silhouette.

The Left Circumflex Artery

The left circumflex artery is the second major branch of the left main coronary artery. It begins at about a 90° angle from the left main coronary artery and enters the left atrioventricular sulcus (Figures 4.1-4.4, 4.7). It usually terminates between the obtuse margin and the crux. At the obtuse margin of the heart it gives off the obtuse marginal artery (Figures 4.7, 4.8).

There are two types of arterial branchings from the circumflex artery: 1) the left marginal arteries supplying the free wall of the left ventricle and 2) the atrial circumflex branches. In Figures 4.18-4.21 are demonstrated variations in the termination of the left circumflex artery as well as variations in the number and branchings of the left marginal arteries. After giving off the obtuse marginal artery, the distal left circumflex artery may become quite a small vessel (Figures 4.18, 4.19). The atrial circumflex branches will be discussed in Chapter 6.

In about 10% of patients the left circumflex artery reaches the crux of the heart and gives off the posterior descending coronary artery (Figures 4.9, 4.13, 4.22). This variation is referred to as a left dominant arterial system.

The right and left anterior oblique views are required for proper examination of the left circumflex artery. In the right anterior oblique view, the artery is seen coursing inferiorly and posteriorly (Figures 4.2, 4.7). In this view, the proximal few centimeters of the left circumflex artery are not as well visualized as the distal portion of this vessel. In the left anterior oblique view (Figures 4.1, 4.3, 4.5, 4.6) the circumflex artery forms the posterior border of the heart. This view is quite useful for assessing the proximal one-third of the left circumflex artery.

References

1. Kronzon, I., Deutsch, P., and Glassman, E.: Length of the left main coronary artery: Its relation to the pattern of coronary arterial distributions. *American Journal of Cardiology,* **34**:787-789, 1974.

2. James, T.N.: *Anatomy of the Coronary Arteries.* Paul B. Hoeber, Inc., New York, 1961.

3. Lespérance, J., Saltiel, J., Petitclerc, R., and Bourassa, M.G.: Angulated views in the sagittal plane for improved accuracy of cinecoronary angiography. *American Journal of Roentgenology, Radium Therapy and Nuclear Medicine,* **121**:565-574, 1974.

4. Sos, T.A., Lee, J.G., Levin, D.C., and Baltaxe, H.A.: New lordotic projection for improved visualization of the left coronary artery and its branches. *American Journal of Roentgenology, Radium Therapy and Nuclear Medicine,* **121**:575-582, 1974.

5. Fulton, W.F.M.: *The Coronary Arteries: Arteriography, Microanatomy and Pathogenesis of Obliterative Coronary Artery Disease.* Charles C. Thomas, Springfield, Ill., 1965.

Figure 4.1:   Left coronary arteriogram; left anterior oblique projection.

A. The left main coronary artery appears in profile as a large vessel originating from the posterior border of the aortic bulb (left coronary sinus of Valsalva). The left anterior descending artery (LAD) partially over-laps itself; the septal arteries (S) are present behind the LAD. The left circumflex artery (CX) is located posteriorly and reaches the crux. The left marginal artery (LM) outlines the posterior border of the heart.

D = diagonal branch of left anterior descending coronary artery.

B. Diagrammatic representation of A.

Figure 4.2:   Left coronary artery; right anterior oblique projection. The distal segment of the left main coronary artery (LCA) is better visualized in this projection. It appears as a short vessel which bifurcates into the left anterior descending (LAD) and left circumflex (CX) arteries. A diagonal artery originates from the LAD and is a tortuous vessel. The left circumflex artery (CX) has a large diameter and gives off three marginal arteries which are of approximately equal size.

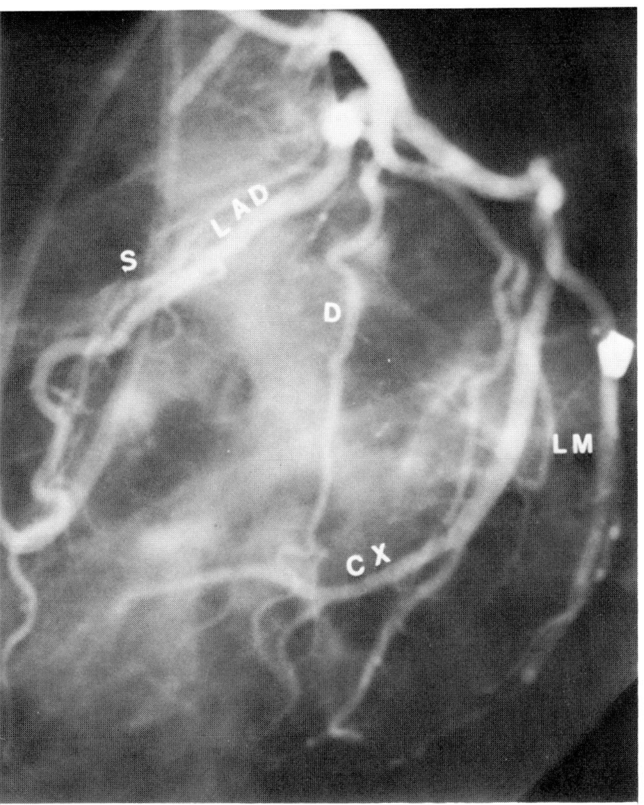

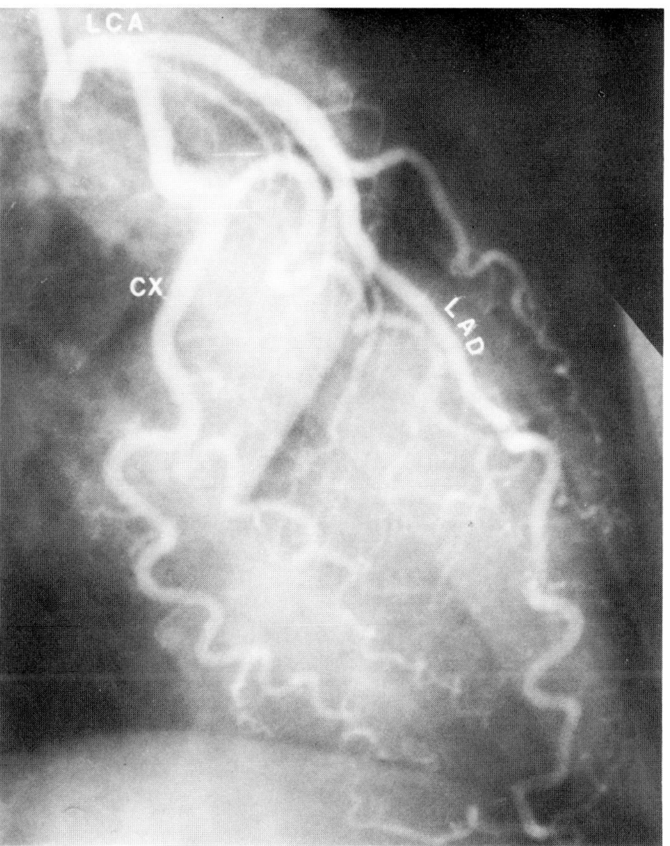

FIGURE 4.2

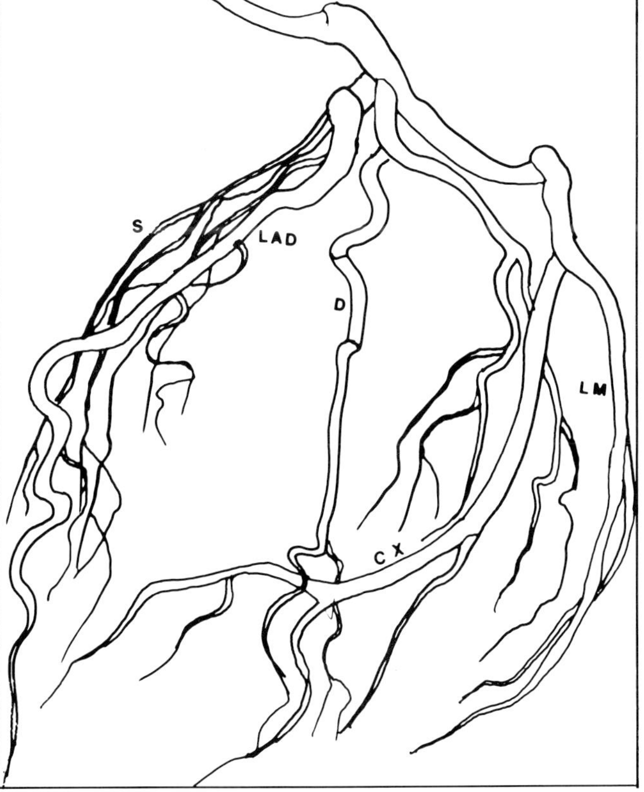

FIGURE 4.1

Figure 4.3:   Left coronary arteriogram; lateral projection. The left main coronary is visualized as a short, oblique channel since it is partially foreshortened in this projection. The entire left anterior descending artery (LAD) runs along the anterior border of the cardiac silhouette, wraps about the apex and ascends a few centimeters up the inferior interventricular sulcus. The left circumflex artery (CX) is located posteriorly; it is partially over-lapped by a left marginal artery (LM).

Figure 4.4:   Left coronary arteriogram; lateral projection. The left main coronary artery is markedly foreshortened. The left anterior descending artery (LAD) is seen outlining the anterior border of the cardiac silhouette. A large diagonal artery (D) is present. The left circumflex artery (CX) and the left marginal artery (LM) outline the posterior and inferior borders of the heart.

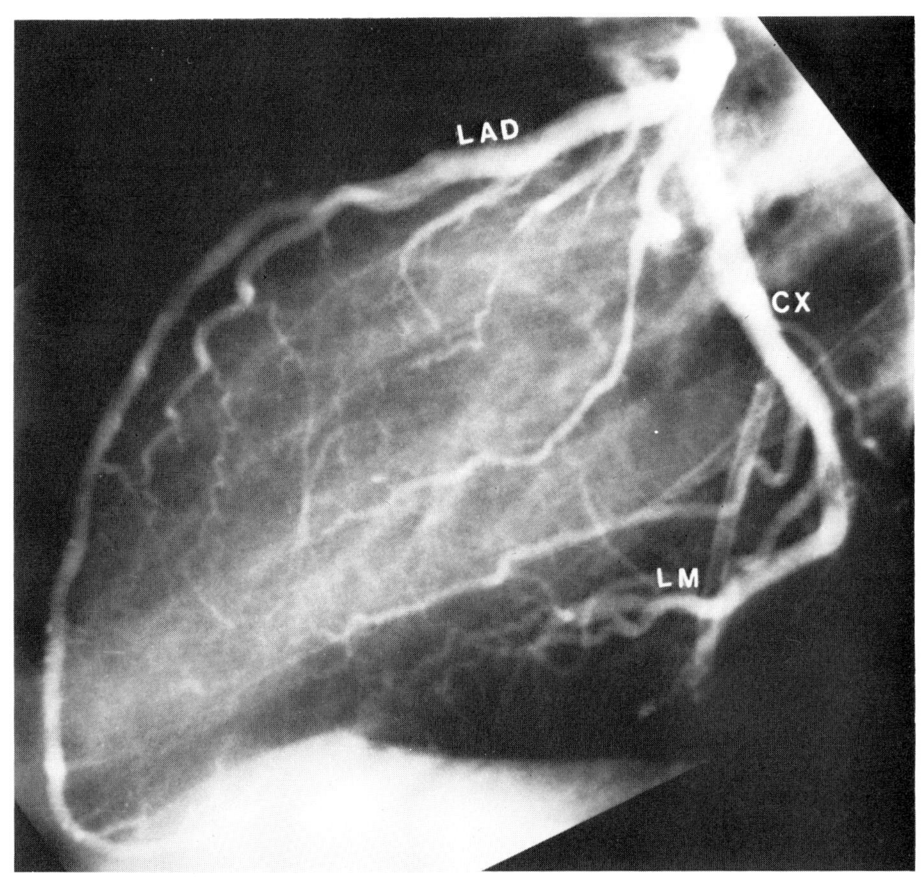

FIGURE 4.3

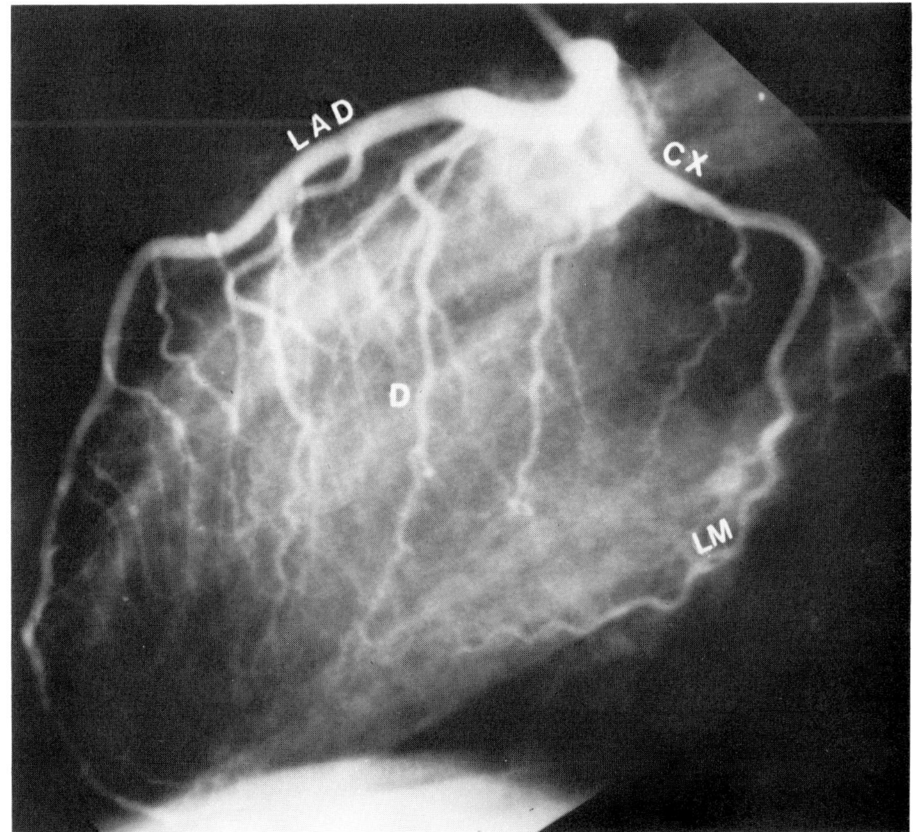

FIGURE 4.4

Figure 4.5:   Left coronary arteriogram; lateral projection. The left main coronary artery is completely obscured in a patient with a horizontal heart. The left anterior descending coronary artery is well visualized. The septal (S) and diagonal (D) arteries are seen originating from the left anterior descending coronary artery. The septals are straight vessels and the diagonals are tortuous channels. The circumflex (CX) and left marginal (LM) arteries course along the posterior border of the heart.

Figure 4.6:   Left coronary arteriogram; left anterior oblique projection. The left main coronary artery is again totally obscured in a patient with a horizontal heart. A diagonal artery (D) courses over the free wall of the left ventricle between the left anterior descending (LAD) and circumflex (CX) arteries.

LM = left marginal branch of circumflex artery.

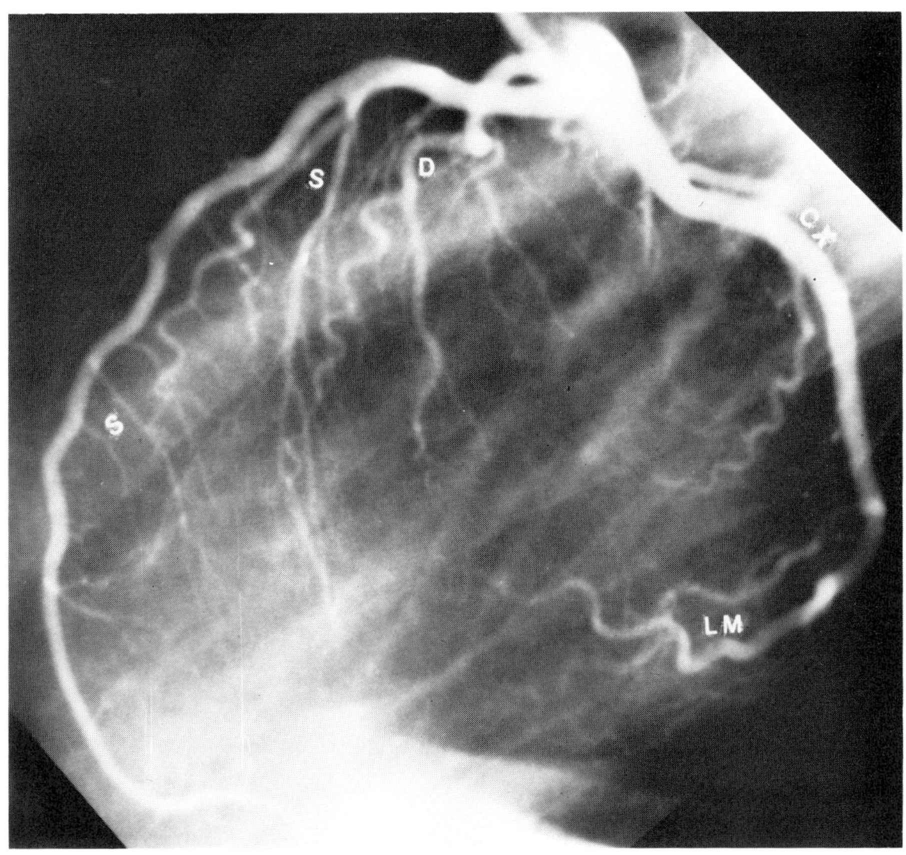

FIGURE 4.5

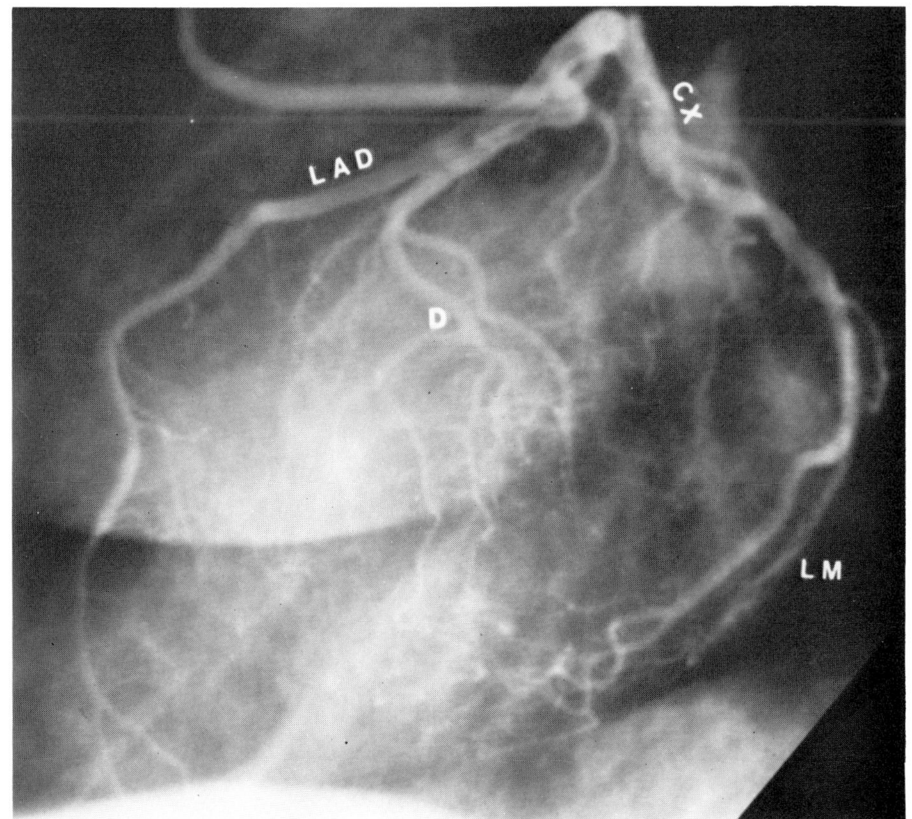

FIGURE 4.6

Figure 4.7:   Left coronary arteriogram; right anterior oblique projection. The left main coronary artery is partially visualized. The left anterior descending artery (LAD) is a large vessel at the anterior border of the cardiac silhouette in the interventricular sulcus. It extends around the cardiac apex to almost the mid-point of the inferior surface of the heart. The first septal artery (S) is a large vessel and originates perpendicularly from the left anterior descending artery. The first diagonal artery (D) is partially over-lapped by the LAD. The circumflex artery (CX) is large and courses posteriorly and inferiorly. A large left marginal artery (LM) lies close to the inferior border of the cardiac silhouette.

Figure 4.8:   Left coronary arteriogram; right anterior oblique projection. The left main coronary artery is a short vessel. The left anterior descending artery (LAD) is a large vessel which courses in the anterior interventricular sulcus and wraps around the apex. The diagonal artery is at the anterior margin of the cardiac silhouette. The left circumflex artery is a short vessel and gives rise to a large left marginal artery (LM) visualized as a continuation of the left circumflex artery. The other large artery branching from the circumflex artery is an atrial vessel, the left atrial circumflex artery (LAC).

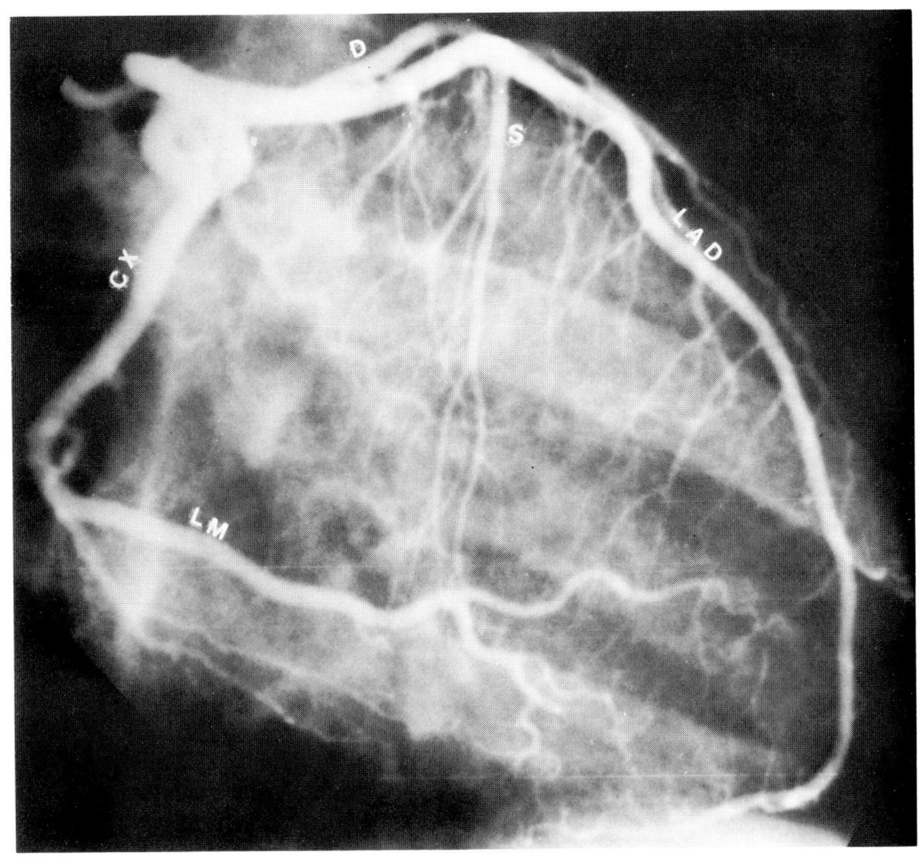

FIGURE 4.7

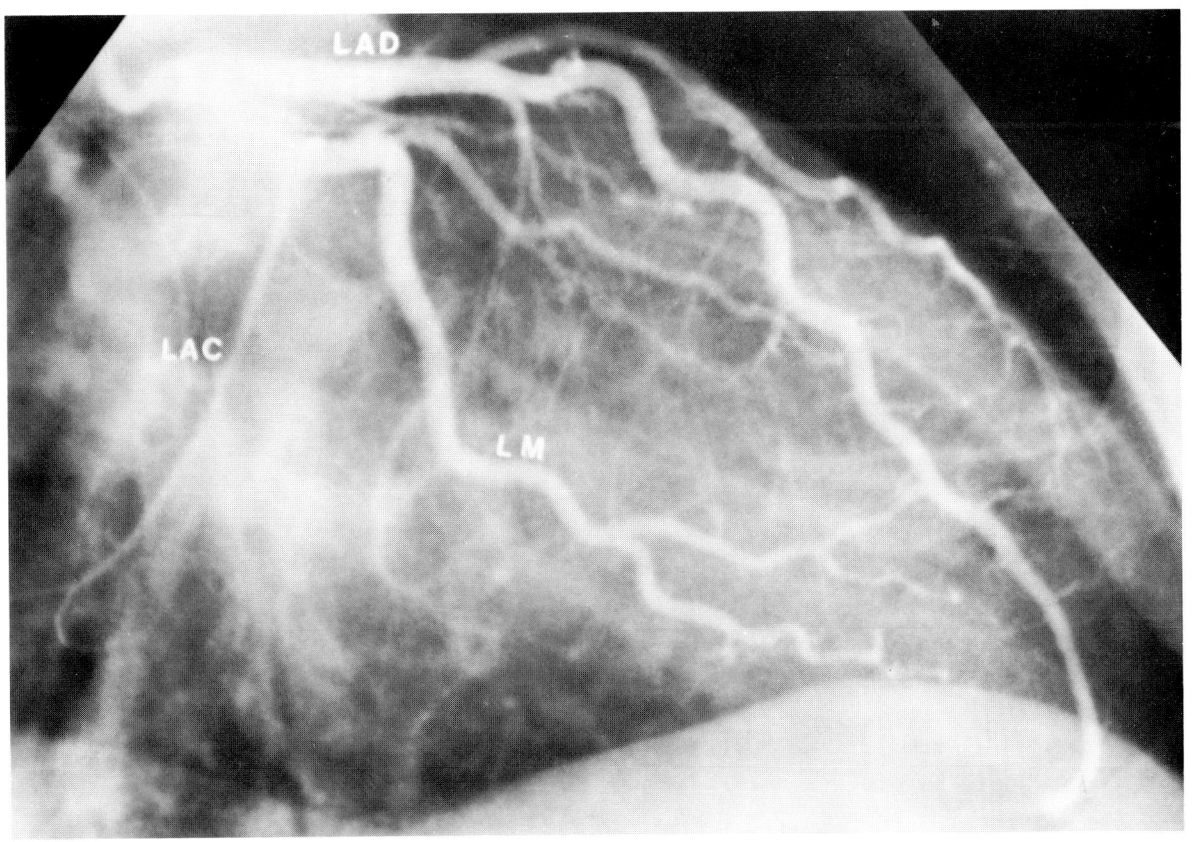

FIGURE 4.8

Figure 4.9:   Left coronary arteriogram; lateral view. A left dominant coronary system is demonstrated. The left anterior descending artery (LAD) and the left circumflex artery (CX) are of the same size. The LAD is on the anterior border of the heart. The CX gives rise to the posterior descending artery (PD). A left marginal artery (LM) and the sinus node artery (SN) are also seen originating from the large CX. Diagonal (D) and septal (S) branches arise from the LAD.

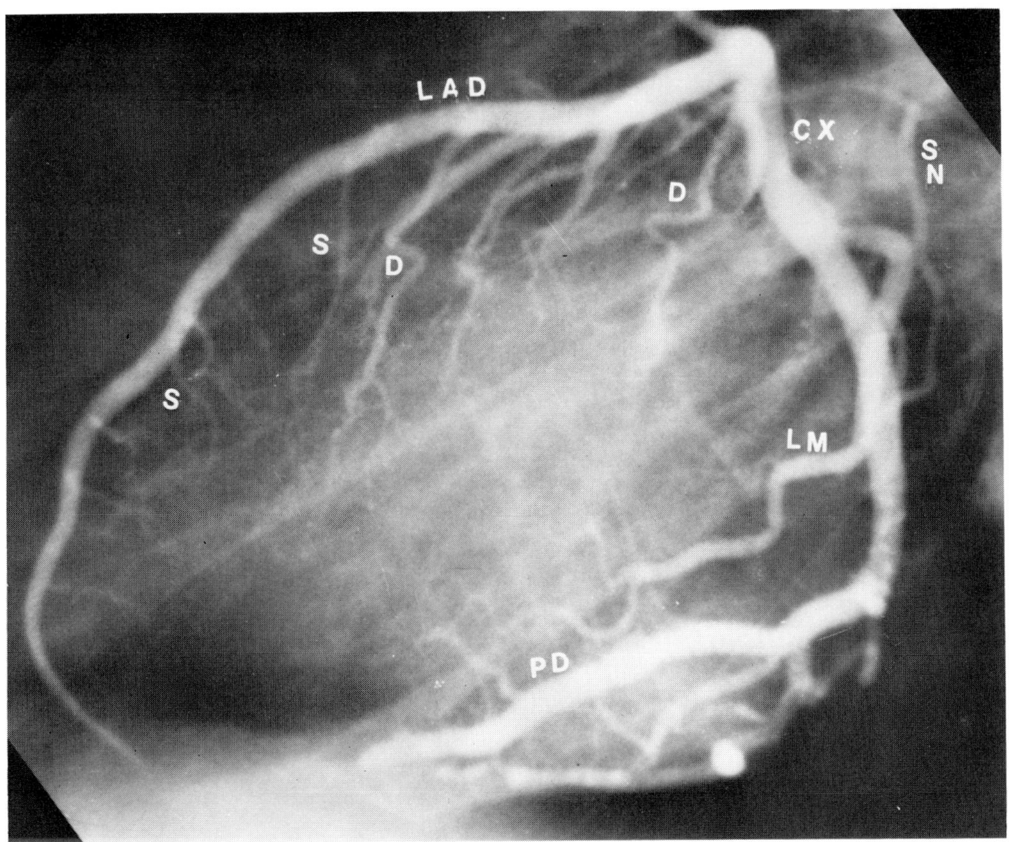

FIGURE 4.9

Figure 4.10:   Left coronary arteriogram; left anterior oblique projection. The left anterior descending artery (LAD) courses near the middle of the cardiac silhouette, reaches the apex and turns up the inferior surface of the left ventricle; in this projection the septial arteries are parallel to the LAD and crowd behind it. The left marginal artery (LM) which is a continuation of the left circumflex artery is present at the posterior and inferior borders of the heart.

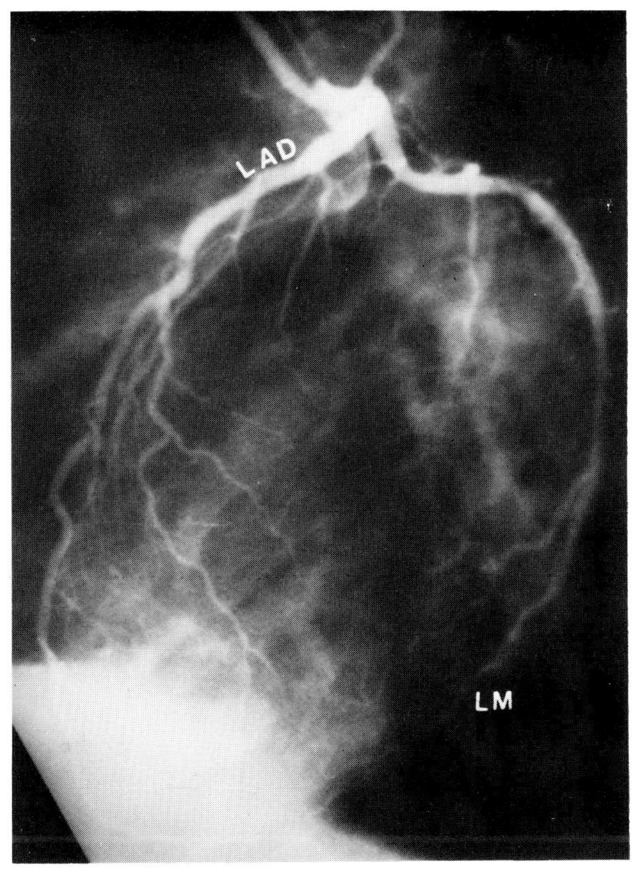

FIGURE 4.10

Figure 4.11: Left coronary arteriogram; right anterior oblique projection. The left anterior descending artery (LAD) is short and does not reach the apex. Overlapping between the LAD and its diagonal branches makes it difficult to identify each vessel in this projection; other views are required. The left circumflex artery (CX) lies in the left atrioventricular groove after giving off the left marginal (LM) artery. The LM is a large vessel in this example.

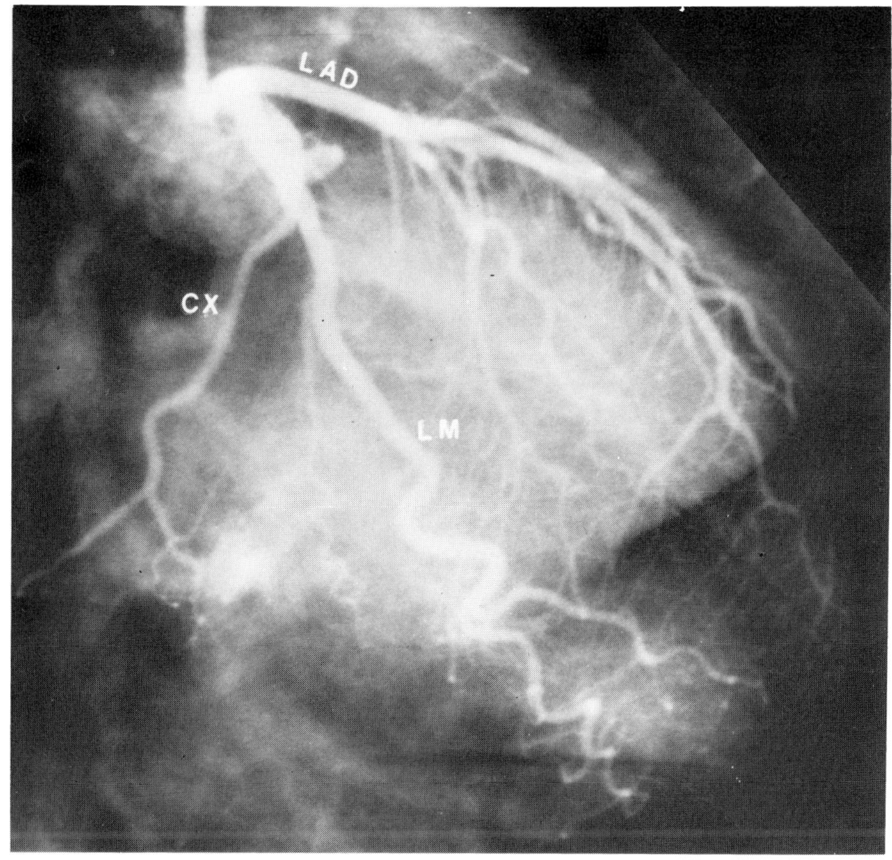

FIGURE 4.11

Figure 4.12:   Left coronary arteriogram; left anterior oblique projection.

A. Another example of a short left anterior descending artery (LAD). It is identified by the presence of septal branches. A large right ventricular diagonal branch (D) supplies the anterior wall of the right ventricle.

CX = circumflex artery.

B. Diagrammatic representation of **A**.

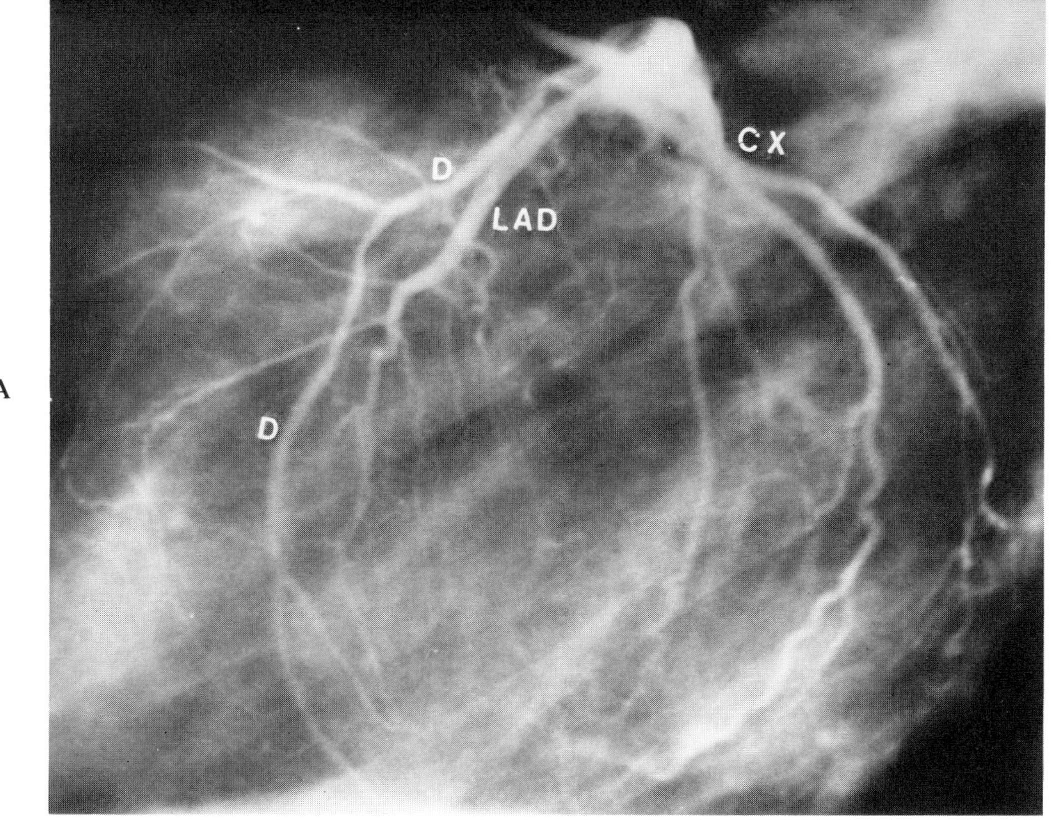

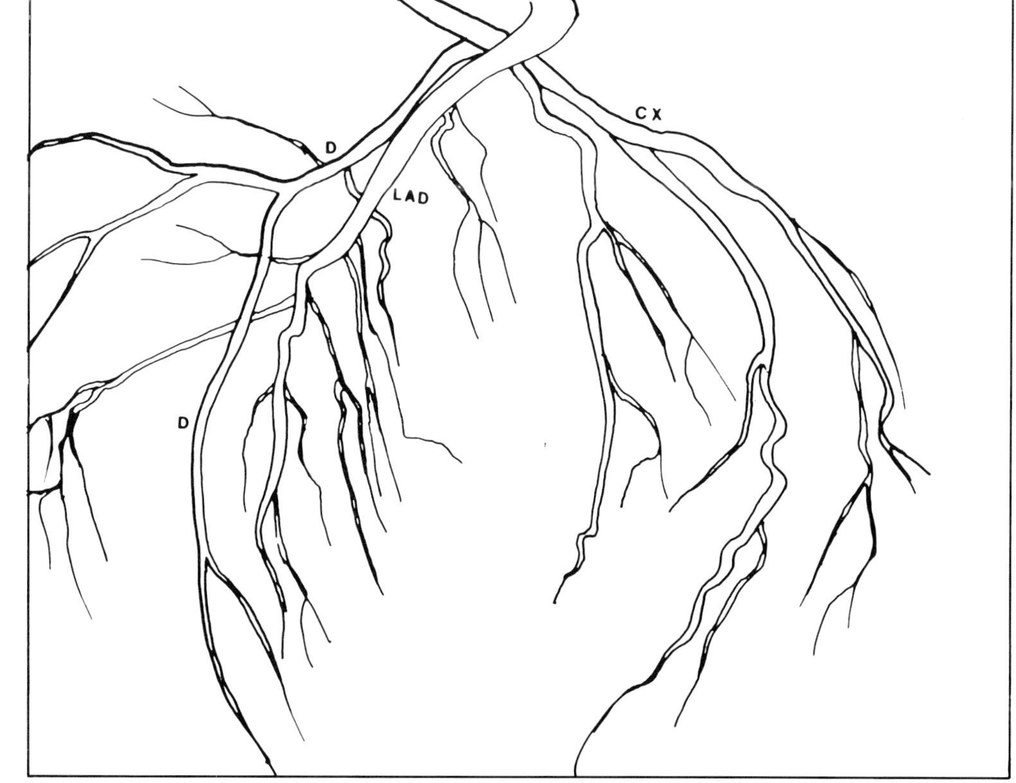

FIGURE 4.12

Figure 4.13: Left anterior descending coronary artery; **A**. Right anterior oblique projection; **B**. Left anterior oblique projection. A left dominant coronary system is visualized in two projections. The left main coronary artery (LC) is easily recognized in the right anterior oblique projection (**A**), but poorly visualized in the left anterior oblique projection (**B**). The left anterior descending artery (LAD) is a direct continuation of the LC and courses in the anterior interventricular groove to the apex. The septal branches (S) of the LAD are easily seen in both projections; the diagonal arteries (D) are better visualized in the left anterior oblique projection. The left circumflex artery (CX) is a large vessel which reaches the crux of the heart after giving off the left marginal branches (LM) and the sinus node (SN) artery. In a left dominant coronary system the posterior descending artery (PD) originates from the CX and courses in the inferior interventricular sulcus.

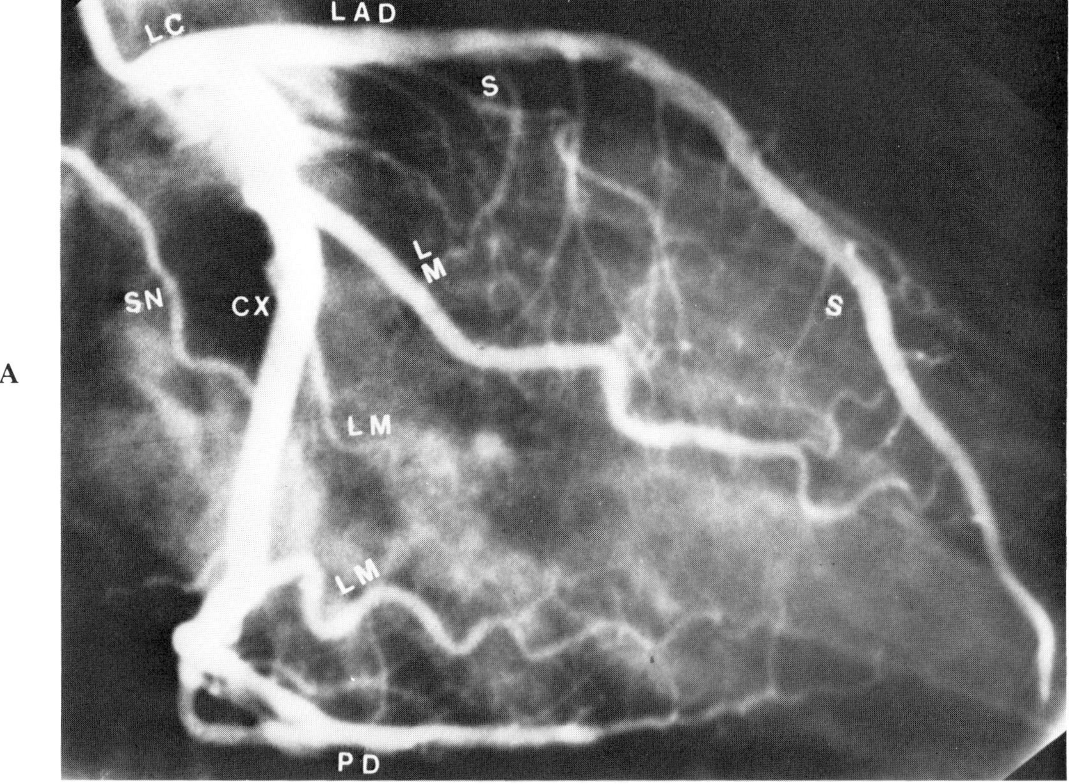

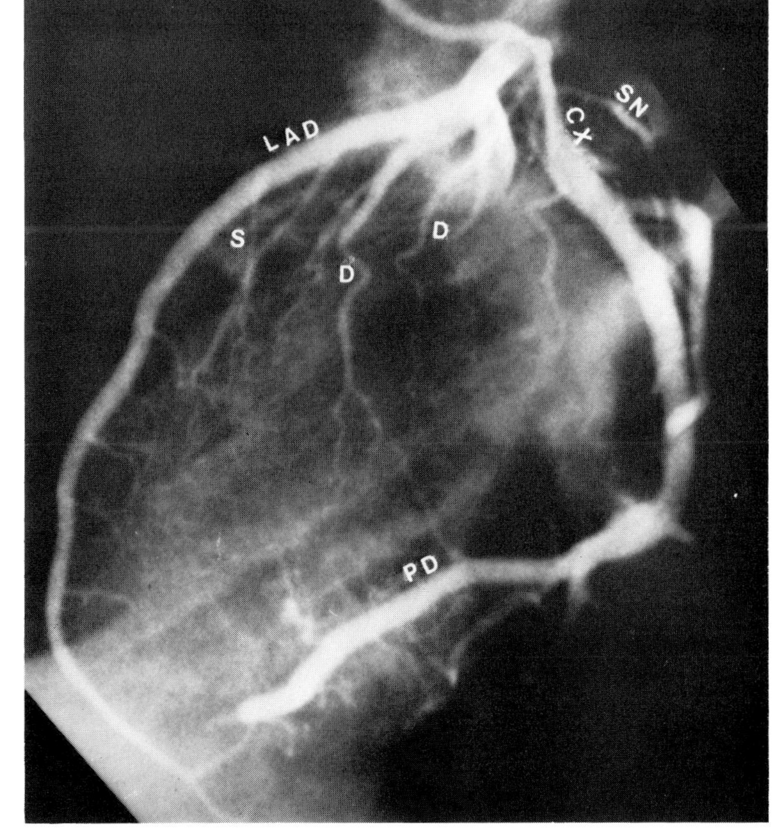

FIGURE 4.13

Figure 4.14:   Left coronary arteriogram; right anterior oblique projection.

A. The left anterior descending artery (LAD) has an unusual angulation; the first septal artery originates at this angulation. The left circumflex artery (CX) is a small vessel after giving off a large left marginal branch (LM).

B. Diagrammatic representation of A.

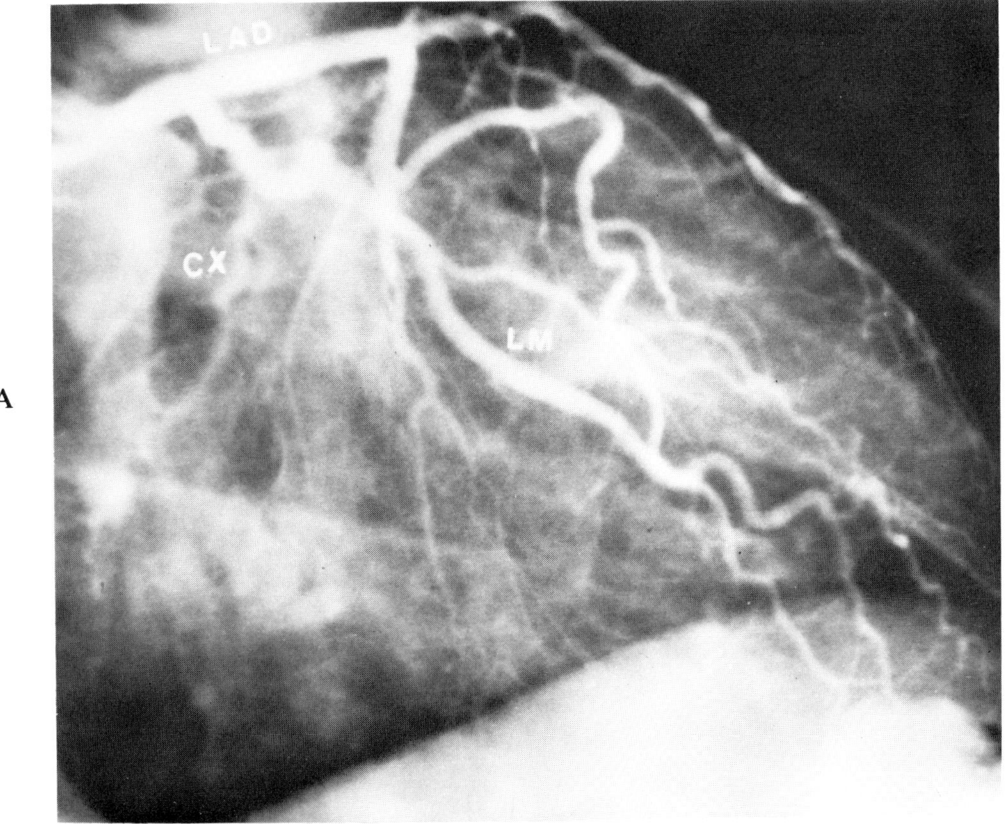

A

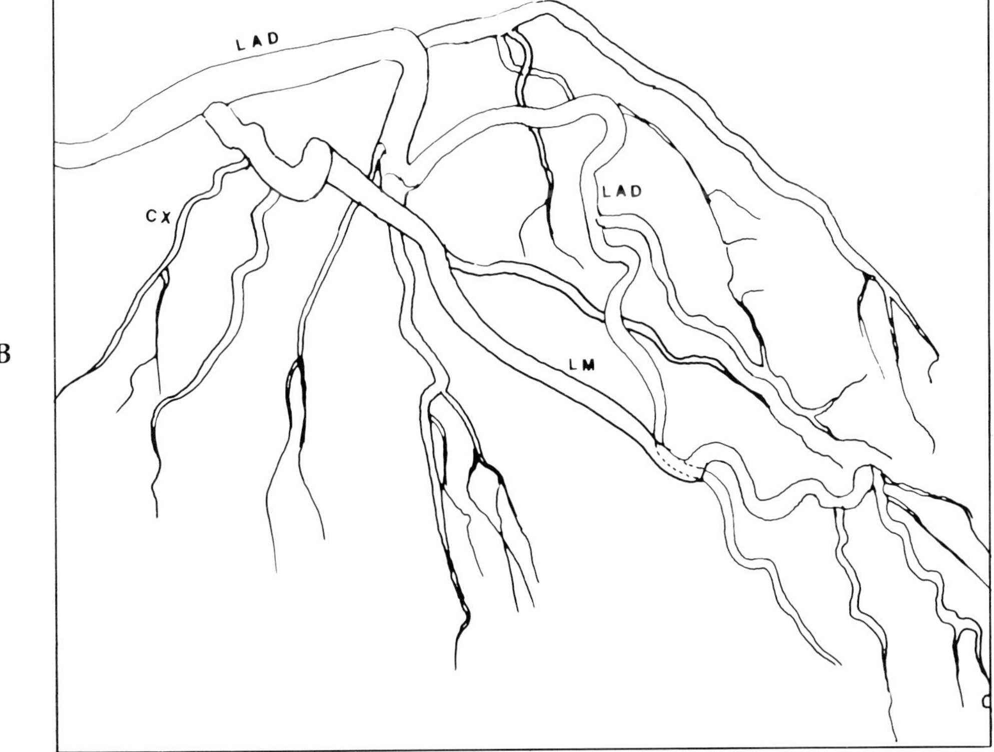

B

FIGURE 4.14

Figure 4.15:   Left coronary arteriogram; lateral projection.

A. The left anterior descending artery (LAD) takes an unusual turn and with its diagonal artery (D) forms a loop. The LAD is recognized by the origin of the septal branches (S). The left circumflex (CX) and left marginal (LM) arteries are present at the posterior and inferior margins of the cardiac silhouette.

B. Diagrammatic representation of **A**.

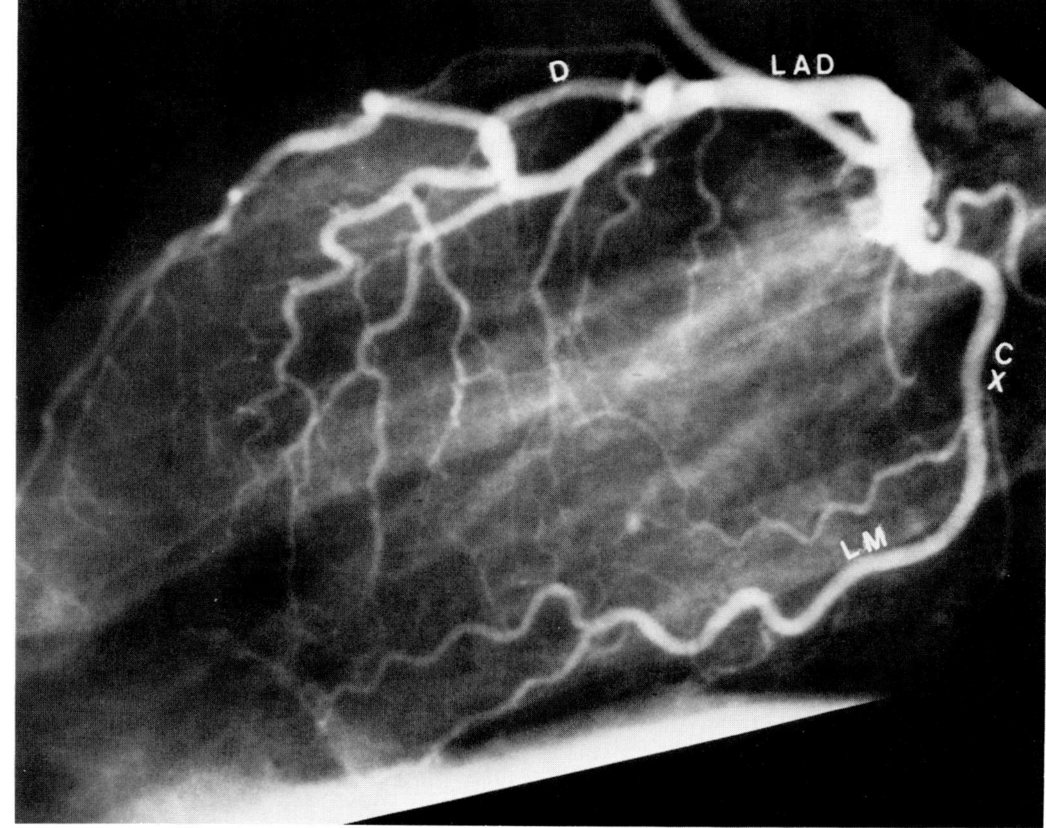

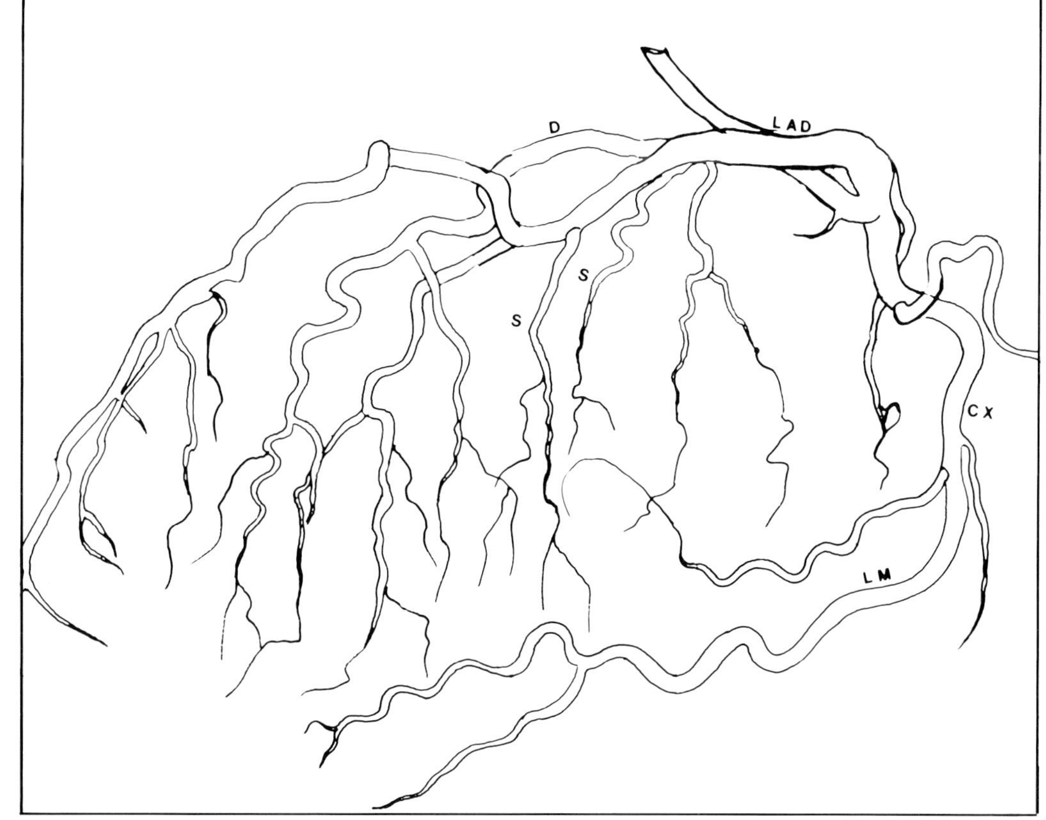

FIGURE 4.15

Figure 4.16:   Left coronary arteriogram; left anterior oblique projection.

A. The left anterior descending artery (LAD) is quite tortuous and forms a loop in the proximal one-half of its course. This loop is crossed by a diagonal branch (D) of the LAD. The diagonal artery is identified by the arrows.

B. Diagrammatic representation of A.

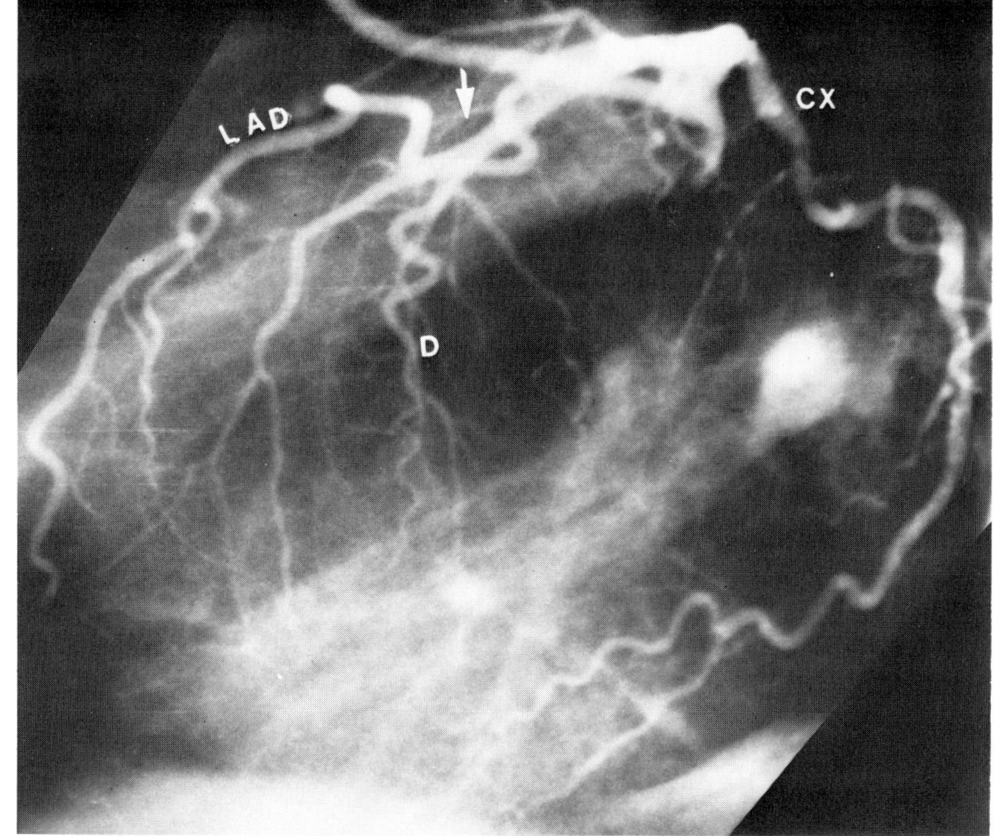

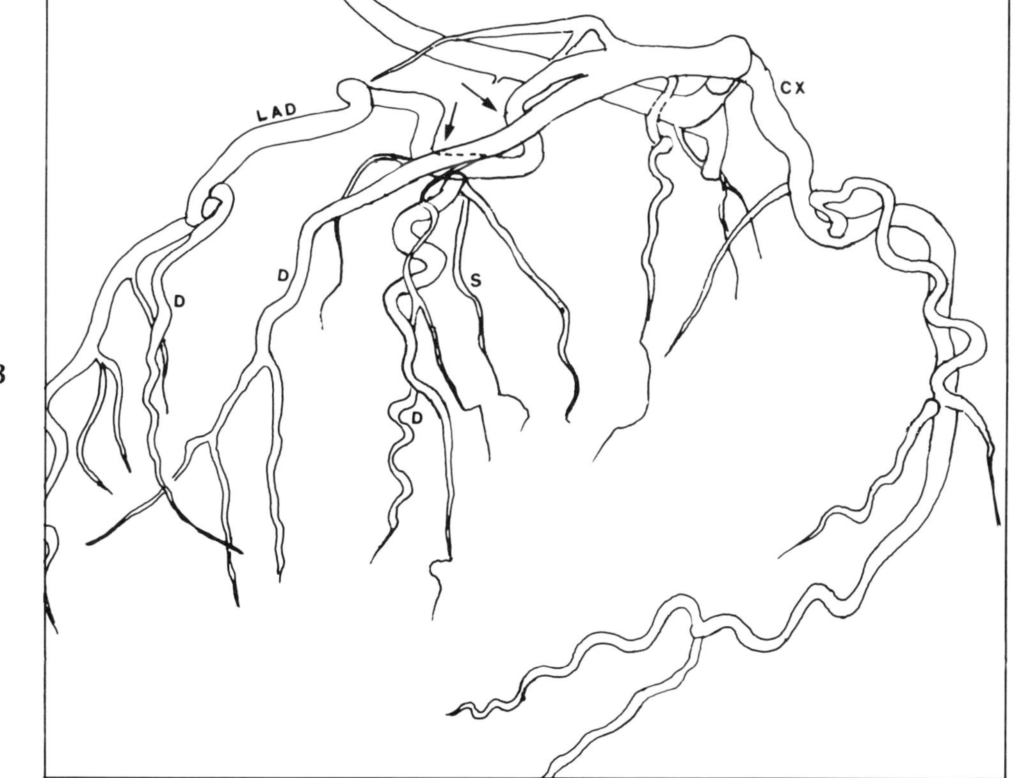

FIGURE 4.16

Figure 4.17:   Left coronary arteriogram; left anterior oblique projection.

A. The left anterior descending artery (LAD) gives off a large diagonal branch (RVD) to the anterior wall of the right ventricle. This is a large right ventricular diagonal branch; they are usually quite small. These vessels may become quite large when functioning as collateral channels.

CX = left circumflex coronary artery. D = diagonal branch (to the left ventricle) of the left anterior descending coronary artery.

B. Diagrammatic representation of **A**.

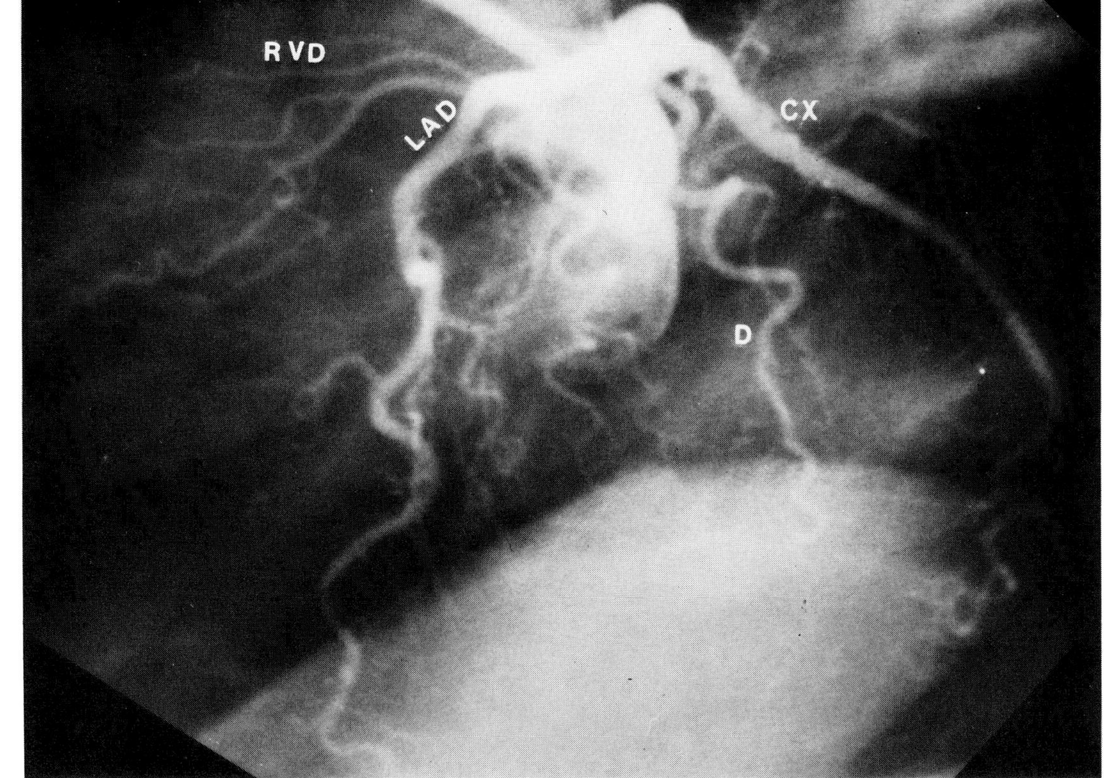

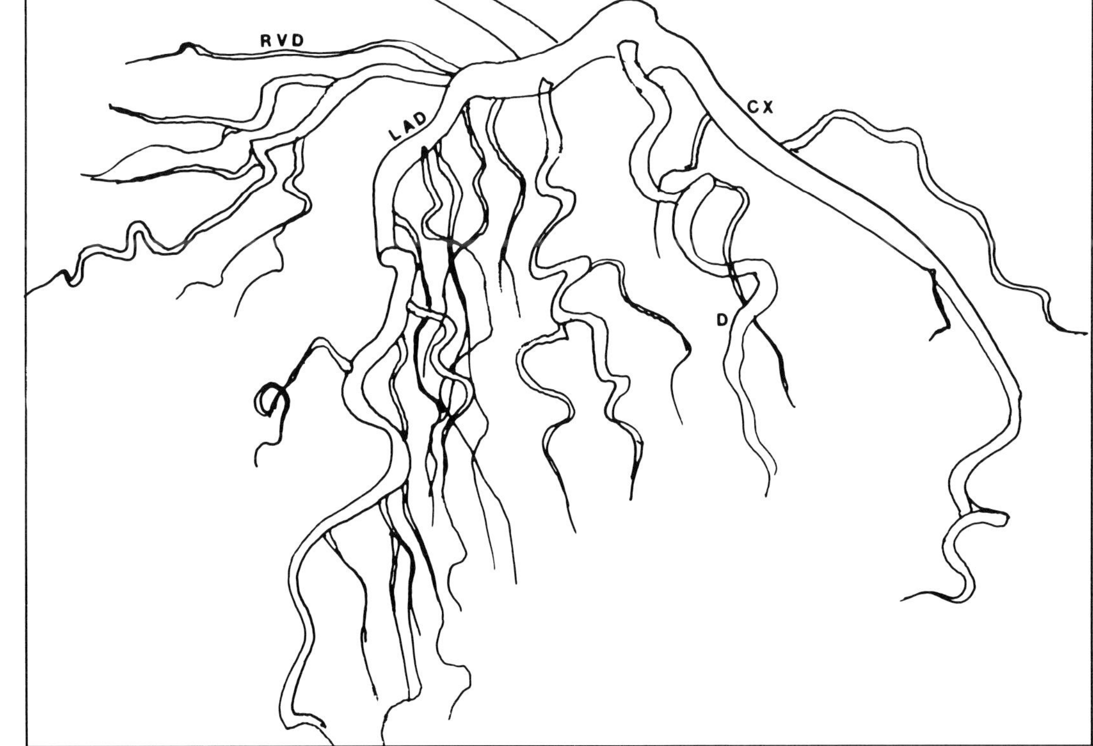

FIGURE 4.17

Figure 4.18:   Left coronary arteriogram; right anterior oblique projection. The left circumflex artery (CX) is a large but short vessel. After giving off a large left marginal branch (LM) near its origin, the CX becomes a very small vessel (arrow).

LAD = left anterior descending coronary artery. D = diagonal branch of left anterior descending coronary artery. S = septal branches of left anterior descending coronary artery.

Figure 4.19:   Left coronary arteriogram; right anterior oblique projection. This left circumflex artery (CX) is much larger than the one seen in Figure 4.18. The left marginal artery (LM) originates as a large trunk and divides into two large branches. After the origin of the LM the distal segment of the CX gives off several atrial branches.

LAD = left anterior descending coronary artery.

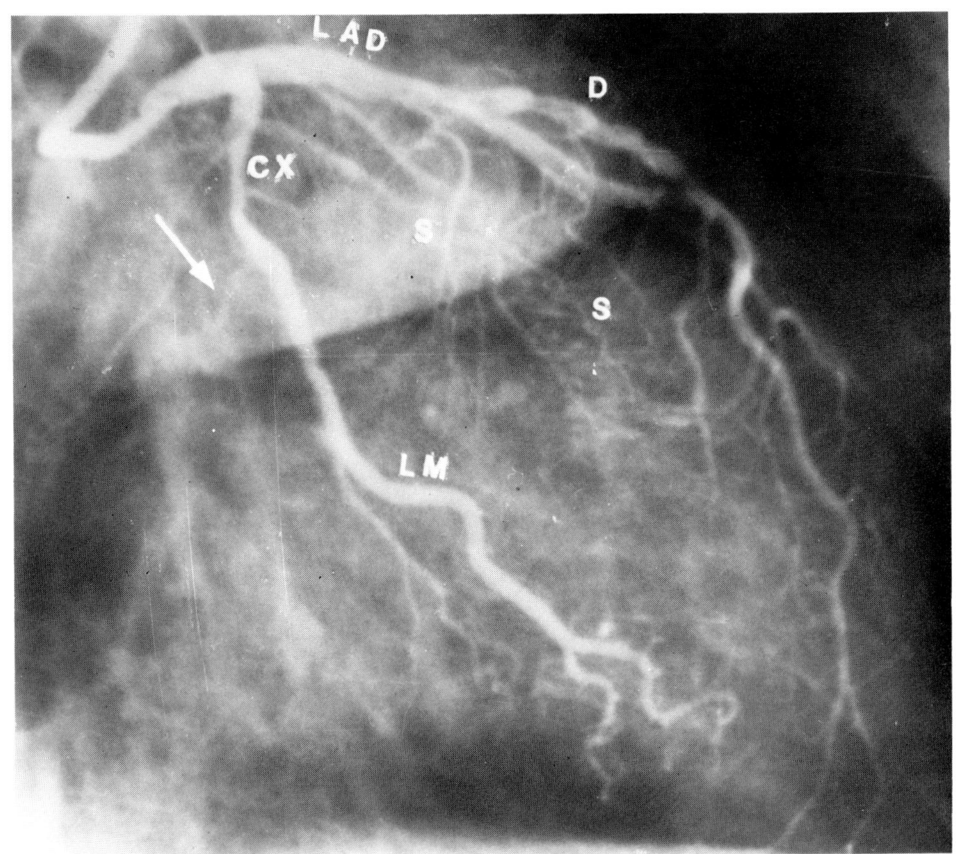

FIGURE 4.18

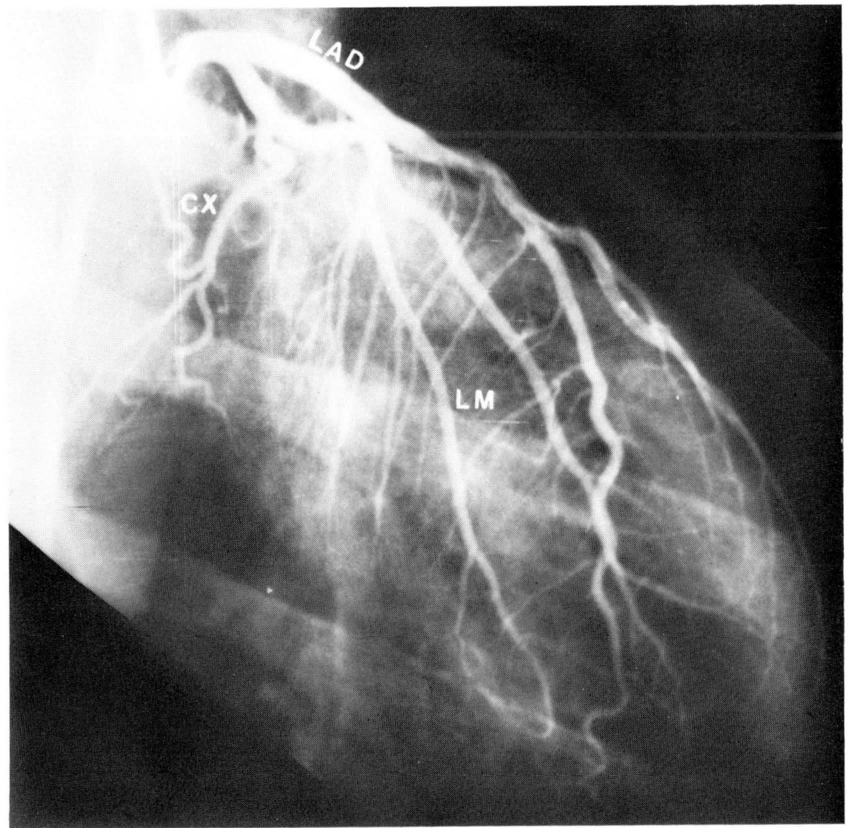

FIGURE 4.19

Figure 4.20:   Left coronary arteriogram; right anterior oblique projection. Left main coronary artery (LCA) is a long vessel. The left circumflex artery (CX) is a large vessel originating at a $90°$ angle from the LCA. The CX becomes quite small after it gives off a large left marginal artery (LM). The CX extends to the middle portion of the left atrioventricular sulcus. The left anterior descending (LAD) coronary artery takes a sharp angulation in the middle of its course to reach the apex of the heart.

Figure 4.21:   Left coronary arteriogram; right anterior oblique projection. The left main coronary artery is not quite as long in this patient and appears to originate in an almost vertical direction from the left coronary sinus of Valsalva. The left circumflex coronary artery (CX) is a large vessel and runs along the entire length of the left atrioventricular sulcus to reach the crux of the heart; during its course it gives off two large left marginal arteries (LM). A smaller marginal vessel is located between the two large marginals. It also supplies blood to the free wall of the left ventricle.

LAD = left anterior descending coronary artery.

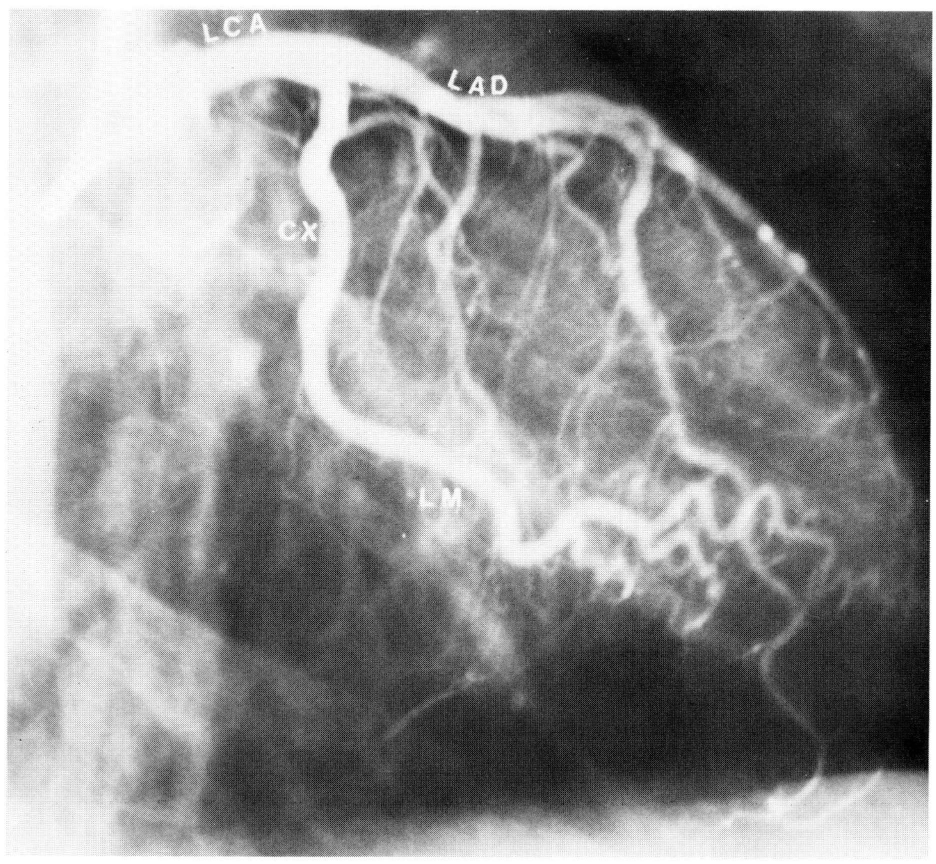

FIGURE 4.20

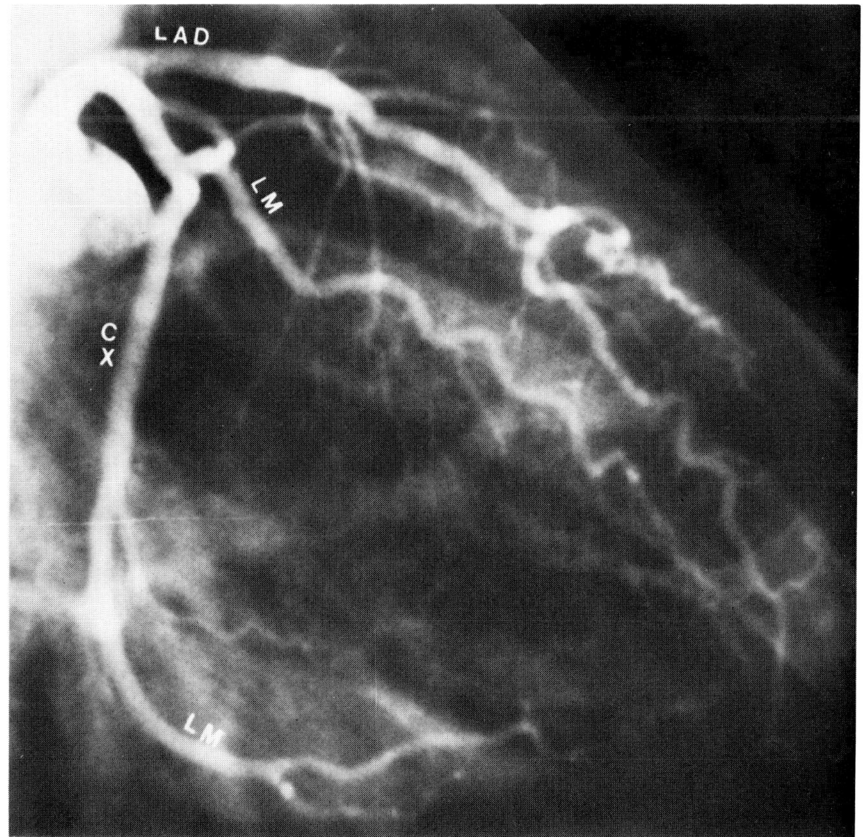

FIGURE 4.21

Figure 4.22: Left coronary arteriogram; right anterior oblique projection. The left circumflex artery (CX) is larger than the left anterior descending artery (LAD). There are several left marginal arteries but only one is quite large (LM). The posterior descending artery (PD) originates from the circumflex artery as is characteristic in a left dominant coronary system.

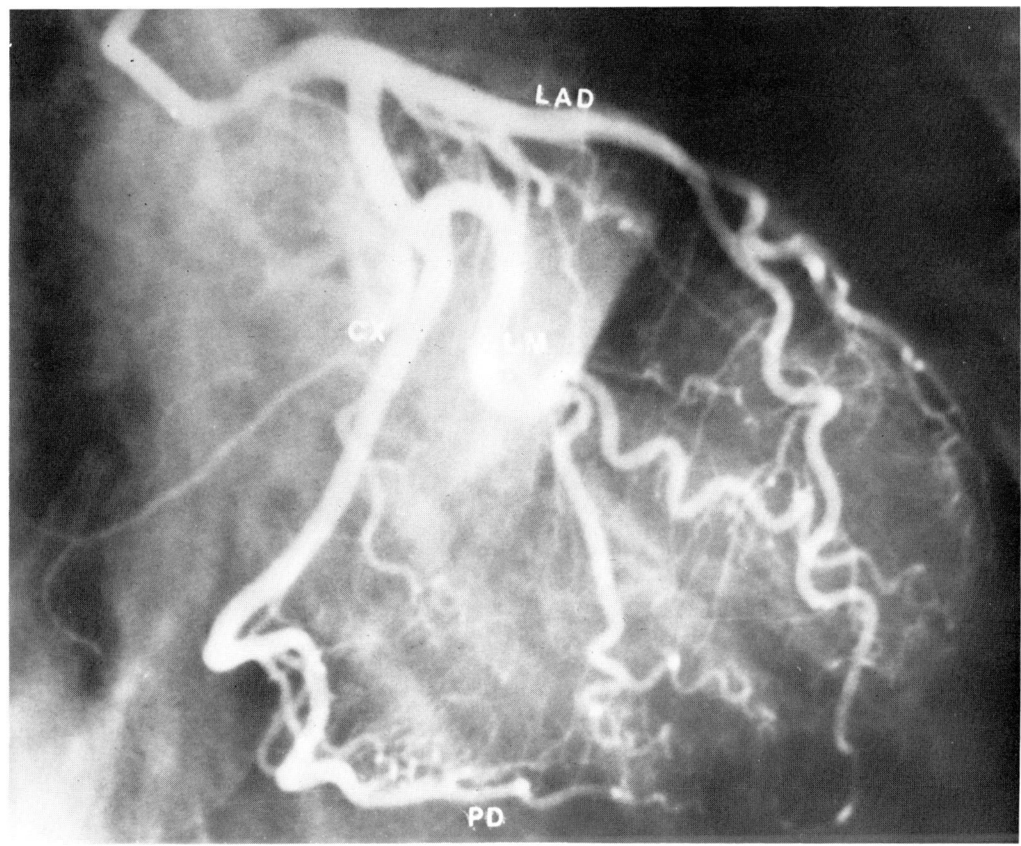

FIGURE 4.22

Chapter 5

The Normal Right Coronary Artery

The right coronary artery originates from the aorta in the right coronary sinus of Valsalva. In 50% of patients the right coronary ostium is unique in that there are two orifices. The second orifice is usually smaller and is the origin of the conus artery.[1] In the antero-posterior projection, the right coronary ostium will be catheterized if the tip of the catheter is oriented anteriorly. In the lateral and left anterior oblique projections, the anterior location of the right coronary ostium is better appreciated and the tip of the catheter is more accurately oriented in an anterior direction.

The origin of the right coronary artery is best visualized in the left anterior oblique projection (Figures 5.1-5.4). In patients with a wide thorax and a horizontal heart, visualization of the first few centimeters of the right coronary artery is improved due to the horizontal direction of the first segment of the right coronary artery (Figure 5.2). In the right anterior oblique and lateral projections, the orifice is overlapped by the first few centimeters of the right coronary artery (Figures 5.5 and 5.6).

The right coronary artery is divided into two portions. The proximal right coronary artery is that portion of the vessel between the orifice and the crux of the heart and represents that portion of the vessel which courses in the right atrioventricular sulcus. The proximal portion of the right coronary artery gives off branches which supply the right ventricle and the right atrium. The right ventricular branches, which are also referred to as the right marginal arteries, supply the free wall of the right ventricle and vary in number between 2 and 6.[2] The first branch of the proximal right coronary artery is called the conus artery. It supplies the anterior wall of the right ventricular outflow tract (parietal band and moderator band). Occasionally, an additional small artery arises from the proximal right coronary artery and supplies the epicardial fat of the pulmonary conus.[2] The origin of the conus artery is best seen in the left anterior oblique projection (Figures 5.1, 5.2), and the proximal segment of this vessel is best appreciated in the right anterior oblique projection (Figure 5.7).

In most patients a large right marginal artery can be visualized originating from the proximal right coronary artery at or near the margo acutus. This artery is frequently called "artery of the margo acutus," and it runs along the free border of the right ventricle to supply the inferior surface of this chamber. This is appreciated in Figures 5.5 and 5.6. Occasionally the origin of this vessel is near the origin of the proximal right coronary artery, and in this situation the artery of the margo acutus runs over the anterior wall of the right ventricle (Figures 5.7, 5.8).

The artery to the sinus node is the most important of the atrial branches of the proximal right coronary artery. It originates generally as the second branch of the proximal right coronary artery and is seen to course posteriorly and superiorly (Figures 5.3-5.5, 5.7). This artery will be discussed in Chapter 6.

Proper angiographic evaluation of the proximal right coronary artery requires visualization in the three basic projections, the left anterior oblique, the right anterior oblique and the lateral projections, each of which demonstrates a different aspect of this vessel and its branches.

The left anterior oblique projection depicts the proximal right coronary artery as a large vessel forming an arch which opens posteriorly. The ostium may be visualized as an evagination of the external border of the right sinus of Valsalva. The posterior descending artery originates at the distal end of the proximal portion of the right coronary artery. The right marginal branches are foreshortened in this projection (Figures 5.1-5.4).

In the right anterior oblique projection, the proximal right coronary artery usually opacifies in an oblique direction from its origin above to the inferior and posterior part of the heart below (Figure 5.5). In this view the proximal and distal thirds of the proximal right coronary artery are foreshortened, but the middle third is well demonstrated, as are the right marginal branches which course in an anterior direction from the main trunk to the apex of the heart (Figures 5.5, 5.6).

When the proximal right coronary artery arrives at the crux of the heart (junction of the atrioventricular groove and the posterior interventricular sulcus)[3] it bifurcates into two arteries: the distal right coronary artery and the posterior descending artery.

The distal right coronary artery is that portion of the right coronary artery lying in the left atrioventricular groove and is actually a continuation of the proximal portion of the right coronary artery. The distal right coronary artery was absent in 18% of hearts studied by James.[1] The length of the distal right coronary artery is variable and is related to the length of the circumflex artery. The branches of the distal right coronary artery vary in number from 1 to 5, as they course from the atrioventricular groove over the inferior surface of the left ventricle to the apex of the heart.

The distal right coronary artery is best visualized in the left anterior oblique projection (Figures 5.1–5.4). In this projection the distal right coronary artery located in the left atrioventricular groove forms a part of the circle, along with the proximal right coronary artery and the left circumflex artery (Figures 3.2, 5.2). In the right anterior oblique projection the distal right coronary artery may be overlapped by the branches supplying blood to the free wall of the left ventricle and will not be well visualized. The arteries will appear as small branches running from the atrioventricular groove to the apex (Figure 5.6).

The posterior descending coronary artery is a relatively large vessel located in the inferior interventricular sulcus running from or prior to the crux towards the apex of the heart. Radiographically the posterior descending coronary artery is best visualized in the right anterior oblique projection. With reference to the circle and loop concept, the posterior descending artery forms the inferior border of the loop. Therefore, in the right anterior oblique projection (Figures 5.5, 5.6, 5.9), it appears as a vessel running along the inferior surface of the heart. Sometimes the posterior descending cannot be easily separated from other vessels which may have the same caliber and lie in close proximity. The presence of septal arteries (Figure 5.9) as well as its restricted motion during the cardiac cycle may help to identify this vessel. Occasionally there are two segments forming the posterior descending coronary artery, one segment originating from the right coronary artery at the crux and the other originating from a right marginal branch (Figure 5.10). At times the posterior descending originates from a right marginal branch (Figures 5.11, 5.12).

The length of the posterior descending is variable and is generally inversely related to the length of the left anterior descending coronary artery which frequently wraps around the apex and ascends on the posterior wall. If the left anterior descending artery is short, the posterior descending is usually long and wraps around the apex ascending a short distance on the anterior wall (Figures 5.9, 5.13). If the posterior descending is short (Figure 5.5), then the left anterior descending is usually a long vessel. According to James,[1] the posterior descending most frequently terminates between one-half to three-quarters of the distance from the crux to the apex down the posterior interventricular sulcus (62%) and in only 26% of cases does the posterior descending terminate at the apex (Figures 5.5, 5.9, 5.13).

The posterior descending artery gives off septal and right and left ventricular branches. With the exception of the artery to the atrioventricular node, which measures 25 mm. in length, the septal arteries are no longer than 15 mm.[1] The arteries to the right ventricle arise in a perpendicular fashion to the course of the posterior descending artery and are parallel to each other. These arteries anastomose with the right marginal branches of the proximal portion of the right coronary artery. The branches to the left ventricle are usually larger than those to the right ventricle and originate at an acute angle from the posterior descending.

In 10% of patients the right coronary artery does not reach the crux of the heart and therefore is considered non-dominant.[1] It divides early in its course giving off one or more branches which represent right marginal arteries (Figure 5.14). Occasionally the artery may reach the margo acutus giving off right marginal branches to the posterior free wall of the right ventricle. Occasionally the appearance of the artery may mimic an occlusion of the right coronary artery. The following criteria are useful in identifying a non-dominant right coronary artery: 1) The non-dominant right coronary system usually consists of small vessels; 2) There is absence of a complete proximal right coronary artery running in the right atrioventricular sulcus and of the bifurcation of the proximal right coronary artery at the crux of the heart; 3) The branches of the proximal right coronary artery leave the atrioventricular sulcus early in its course and run toward the inferior surface of the right ventricle instead of to the crux of the heart; 4) The absence of collateral filling of a distal right coronary artery or posterior descending artery favors the presence of a non-dominant system rather than an occluded vessel.

References

1. James, T.N.: *Anatomy of the Coronary Arteries*. Paul B. Hoeber, Inc., New York, 1961.
2. Paulin, S.: Coronary angiography. A technical, anatomic and clinical study. *Acta Radiologica Supplementum*, **233**, 1964.
3. James, T.N.: Anatomy of the coronary arteries in health and disease. *Circulation*, **32**:1020-1033, 1965.

Figure 5.1:   Right coronary arteriogram; left anterior oblique projection, during systole. The coronary ostium, the entire proximal right coronary artery (RC) and the distal right coronary artery (DRC) are well visualized. The first branch of the right coronary artery, the conus artery, runs superiorly and anteriorly; the second branch of the right coronary artery is the artery to the sinus node (SN) which courses posteriorly and superiorly. The right marginal arteries are seen end on as they course over the right ventricular free wall. The posterior descending artery (PD) is not well visualized as it courses along the inferior surface of the right ventricle towards the observer.

Figure 5.2:   Right coronary arteriogram; left anterior oblique projection, during systole. The proximal right coronary artery (RC) which is tortuous and the distal right coronary artery (DRC) are well demonstrated. The posterior descending artery (PD) is still not completely visualized.

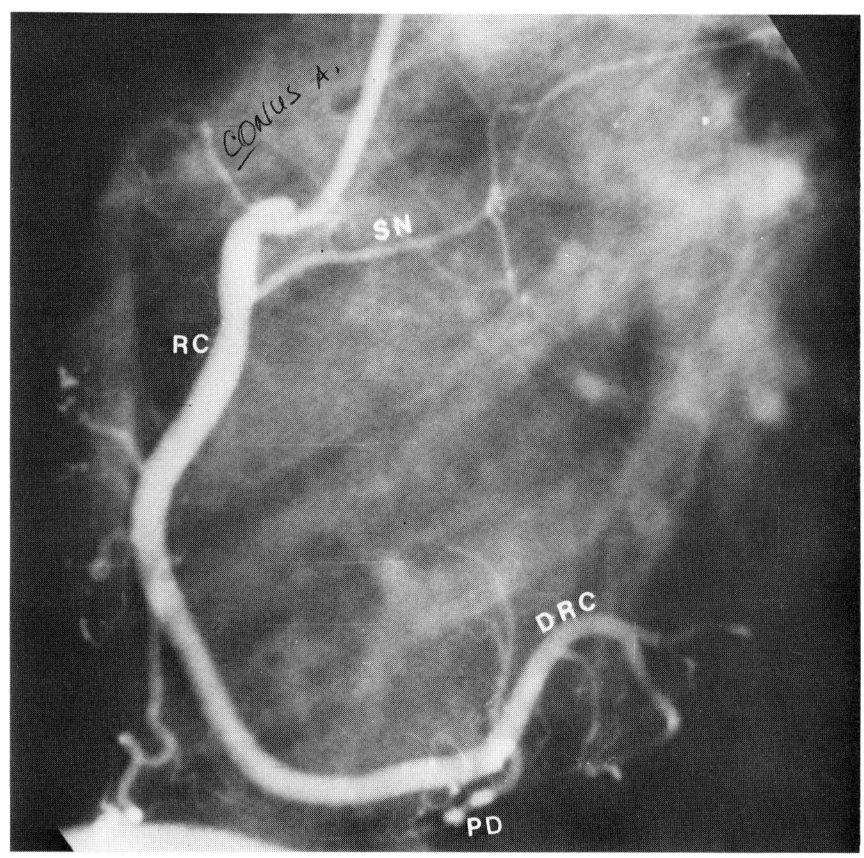

FIGURE 5.1

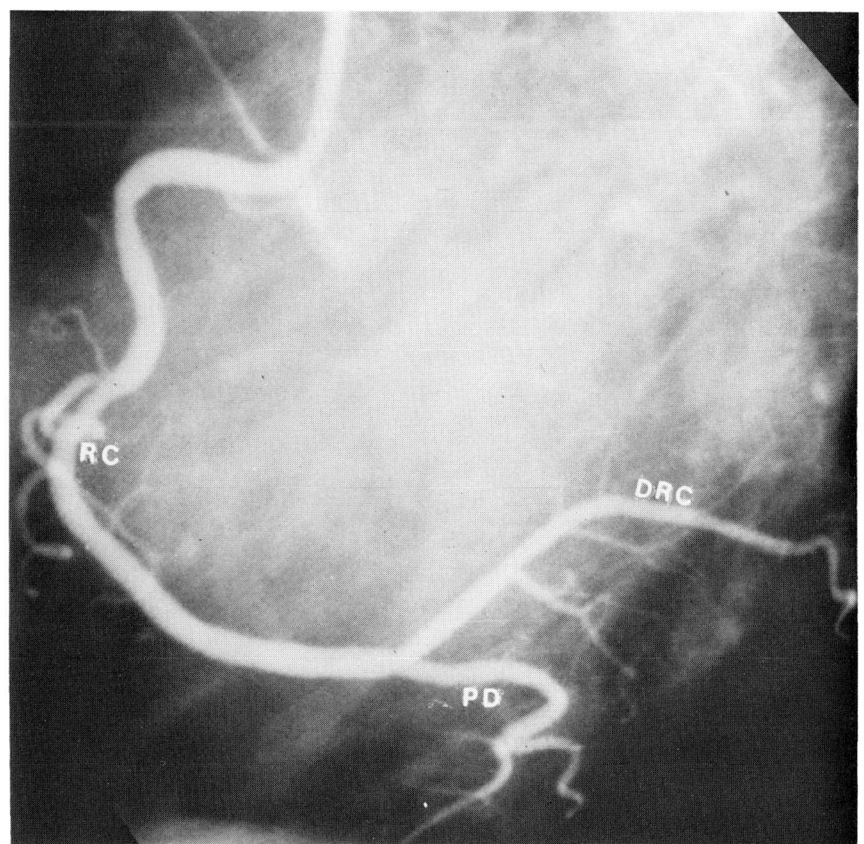

FIGURE 5.2

Figure 5.3:   Right coronary arteriogram; left anterior oblique projection. The proximal right coronary artery (RC), a right marginal branch (RM) and the distal right coronary artery (DRC) are well visualized. The sinus node artery (SN) is seen running posteriorly and superiorly toward the SA node. The posterior descending is very poorly seen due to the horizontal position of the heart.

Figure 5.4:   Right coronary arteriogram; left anterior oblique projection. Proximal right coronary artery (RC) and the sinus node artery (SN) are well seen. The proximal right coronary artery describes a posteriorly directed concavity. The distal right coronary artery (DRC) appears foreshortened at the posterior aspect of the heart.

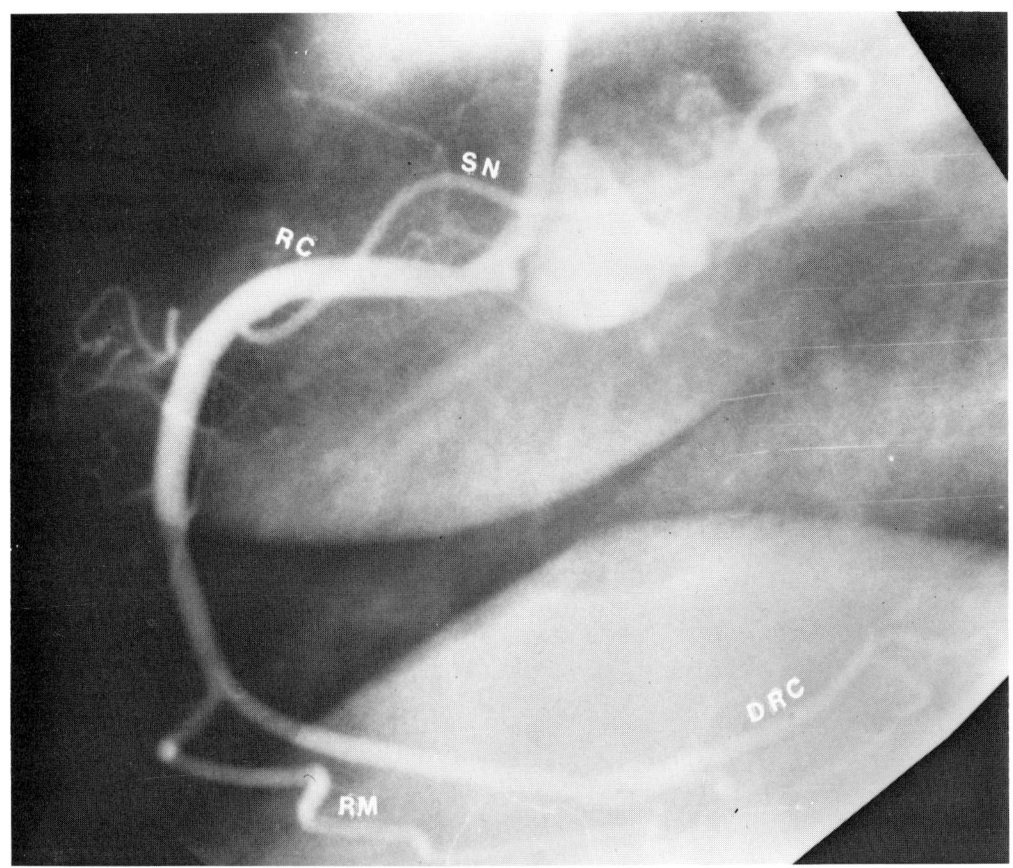

FIGURE 5.3

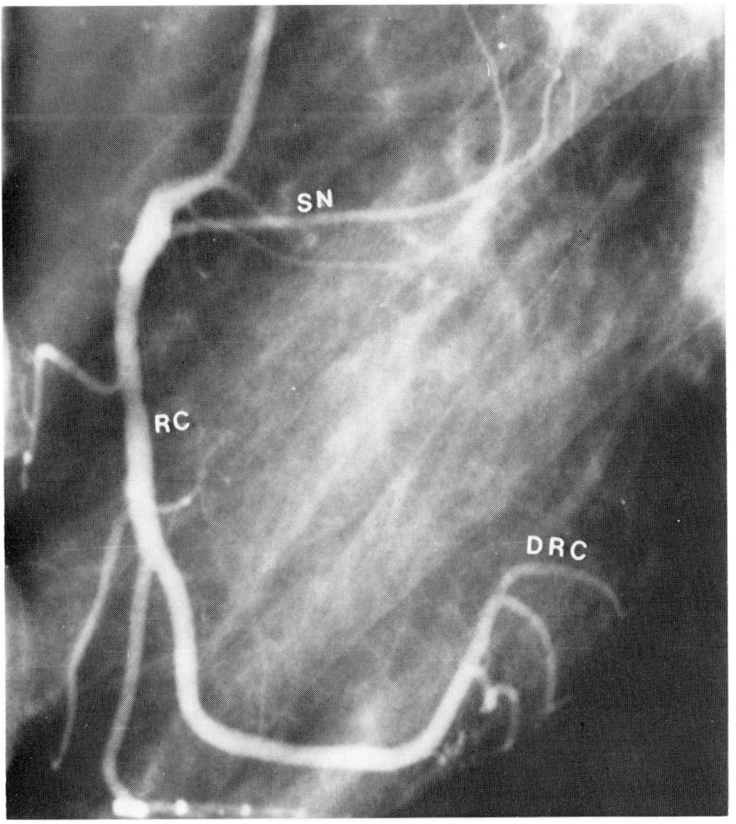

FIGURE 5.4

Figure 5.5:   Right coronary arteriogram; right anterior oblique projection, during systole. The middle segment of the proximal right coronary artery (RC) is well visualized. The proximal few centimeters and the distal segment of the proximal right coronary artery near the crux are not well visualized in this projection. There are four right marginal branches coursing anteriorly over the right ventricular free wall. Atrial branches are seen running in a posterior direction from the proximal right coronary artery. The sinus node artery (SN) and a large atrial branch (A) are present. The posterior descending artery (PD) is now seen along the inferior surface of the heart.

Figure 5.6:   Right coronary arteriogram; right anterior oblique projection, during diastole. The proximal right coronary artery (RC) appears displaced posteriorly and the proximal and distal segments of this vessel are better visualized. There are four right marginal arteries (RM) coursing anteriorly. The posterior descending (PD) branch is well seen and gives off septal branches.

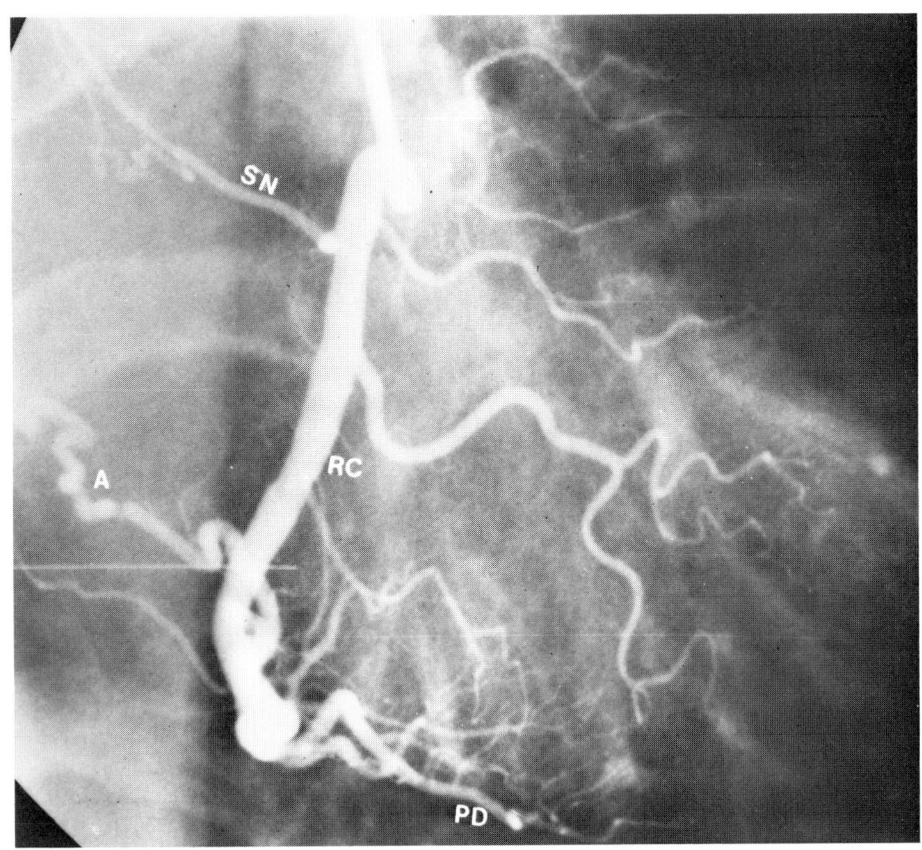

FIGURE 5.5

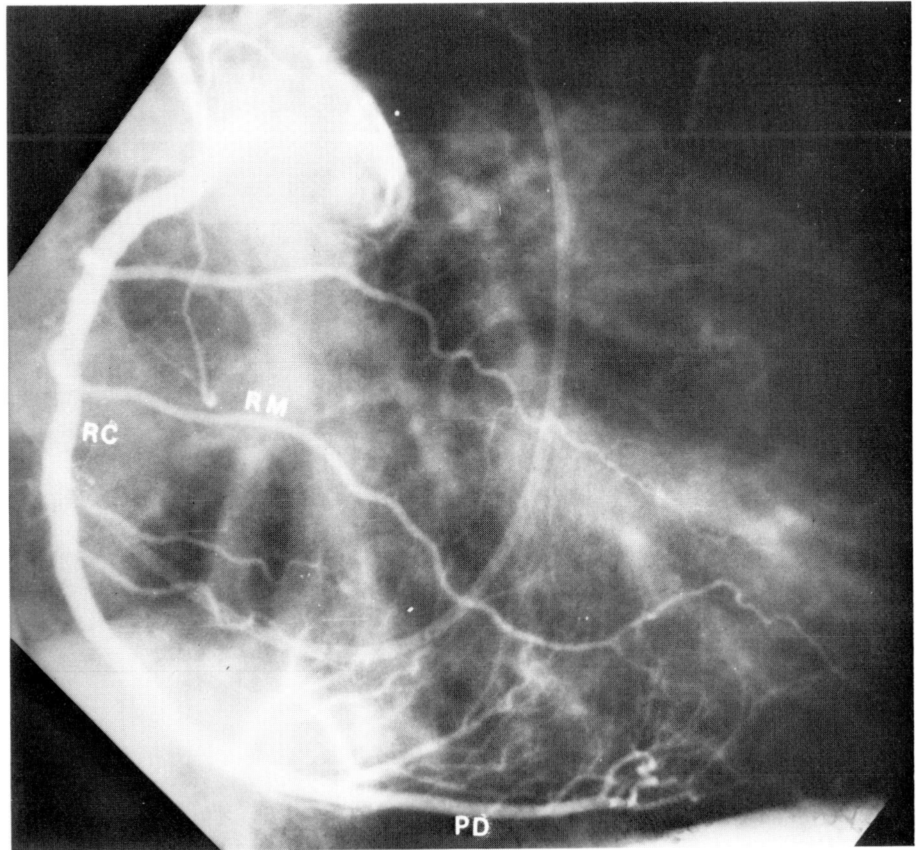

FIGURE 5.6

Figure 5.7:   Right coronary arteriogram; right anterior oblique projection. The right marginal artery (RM) is seen originating
near the origin of the proximal right coronary artery (RC).
The proximal portion of the conus artery (C) is well visualized.

SN = sinus node artery. PD = posterior descending
artery.

Figure 5.8:   Right coronary arteriogram; left anterior oblique projection. This figure again demonstrates an unusually high
origin of the right marginal artery (RM) from the proximal
right coronary artery (RC).

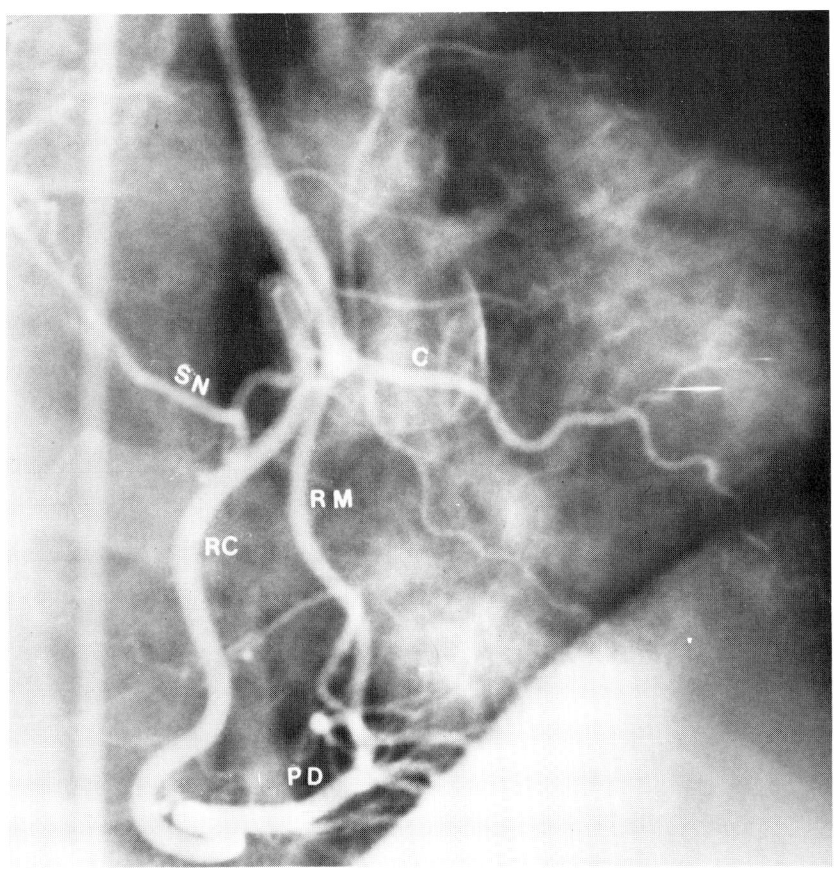

FIGURE 5.7

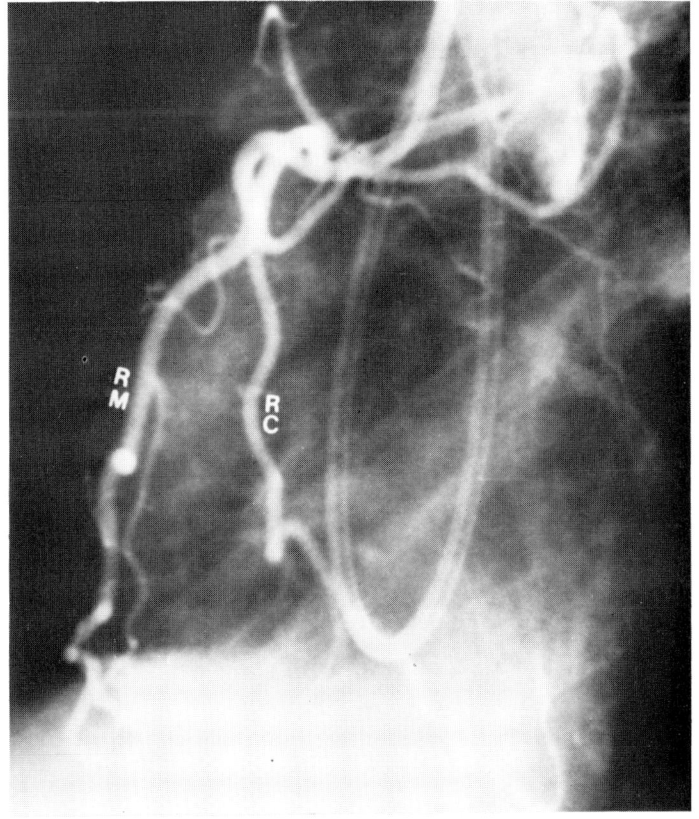

FIGURE 5.8

Figure 5.9:   Right coronary arteriogram; right anterior oblique projection. The posterior descending coronary artery (PD) is a large vessel located in the inferior interventricular sulcus coursing from crux to apex. The posterior descending wraps around the apex of the heart in this patient. The septal branches of the posterior descending artery are well seen.

AV = atrioventricular node branch of the right coronary artery. RM = right marginal artery.

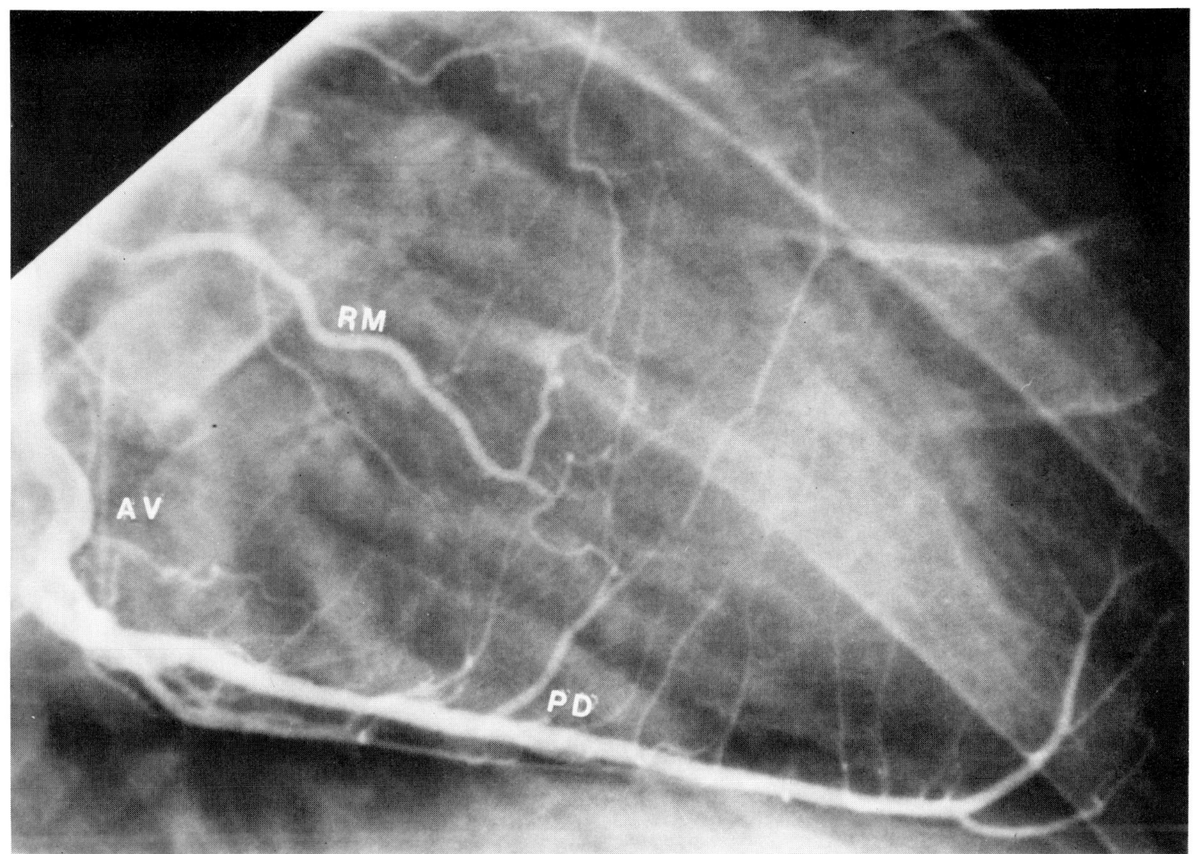

FIGURE 5.9

Figure 5.10:   Right coronary arteriogram:

A. Lateral projection; two posterior descending coronary arteries are easily appreciated (PD). The proximal segment of the posterior descending artery originates from the right coronary artery (RC) at the level of the crux. At this point, one sees the distal right coronary artery (DRC) as a short vessel. The distal segment of the posterior descending artery arises from the right marginal artery (RM).

B. Left anterior oblique projection; the posterior descending vessels are now foreshortened. The sinus node artery (SN) is well seen.

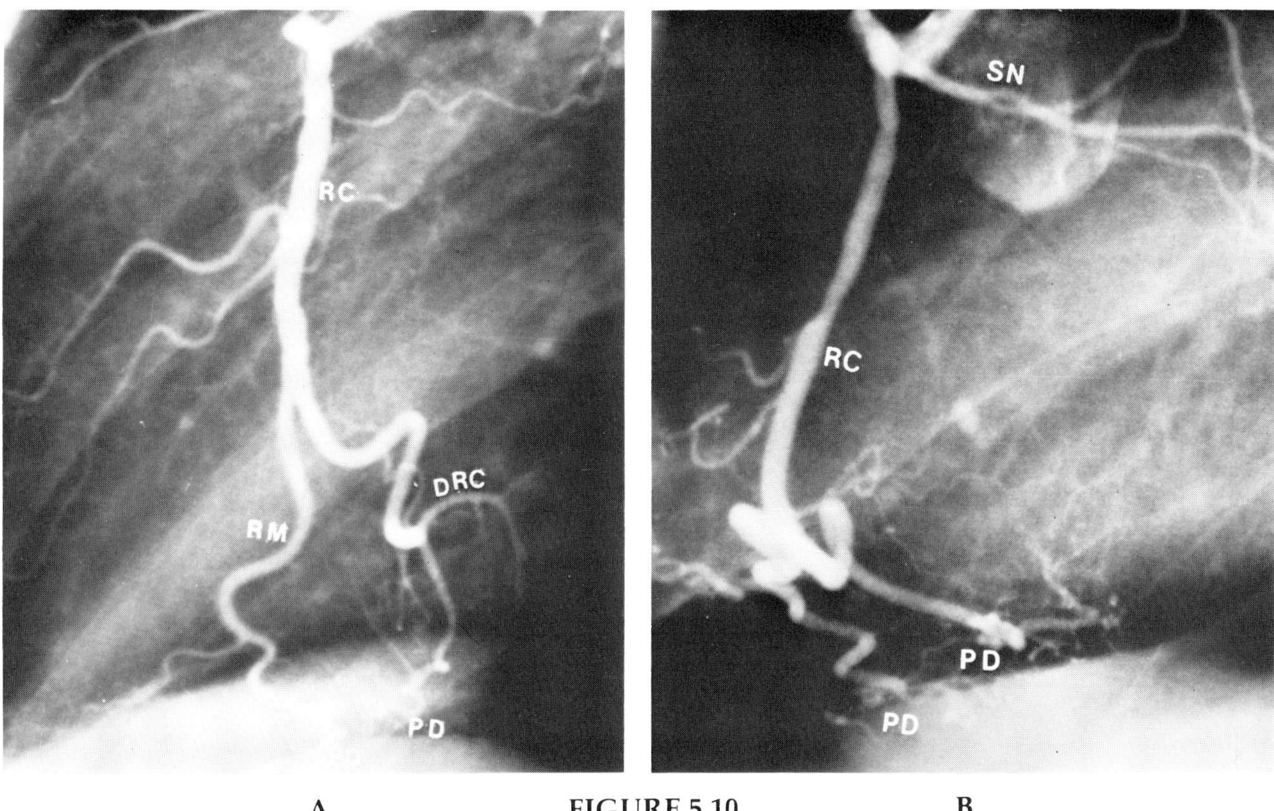

A   **FIGURE 5.10**   B

Figure 5.11:   Right coronary arteriogram; right anterior oblique projection. In **A** and **B** the posterior descending coronary artery (PD) is seen originating from the right marginal artery (RM). In **B** the origin of the right marginal artery is seen very near the origin of the proximal right coronary artery (RC).

Figure 5.12:   Right coronary arteriogram; left anterior oblique projection. Another example of the posterior descending artery originating from a right marginal branch of the right coronary artery (RC). The sinus node artery (SN) is well visualized and encircles the base of the superior vena cava.

AV = atrioventricular node branch of the right coronary artery.

PD = posterior descending coronary artery.

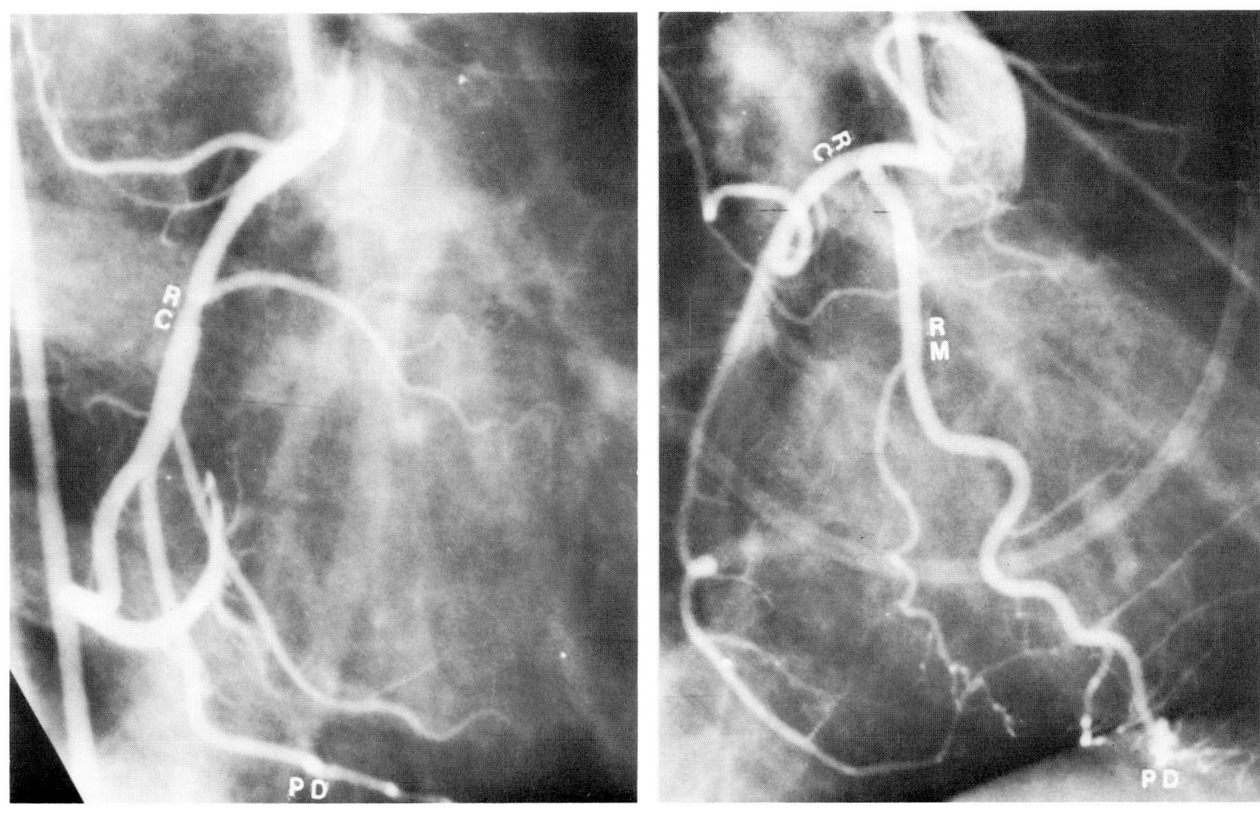

FIGURE 5.11

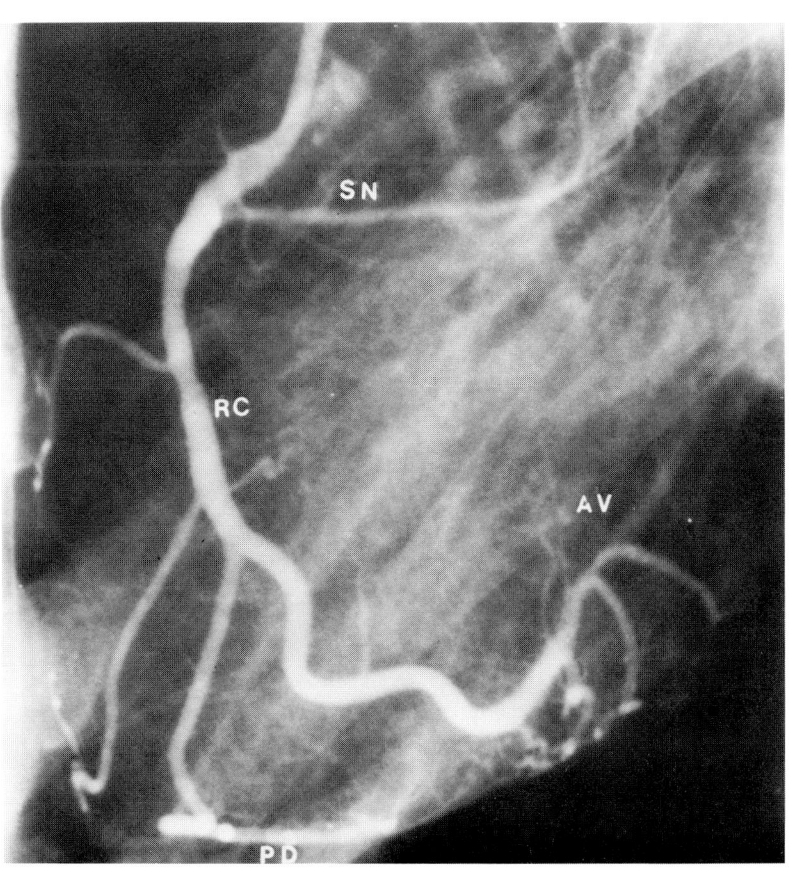

FIGURE 5.12

Figure 5.13:   Right coronary arteriogram; left anterior oblique projection. The large posterior descending coronary artery (PD)
which wraps around the apex is foreshortened in this projection. The distal right coronary artery (DRC) and its left
ventricular branches are well visualized.

RC = right coronary artery. SN = sinus node branch
of right coronary artery.

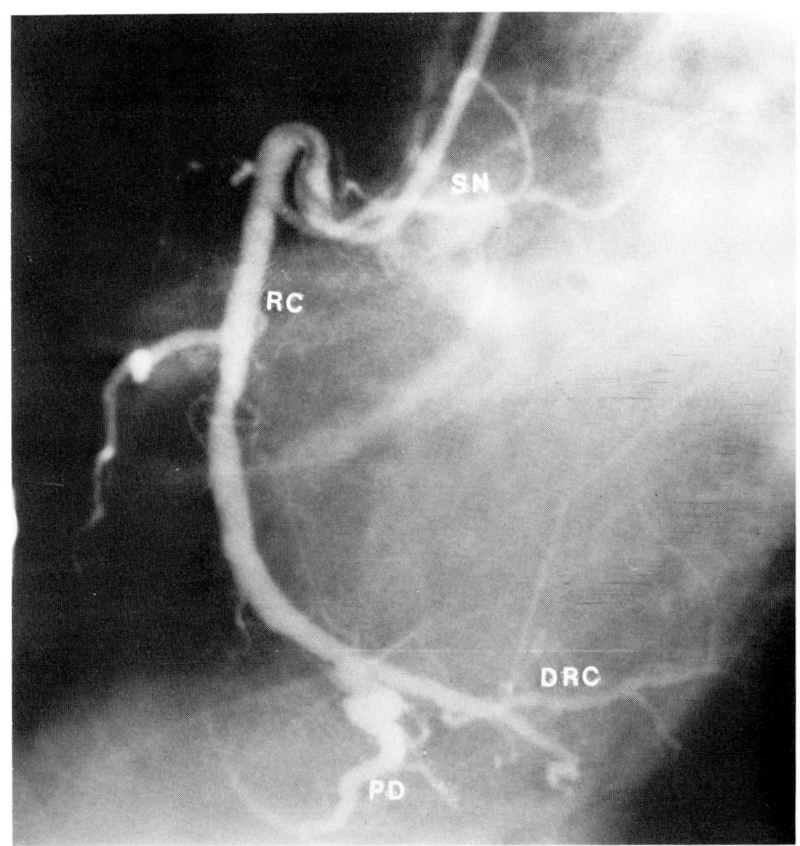

FIGURE 5.13

Figure 5.14:   Right coronary arteriogram; **A**. Left anterior oblique projection; **B**. Lateral projection; **C**. Right anterior oblique projection. The right coronary artery (RC) is nondominant. It divides early giving off a large right marginal branch (RM). The main right coronary artery tapers rapidly and terminates at the margo acutus. No right coronary artery is present in the distal one-half of the right atrioventricular sulcus. The distal right coronary and the posterior descending arteries are not present.

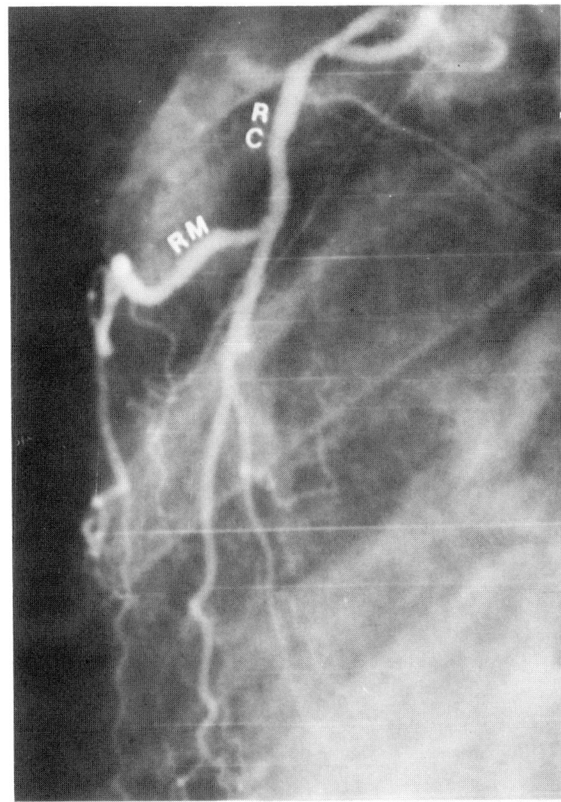

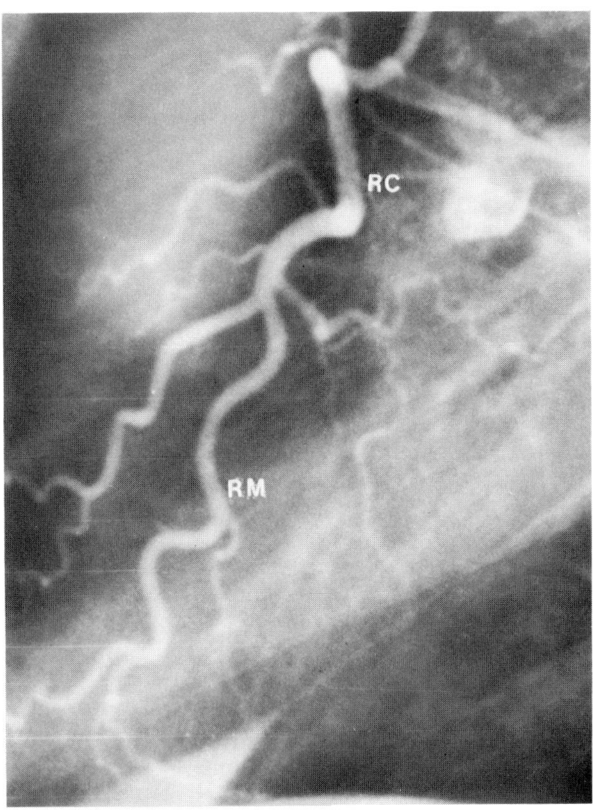

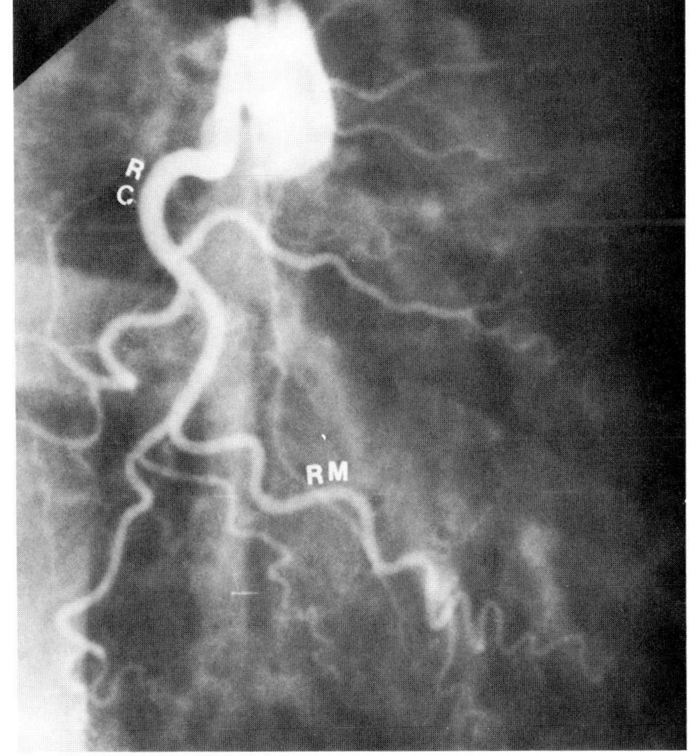

FIGURE 5.14

Chapter 6

The Arteries to the Conduction System of the Heart. Other Atrial Branches

The Sinus Node Artery

The blood supply to the sinus node is provided by the sinus node artery. This vessel originates from the right coronary artery in 60% of hearts (Figures 6.1, 6.2, 6.3 D, C, 6.4).[1] In 40% of hearts the sinus node artery originates from the left coronary artery (Figures 4.13, 6.5).[1]

When the sinus node artery originates from the right coronary artery, it courses posteriorly and superiorly over the anterior wall of the right atrium, through the anterior portion of the interatrial septum to the base of the superior vena cava (Figures 6.1, 6.2, 6.4). When the sinus node artery originates from the left coronary artery, it usually does so from the left circumflex artery (Figure 6.5), but occasionally it may originate from the left main coronary artery.

When the sinus node artery originates from the middle portion of the left circumflex artery, it turns superiorly from the atrioventricular sulcus (Figure 6.5 D). In such instances, the sinus node artery is located over the posterior wall of the left atrium. At the base of the superior vena cava, the artery sends two branches which encircle the superior vena cava (Figure 6.4). It may proceed as a common trunk and encircle the superior vena cava in a clockwise direction as it passes through the crista supraventricularis (Figures 5.3, 5.12).

The artery to the sinus node is almost always visualized. Either the right or left anterior oblique view is adequate for examining this vessel regardless of whether it arises from the right or left coronary artery. On occasion two arteries to the sinus node may be identified in post-mortem studies and occasionally two vessels to the sinus node may be identified by arteriography as well.

The Atrioventricular Node Artery

This small vessel arises from the artery which crosses the crux of the heart and accordingly originates from the right coronary artery in 90% of hearts and from the left circumflex artery in the remainder.[1] It is usually easily recognized as it originates from the apex of a characteristic arch in the right coronary artery at the crux. From that point it runs superiorly and anteriorly toward the non-coronary sinus of Valsalva and terminates with a distinctive angulation (Figures 6.3, 6.4). This vessel is best visualized in the lateral and left anterior oblique projections. In the right anterior oblique projections it may be obscured by the distal right coronary artery.

Other Atrial Branches

Other atrial branches include: 1) the right intermediate atrial artery; 2) the left atrial circumflex artery and 3) the arteria anastomotica auricularis magna, or Kugel's artery.

The right intermediate atrial artery originates from the right coronary artery near the margo acutus and courses in the direction opposite to the right marginal artery (Figure 6.6). Frequently, this vessel is small and is not visualized.

The left atrial circumflex artery originates from the left circumflex artery near the margo obtusus. The size of the vessel is variable although it is usually smaller than the left circumflex artery (Figures 4.8, 6.7, B, D). It runs posteriorly from the atrioventricular groove. Occasionally the vessel may be larger than the left circumflex artery (Figure 6.8).

Kugel's artery, the arteria anastomotica auricularis magna, originates from the proximal segment of either the right coronary artery or the left circumflex artery. It courses on the anterior wall of the atrium close to the aorta, proceeds through the interatrial septum along its base to the inferior surface of the heart and anastomoses with the atrioventricular node artery. Figure 6.9 demonstrates this vessel anastomosing the proximal with the distal right coronary artery. It is an important anastomotic channel for blood supply to the atrioventricular node.

Reference

1.   James, T.N.: *Anatomy of the Coronary Arteries*. Paul B. Hoeber, Inc., New York, 1961.

Figure 6.1:   Right coronary arteriogram; left anterior oblique projection. The sinus node artery (SN) originates from the proximal segment of the right coronary artery (RCA) and courses posteriorly and superiorly. At its distal end the sinus node artery divides into several branches which course around the base of the superior vena cava (arrows). The left anterior oblique projection is optimal for visualizing the sinus node artery when it originates from the right coronary artery.

DD = double posterior descending coronary artery.

B. Diagrammatic representation of **A**.

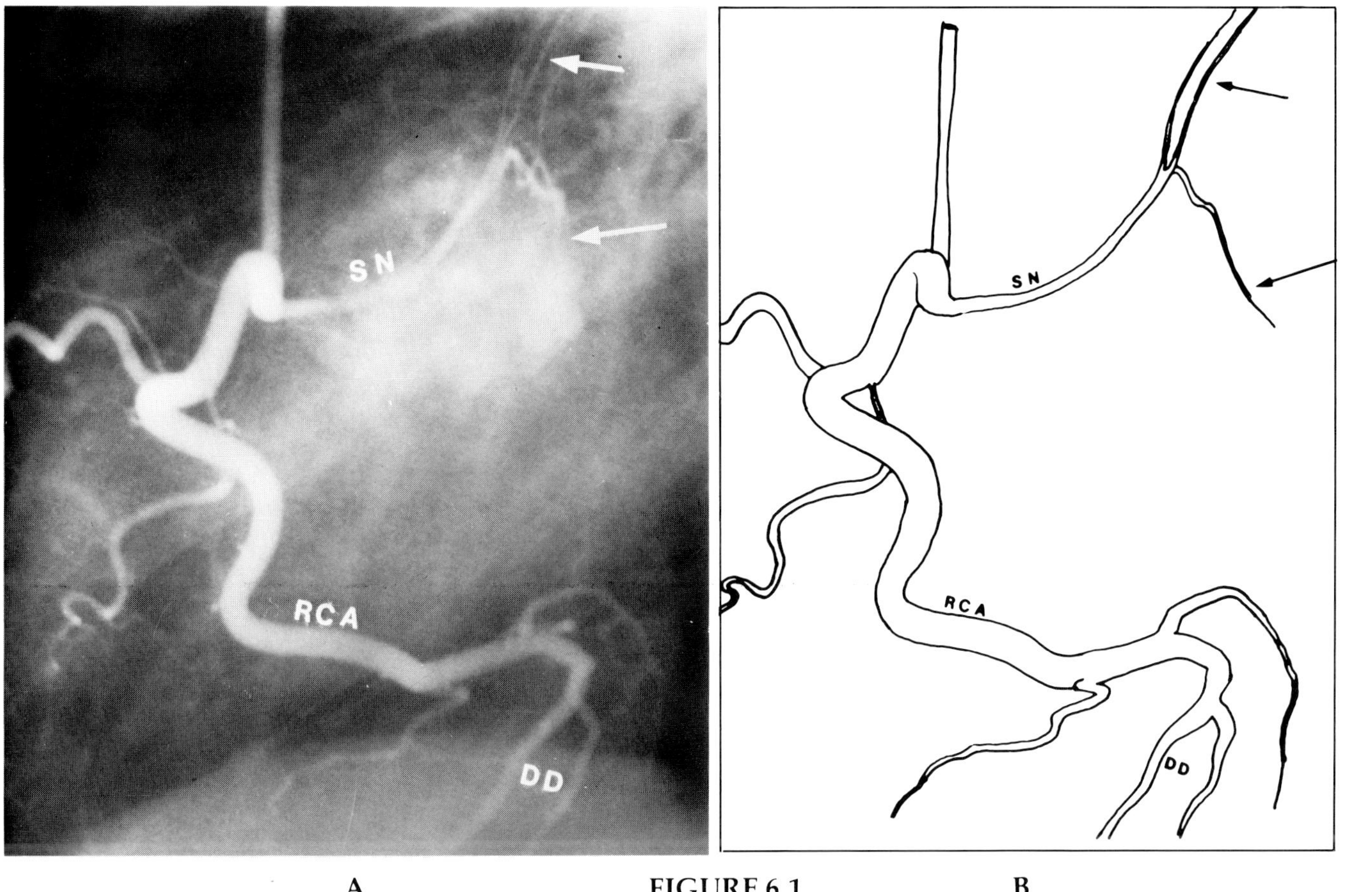

FIGURE 6.1

Figure 6.2:   Right coronary arteriogram; right anterior oblique projection.

A and C. The sinus node artery (SN) originates from the right coronary artery (RCA and RC) and courses posteriorly and superiorly toward the sinus node. At its termination the SN divides into a characteristic "Y" as it wraps around the base of the superior vena cava.

RM = right marginal branches. A = atrial branch of right branch of right coronary artery. AV = atrioventricular node branch of the right coronary artery.

B and D. Diagrammatic representation of A and C, respectively.

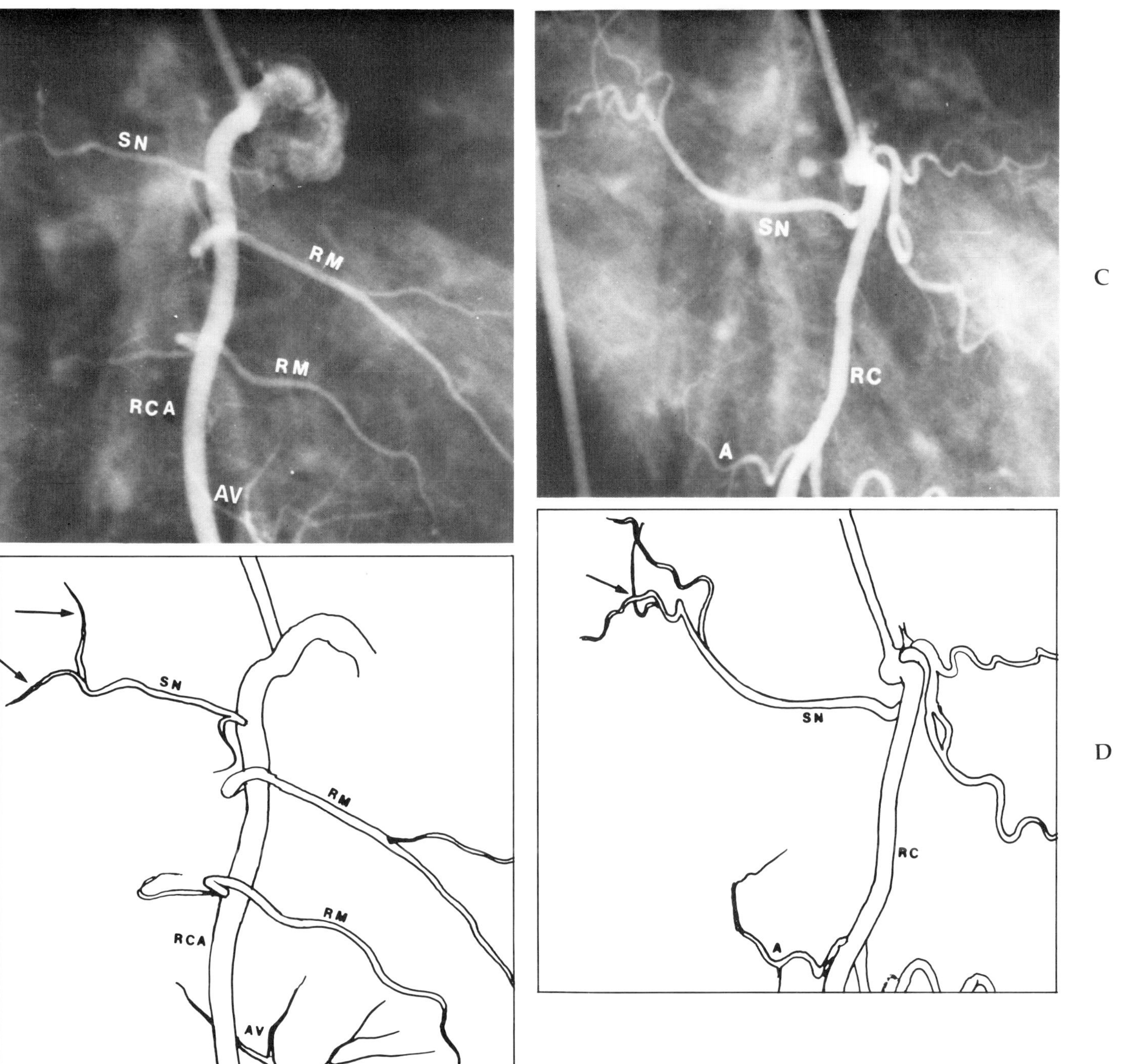

FIGURE 6.2

Figure 6.3:   Right coronary arteriogram; **A**. Left anterior oblique projection; **C**. Right anterior oblique projection. In the left anterior oblique projection (**A**) the artery to the atrioventricular node (AV) is a narrow vessel running superiorly and anteriorly from the crux of the heart towards the middle of the cardiac silhouette. Its characteristic termination is easily appreciated. In this patient the AV node artery does not arise from the apex of the arch of the vessel as it passes the crux. In the right anterior oblique projection (**C**) the artery to the atrioventricular node (AV, at pointers) lies almost behind the proximal segment of the right coronary artery.

RCA = right coronary artery. RM = right marginal arteries. PD = posterior descending artery. SN = sinus node artery.

B and **D**. Diagrammatic representation of **A** and **C**, respectively.

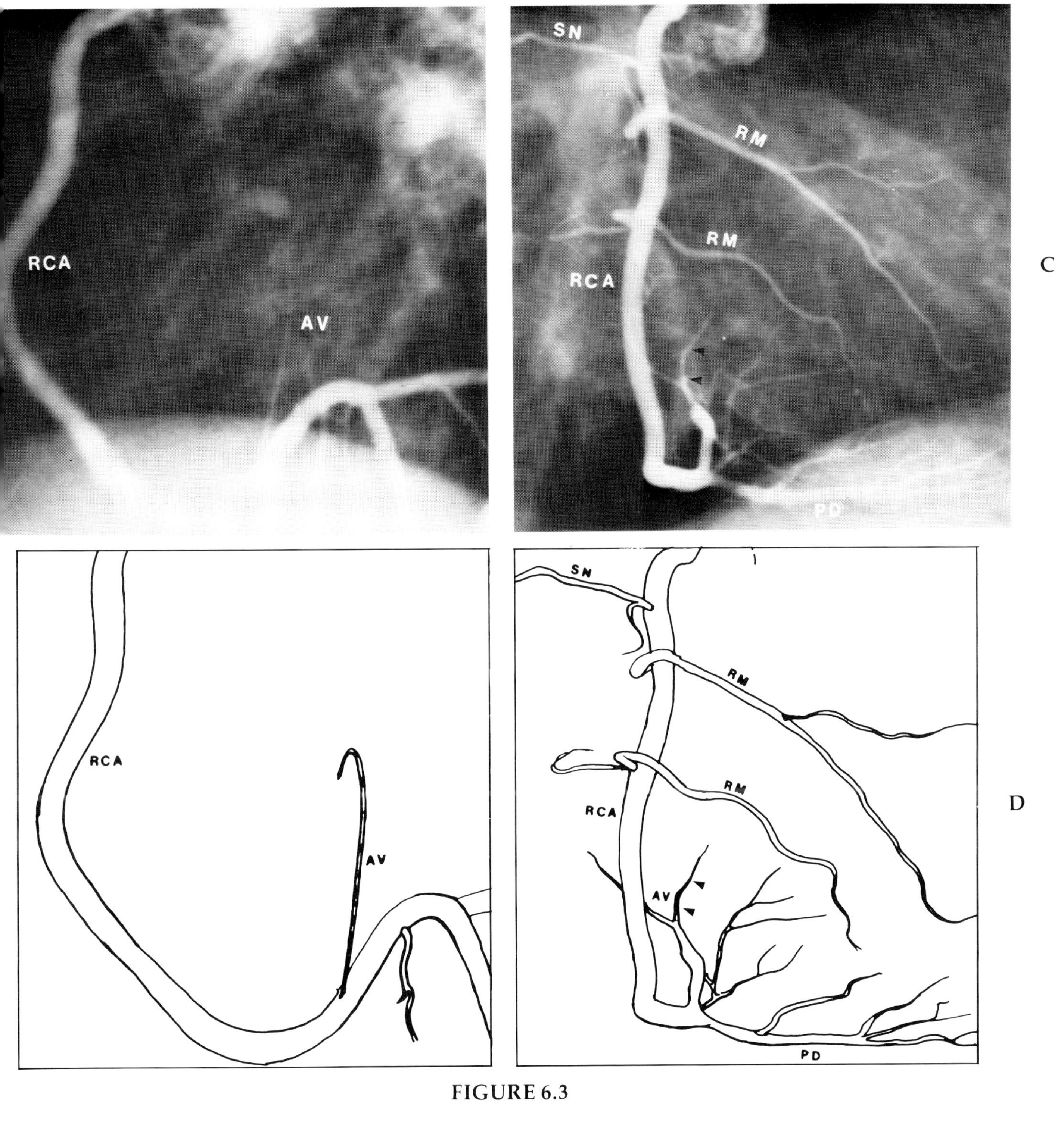

FIGURE 6.3

Figure 6.4:   Right coronary arteriogram; lateral projection. In this projection the artery to the sinus node (SN) terminates in a "C" shape about the base of the superior vena cava (arrows). The artery to the atrioventricular node (AV) arises from the apex of the arch of the right coronary artery as it crosses the crux. The AV node artery follows a superior and anterior direction to the middle of the cardiac silhouette. Again, the distinctive terminal angulation of the AV node artery is recognized.

RCA = right coronary artery.

B. Diagrammatic representation of **A**.

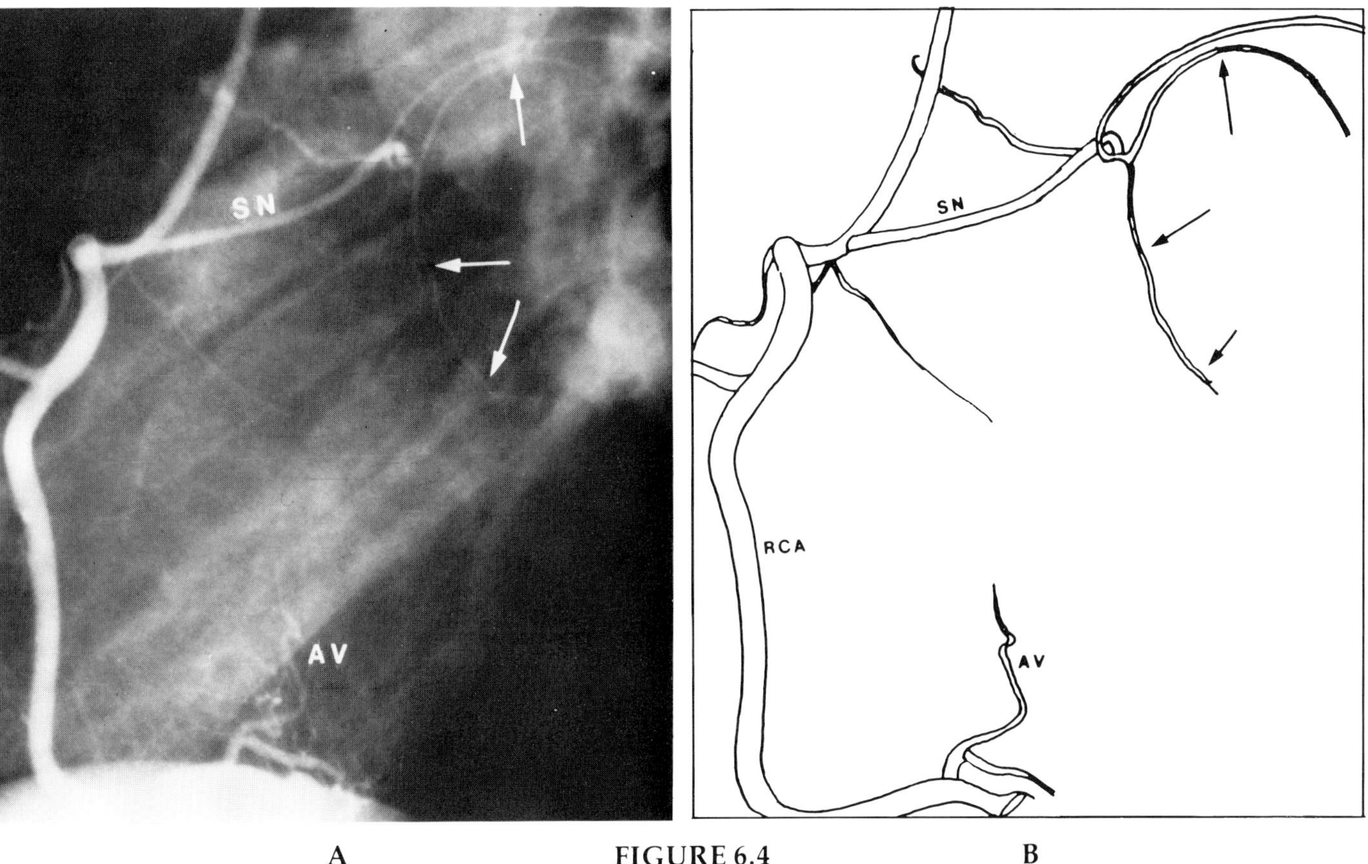

FIGURE 6.4

Figure 6.5:   Left coronary arteriogram; **A** and **B**. Right anterior oblique projection. **C** and **D**. Lateral projection. The artery to
the sinus node (SN) may originate from different sites on
the left coronary artery. It usually originates in the proximal one-third of the left circumflex artery (CX) but
ocasionally may originate near the crux or from the left
main coronary artery.

LAD = left anterior descending coronary artery. D =
diagonal branches of left anterior descending coronary
artery.

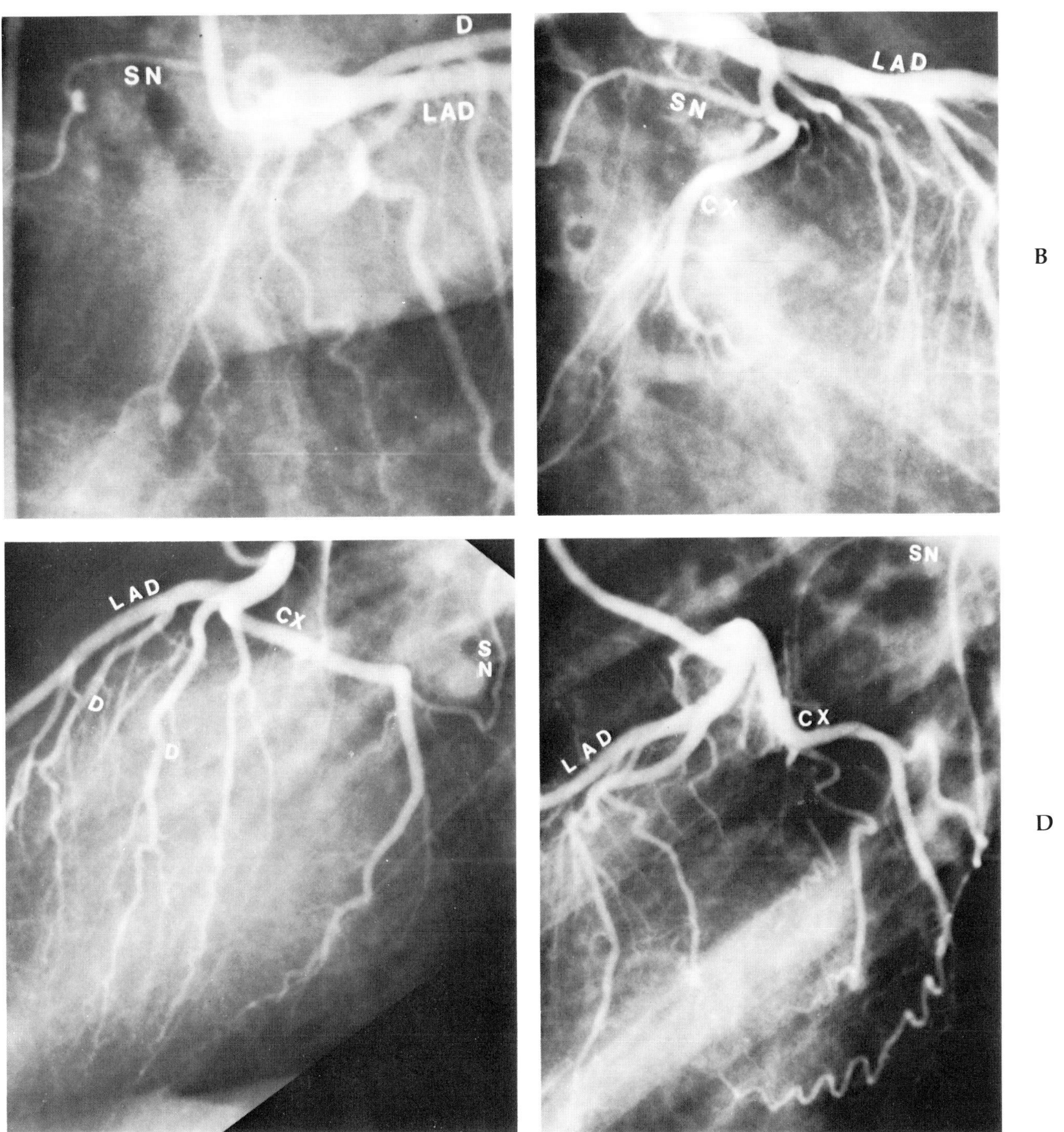

FIGURE 6.5

Figure 6.6:   Right coronary arteriogram; right anterior oblique projection.

A. Two atrial branches (A) originate from the right coronary artery and supply the right atrium. These branches are usually small and short. The right intermediate atrial artery is the second atrial (lower A) branch.

B. Only one atrial branch is present.

RCA = right coronary artery. RM = right marginal branch. PD = posterior descending coronary artery.

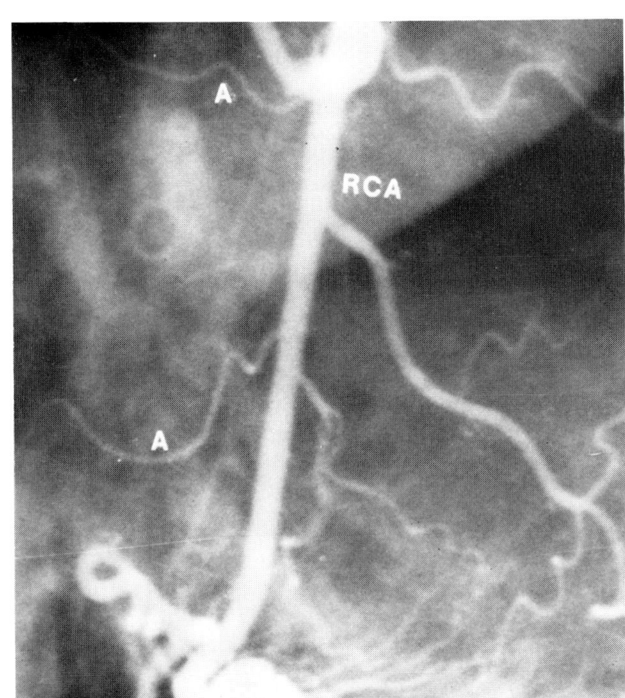

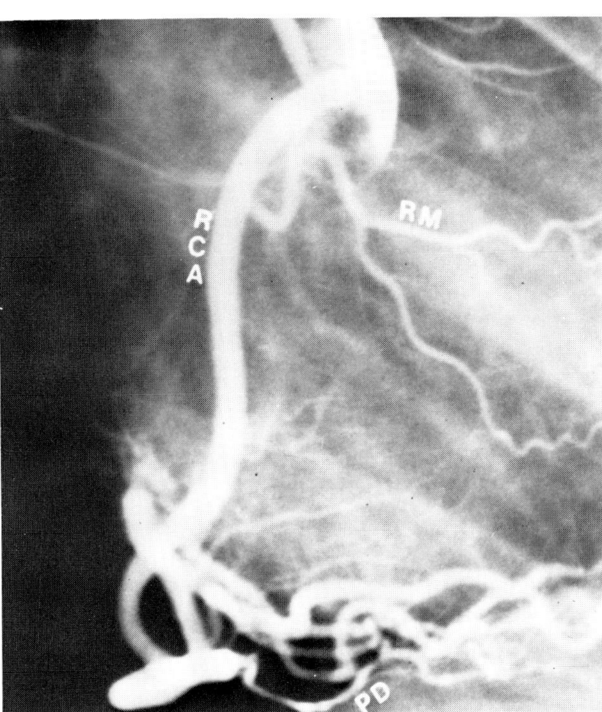

FIGURE 6.6

Figure 6.7:   Left coronary arteriogram; **A** and **B**. Lateral projection. **C** and **D**. Right anterior oblique projection.

A and **C**. Several atrial branches are present.

B and **D**. The left atrial circumflex artery (LAC) is the atrial branch most frequently present and also the largest atrial branch from the left circumflex artery.

LAD = left anterior descending coronary artery. CX = left circumflex coronary artery. LM = left marginal branch of the left circumflex coronary artery.

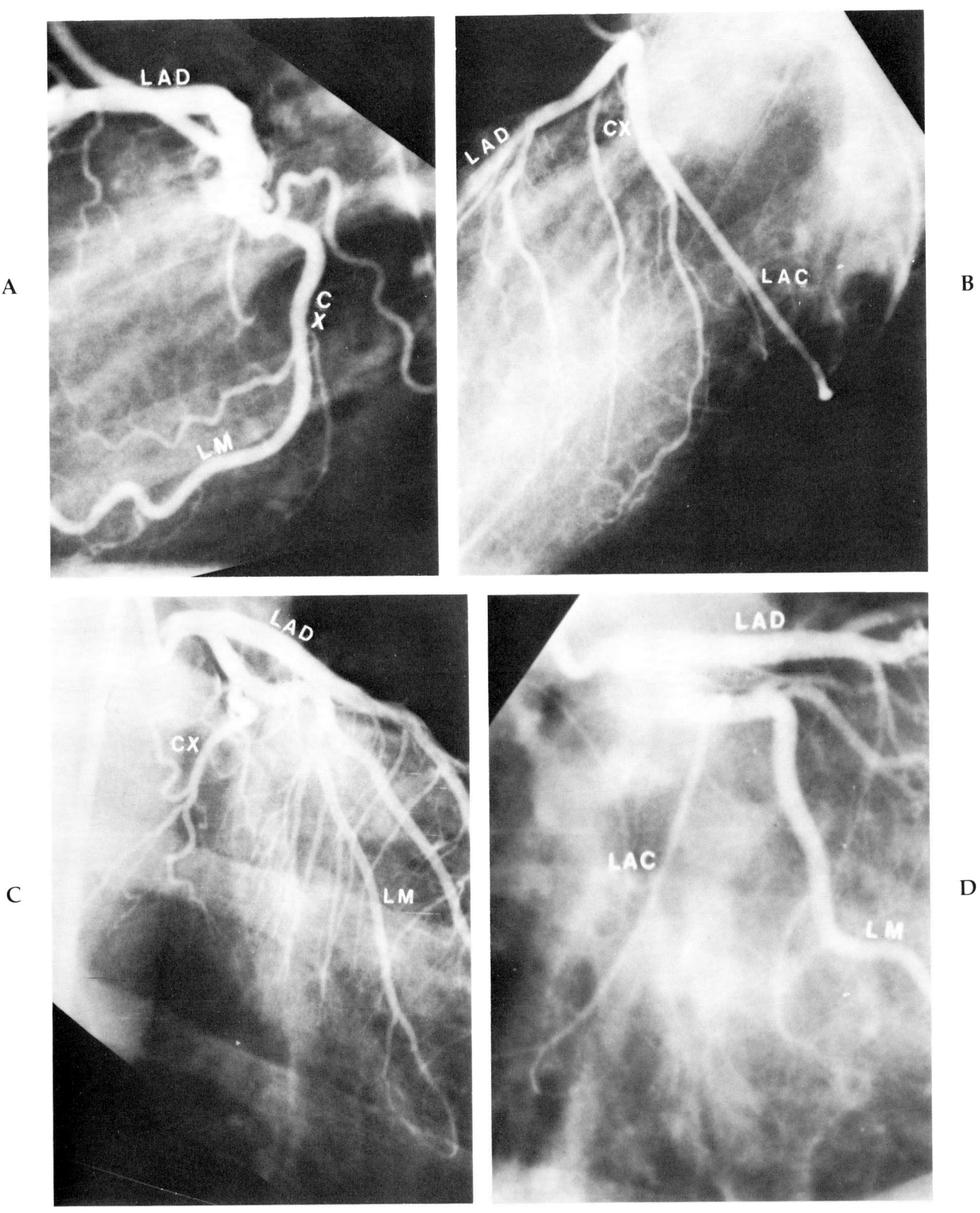

FIGURE 6.7

Figure 6.8:   Left coronary arteriogram; **A**. Right anterior oblique projection; **B**. Lateral projection. The left atrial circumflex artery (LAC) is larger than the left circumflex artery (CX) indicated by the arrow. At its distal end the left atrial circumflex artery (LAC) gives off a large atrial vessel which runs over the right atrial wall (pointers).

LAD = left anterior descending artery. D = diagonal branches of the LAD.

C. Diagrammatic representation of **A**.

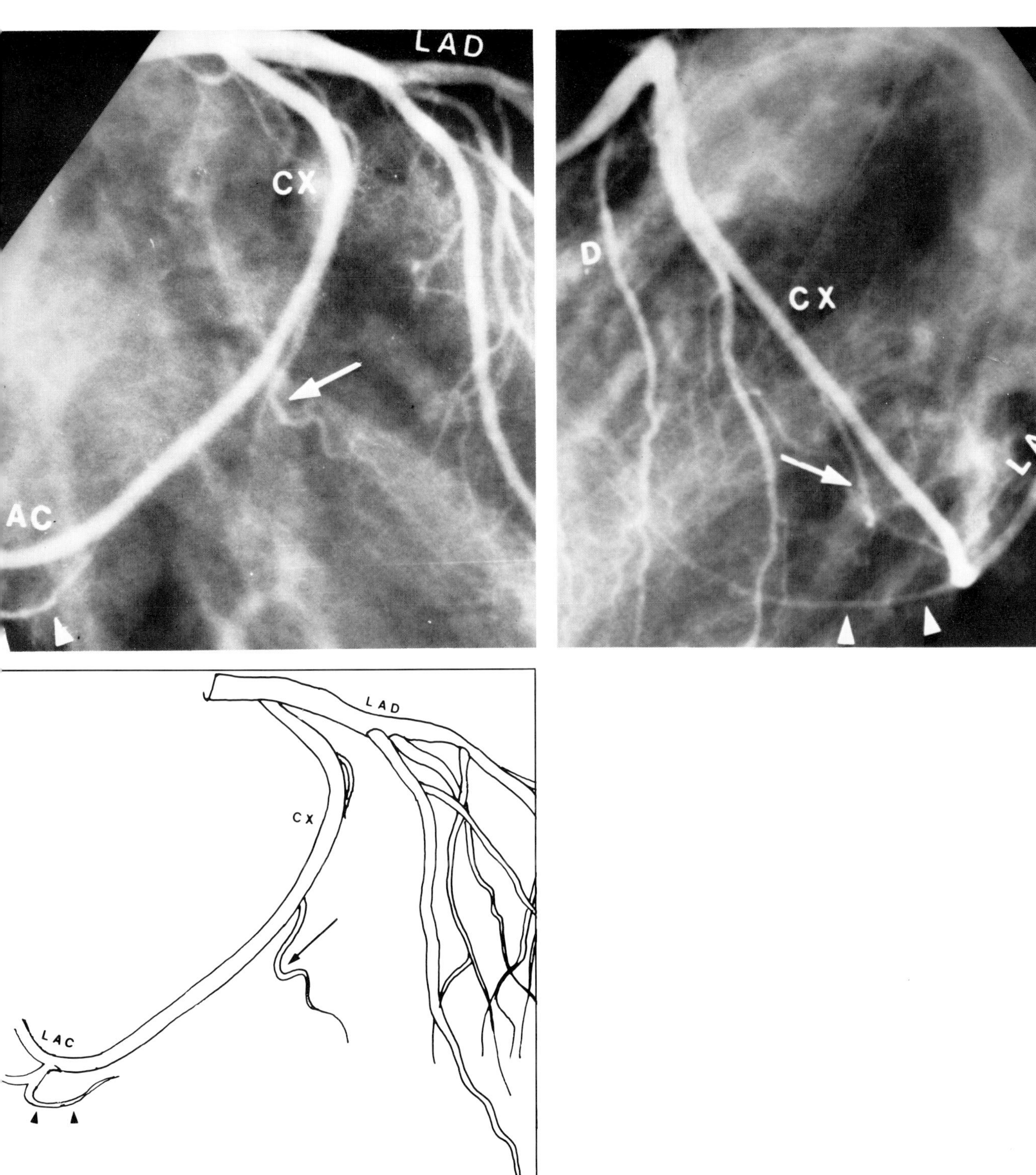

FIGURE 6.8

Figure 6.9:   Right coronary arteriogram; left anterior oblique projection.

A. Kugel's artery (KA) originates from the proximal right coronary artery (RC) and anastomoses with the distal right coronary atery (DRC). Kugel's artery is occasionally seen in patients with normal coronary arteriograms, but most frequently is found in association with occlusion of the right coronary or circumflex arteries.

(From Soto, B., Jochem, W., Karp, R.B., and Barcia, A.: Angiographic anatomy of Kugel's artery. *American Journal of Roentgenology, Radium Therapy and Nuclear Medicine,* **119**:503-507, 1973. Published with permission.)

PD = posterior descending coronary artery.

B. Diagrammatic representation of **A**.

A

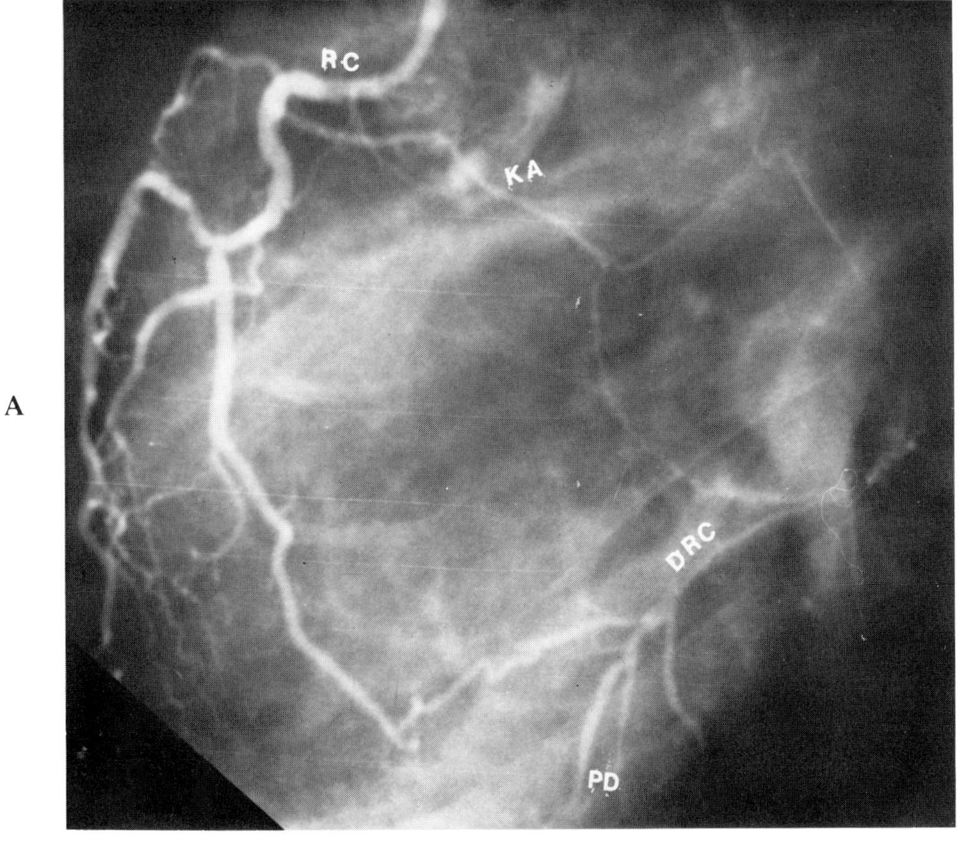

B

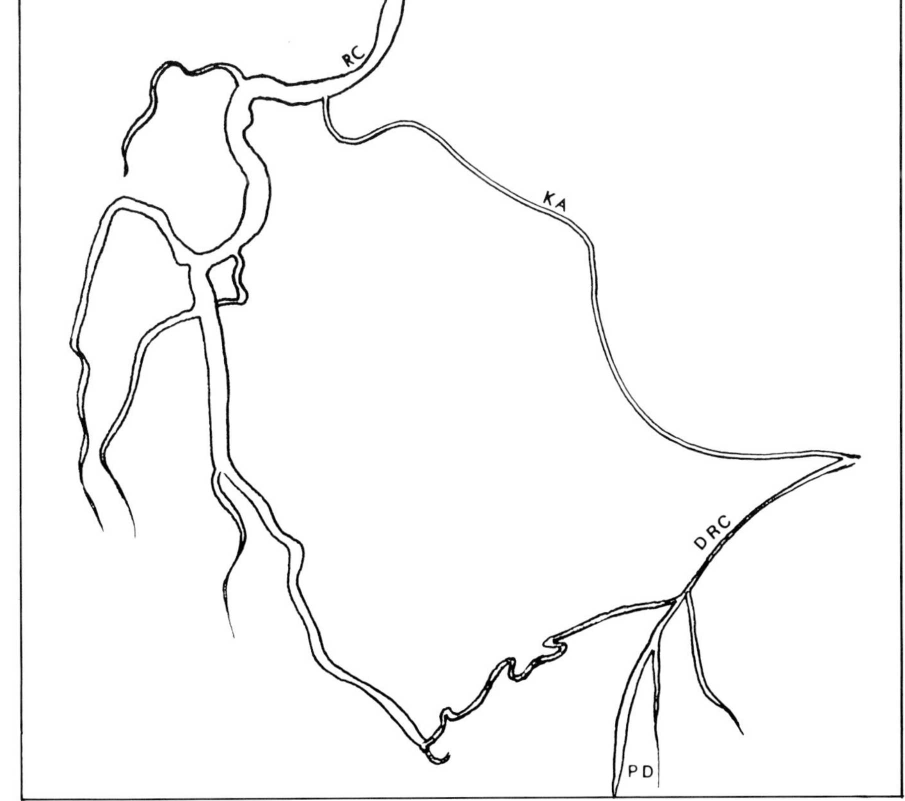

FIGURE 6.9

PART III

ABNORMAL CORONARY ANATOMY

Chapter 7

Obstructive Disease of the Left Coronary Artery

Atherosclerotic obstructive disease of the coronary arteries is the most common cause of ischemic heart disease. The widespread clinical spectrum of this disorder necessitates angiographic definition in order to accurately determine the extent and severity of the disease. In this chapter, the radiographic appearance of obstructive lesions in the left coronary artery will be demonstrated.

The Left Main Coronary Artery

Stenosis of the left main coronary artery prior to its bifurcation into the left anterior descending and circumflex arteries occurs in about 10-15% of patients with coronary artery disease.[1] (Figures 7.1—7.5). Rarely is it an isolated lesion, and it is unusual to find the vessel completely obstructed[2] (Figure 7.5).

The over-all prognosis of patients with involvement of the left main coronary artery is poor.[3] Since the left anterior descending and circumflex arteries provide blood flow to the anterior and lateral walls of the left ventricle, to its apex and to the interventricular septum, a significant portion of the left ventricular myocardium is at jeopardy from a stenosis or occlusion prior to the origin of these vessels. Although arteriography in patients with obstructive disease in the left main coronary artery carries an increased risk,[4] recent data has shown improved survival in patients receiving saphenous vein bypass grafts.[5,6] Thus, the presence of such a lesion needs to be detected. Various precautions and techniques have been recommended for proper and safe examination of this vessel.[4,6,7]

The Left Anterior Descending Coronary Artery

Significant coronary artery disease occurs most frequently in the left anterior descending coronary artery.[1] Such disease may be isolated

(Figures 7.6-7.13) or in combination with occlusive lesions in other vessels (Figures 7.14-7.16, Chapter 9). Complete occlusion is frequently seen (Figures 7.16-7.23).

Stenosis may occur in the proximal, middle and distal segments of the artery. The most siginficant lesions occur in the proximal segment (Figures 7.6-7.12). There may be an associated stenosis in the middle segment (Figure 7.13). Isolated lesions are not as frequent in the middle segment (Figure 7.15). In complete proximal occlusion of the left anterior descending artery, the middle segment may not be visualized at all (Figures 7.21-7.23). Isolated stenosis in the distal segment of the left anterior descending artery is infrequent.

Stenosis or occlusions in the proximal segment of the left anterior descending artery may be associated with lesions in the diagonal and/or septal vessels as well (Figure 7.15).

There are significant variations in the appearance of the lesions or stenoses. Some are circumscribed (Figures 7.2, 7.8, 7.14) but the majority involve segments of various lengths of the vessel (Figures 7.1 B, 7.6, 7.9, 7.10, 7.15). The lesions may also appear ulcerated, with a roughened appearance or a central crater filled with contrast material (Figures 7.1, 7.7), or as plaques (Figure 7.12).

The Left Circumflex Artery

Coronary disease in the left circumflex artery occurs less frequently than in the left anterior descending coronary artery, and disease isolated to the left circumflex artery is unusual.[1] Stenosis in the proximal circumflex artery prior to the origin of the first or obtuse left marginal branch (Figures 7.24, 7.25) is more significant than a lesion beyond this bifurcation (Figures 7.26 A, 7.27), as such a proximal lesion can be bypassed by a graft into the left marginal branch. If more than one large left marginal artery is present, then a lesion between the two marginal vessels would also be surgically significant (Figure 7.26 C). Of course, when the system is left dominant, a lesion located beyond the left marginal branch would be of surgical significance since it would be located prior to the origin of the posterior descending artery (Figure 7.28). Disease located in the obtuse left marginal artery near its origin is surgically significant since this artery is capable of receiving a saphenous vein bypass graft (Figure 7.29).

References

1. Proudfit, W.L., Shirey, E.K., and Sones, F.M. Jr.: Distribution of arterial lesions demonstrated by selective cinecoronary arteriography. *Circulation*, **36**:54-62, 1967.

2. Kerschbaum, K.L., Manchester, J.H., and Shelburne, J.C.: Complete left coronary artery obstruction. *Chest*, **64**:539-540, 1973.

3. Bruschke, A.V.G., Proudfit, W.L., and Sones, F.M. Jr.: Progress study of 590 consecutive nonsurgical cases of coronary disease followed 5-9 years. I. Arteriographic correlations. *Circulation*, **47**:1147-1153, 1973.

4. Lavine, P., Kimbiris, D., Segal, B.L., and Linhart, J.W.: Left main coronary artery disease: Clinical, arteriographic and hemodynamic appraisal. *American Journal of Cardiology*, **30**:791-796, 1972.

5. Harrell, R.R., Oberman, A., Russell, R.O., Kouchoukos, N.T., Holt, J.H., and Rackley, C.E.: Left main coronary disease: Predictability and survival in medical versus surgical groups. *Circulation*, **50**:III-35, 1974. (Abstract)

6. Zeft, H.J., Manley, J.C., Huston, J.H., Tector, A.J., Auer, J.E., and Johnson, W.D.: Left main coronary artery stenosis: Results of coronary bypass surgery. *Circulation*, **49**:68-76, 1974.

7. Rösch, J., DeMots, H., Antonovic, R., Rahimtoola, S.H., Judkins, M.P., and Dotter, C.T.: Coronary arteriography in left main coronary artery disease. *American Journal of Roentgenology, Radium Therpay and Nuclear Medicine*, **121**:583-590, 1974.

Figure 7.1:   Left coronary arteriogram; right anterior oblique projection. Two examples of stenosis in the left main coronary artery (LCA) are shown.

A. The arrow points to the stenotic segment and ulceration is seen on the wall opposite the arrow.

B. A long segment of stenosis (arrow) involves almost the entire length of the left main coronary artery.

CX = left circumflex artery. LM = left marginal branch of circumflex artery. LAD = left anterior descending artery.

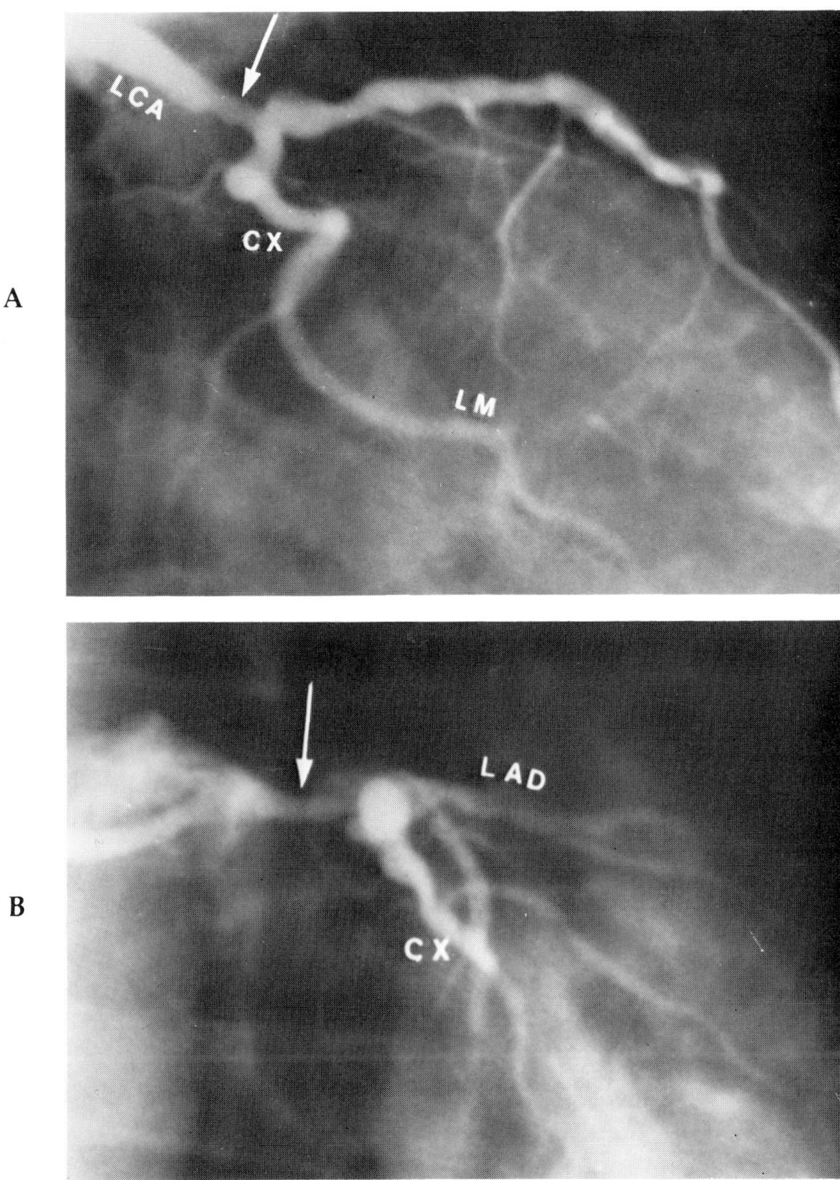

FIGURE 7.1

Figure 7.2:   Left coronary arteriogram; left anterior oblique projection. Two examples of severe and circumscribed stenosis in the left main coronary artery.

A. 70-90% stenosis of the left main coronary artery (arrow) 10 mm. proximal to its bifurcation.

B. 90% stenosis (arrow) at the distal end of the left main coronary artery just before its bifurcation. Additional stenoses in the left anterior descending artery (LAD) and its diagonal branch (D) are present.

S = septal branches of left anterior descending. CX = left circumflex artery.

Figure 7.3:   Left coronary arteriogram; **A**. Left anterior oblique projection. **B**. Lateral projection. A severe (greater than 90%) stenosis (arrow) in the left main coronary artery is shown in two projections.

CX = left circumflex artery. D = diagonal branch of left anterior descending. LM = left marginal branch of circumflex artery. LAD = left anterior descending coronary artery.

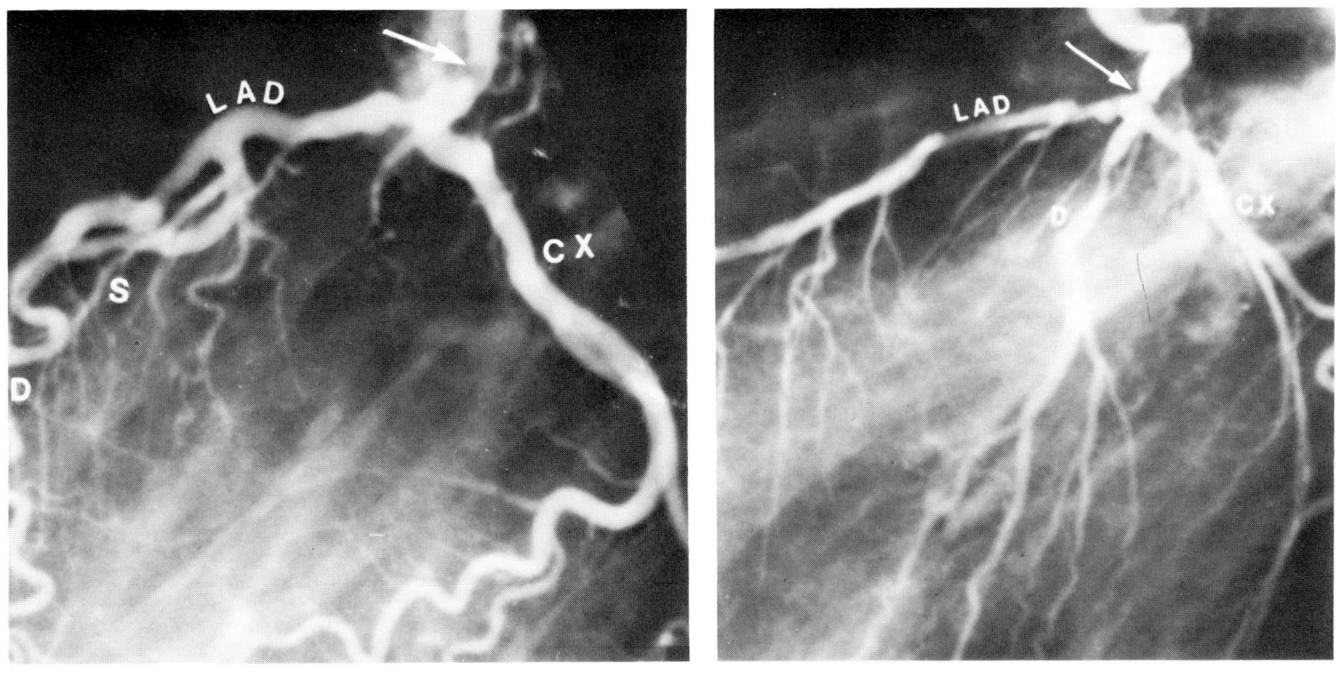
LAD
S
D
CX
A   FIGURE 7.2   B
LAD
D
CX

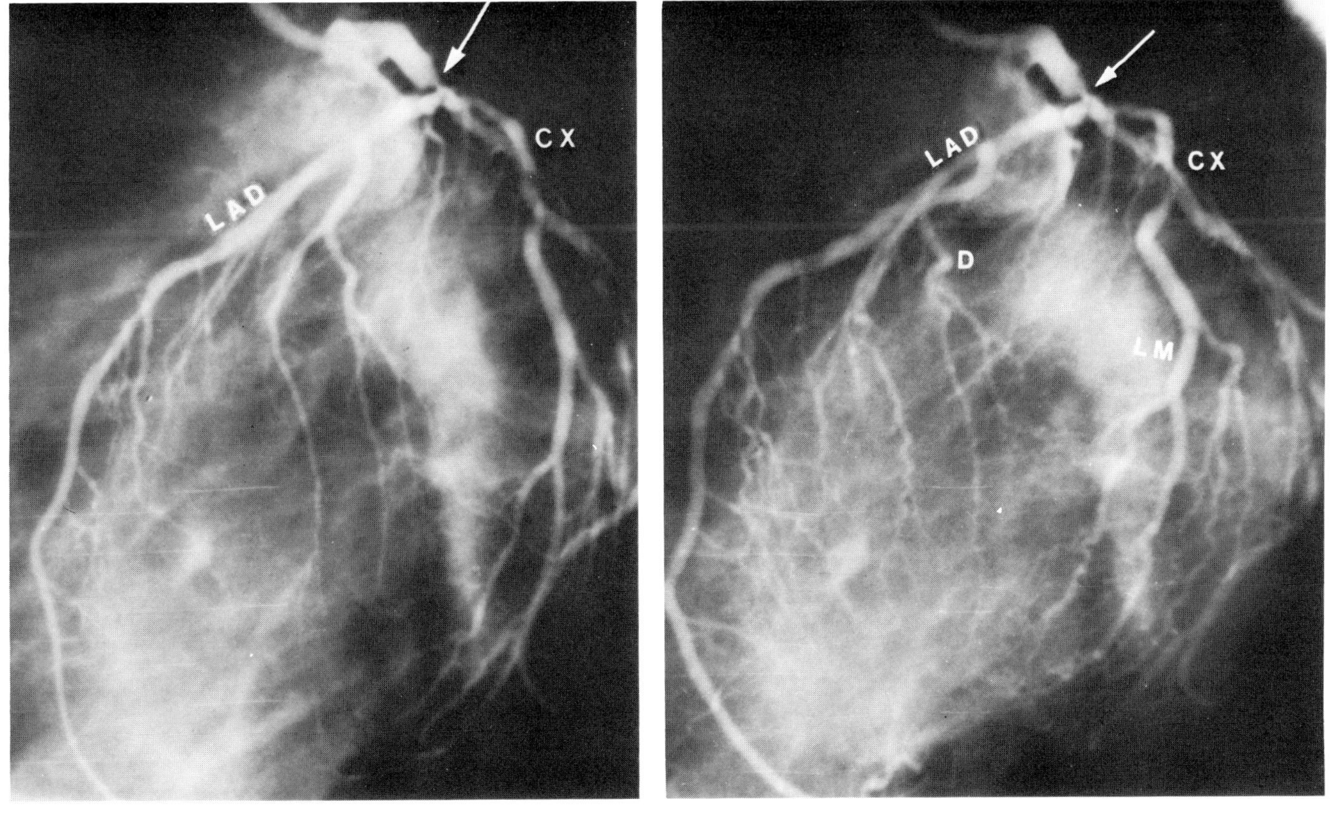
CX
LAD
LAD
CX
D
LM
A   FIGURE 7.3   B

Figure 7.4:   Left coronary arteriogram; right anterior oblique projection. There is a severe (70-90%) lesion (uppermost arrow) in the left main coronary artery. Also demonstrated is a lesion (arrow) in the proximal one-third of the left anterior descending artery (LAD) before the first septal (S) and diagonal branches. Following another stenosis in the middle one-third of the LAD (arrow), the distal vessel is size "B". A long stenotic segment (between arrows) is present in the left circumflex artery (CX) before the obtuse marginal (LM) branch. Left main coronary artery stenosis is usually associated with obstructive lesions in other coronary arteries.

(Refer to pages 6 and 7 for grading of vessels.)

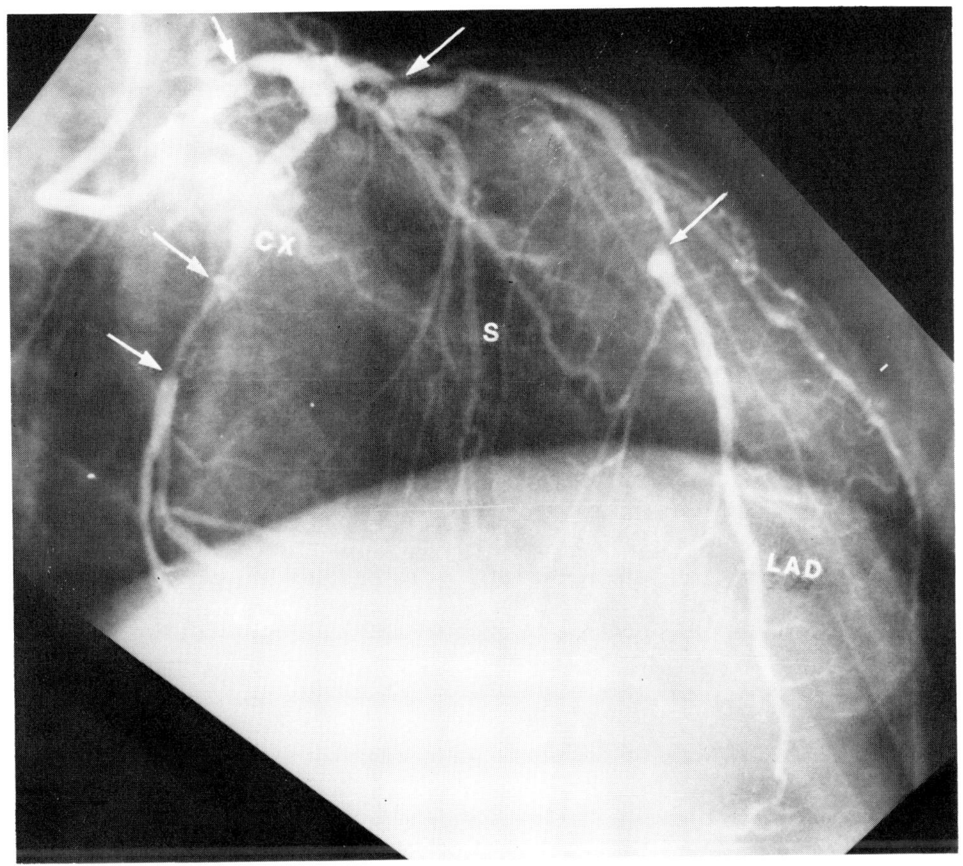

FIGURE 7.4

Figure 7.5:   A rare example of complete occlusion of the left main coronary artery is shown.

A. Selective injection into the left main coronary artery demonstrates the occlusion a few millimeters distal to its ostium.

B. Right coronary arteriogram; lateral projection. A normal vessel with a well developed collateral network is present in this patient with the occluded left main coronary artery.

SN = sinus node artery. RCA = right coronary artery. S = septal branches connecting posterior descending (PD) branch of right coronary artery and left anterior descending artery. DRCA = distal right coronary artery.

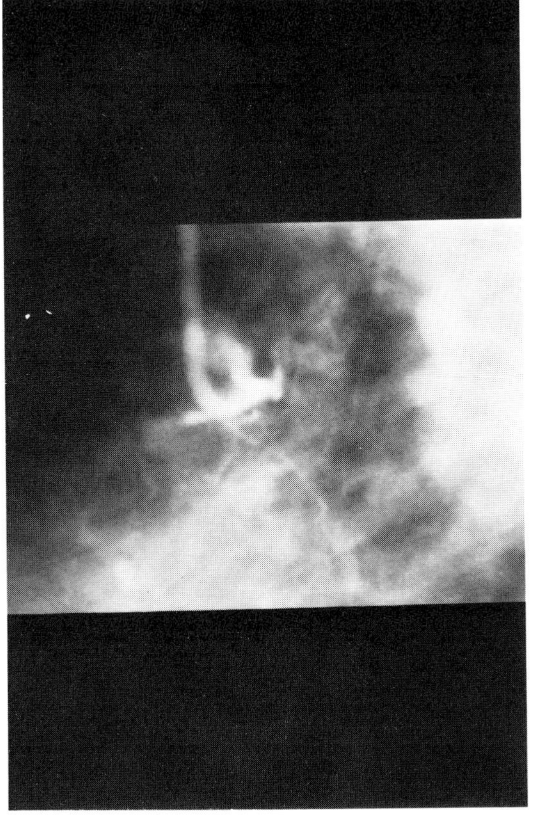

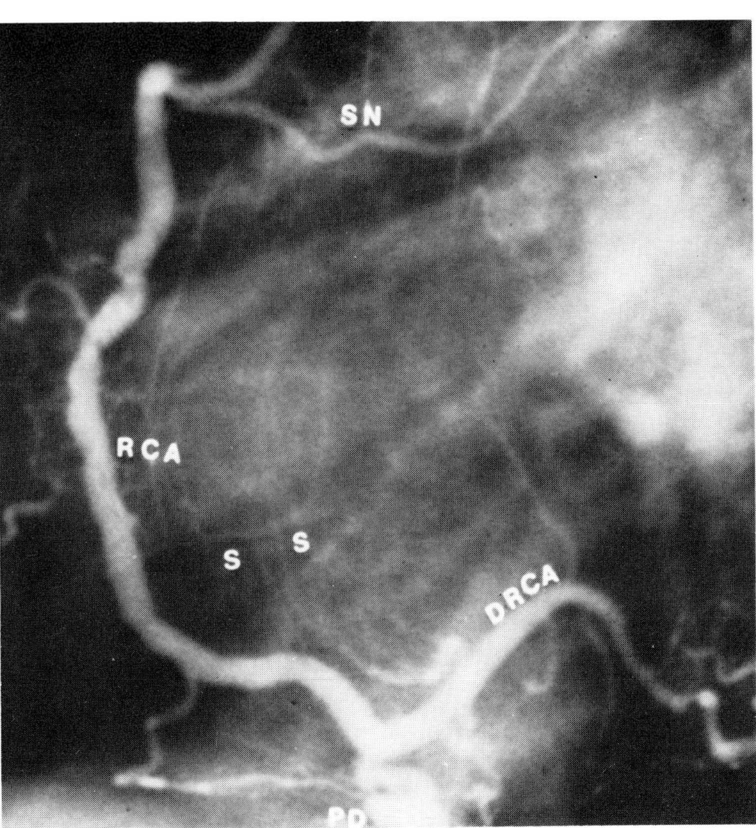

A   FIGURE 7.5   B

Figure 7.6:   Left coronary arteriogram; lateral projection. 50-70% stenosis (arrow) is present in the proximal segment of the left anterior descending artery (LAD) immediately after the origin of the first septal artery (S). The post-stenotic segment is size "A". This is the only stenosis detected in this patient.

CX = left circumflex artery.

(Refer to pages 6 and 7 for grading of vessels.)

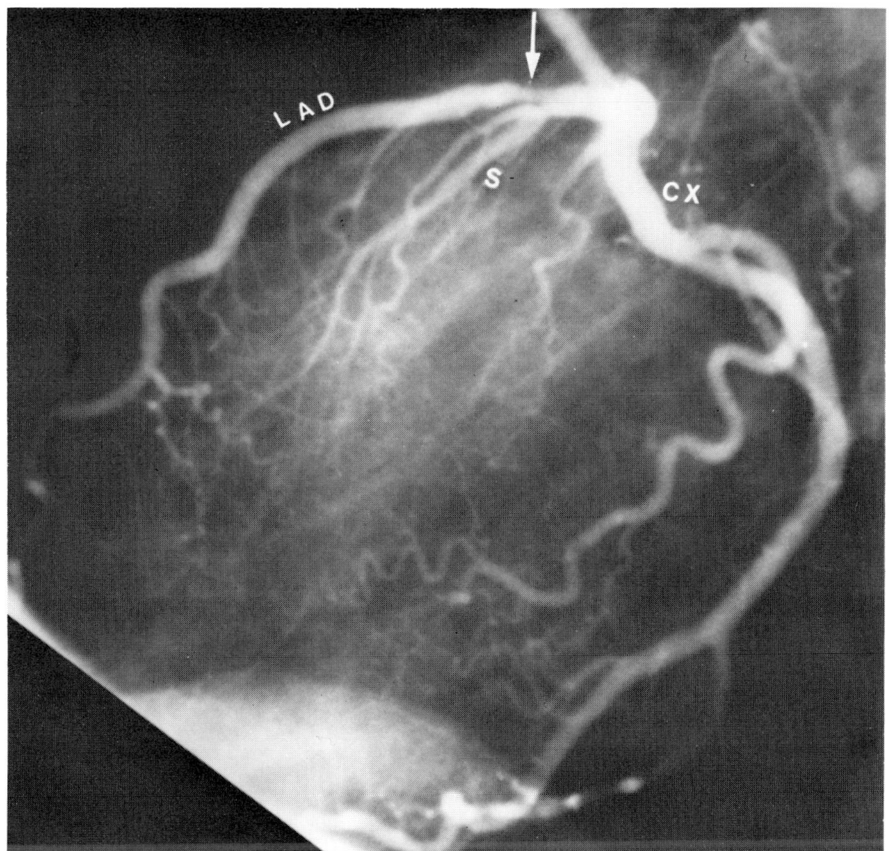

**FIGURE 7.6

Figure 7.7:   Left coronary arteriogram; right anterior oblique projection. Severe (70-90%) stenosis (arrow) in the proximal one-third of the left anterior descending artery (LAD) just before the origin of the first septal and first diagonal arteries. The borders of the stenotic segment are irregular suggesting ulceration. The post-stenotic segment is size "A".

CX = left circumflex artery.

(Refer to pages 6 and 7 for grading of vessels.)

Figure 7.8:   Left coronary arteriogram; left anterior oblique projection. A circumscribed 50-70% stenosis (arrow) with smooth borders is present in the proximal one-third of the left anterior descending (LAD) artery after the origin of the first diagonal branch. The distal LAD is size "A".

CX = left circumflex artery.

(Refer to pages 6 and 7 for grading of vessels.)

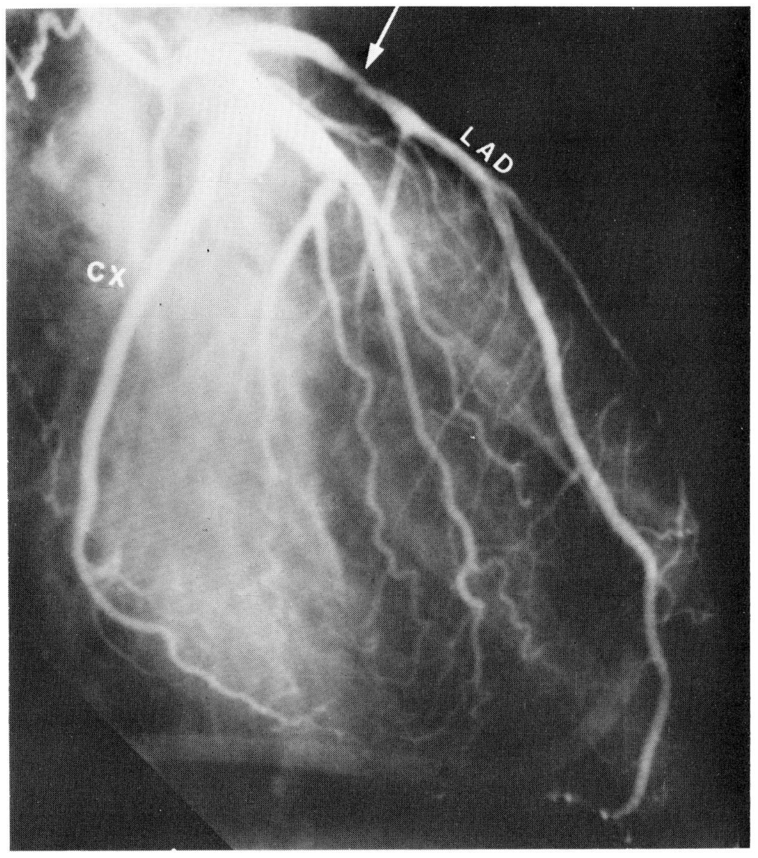

FIGURE 7.7

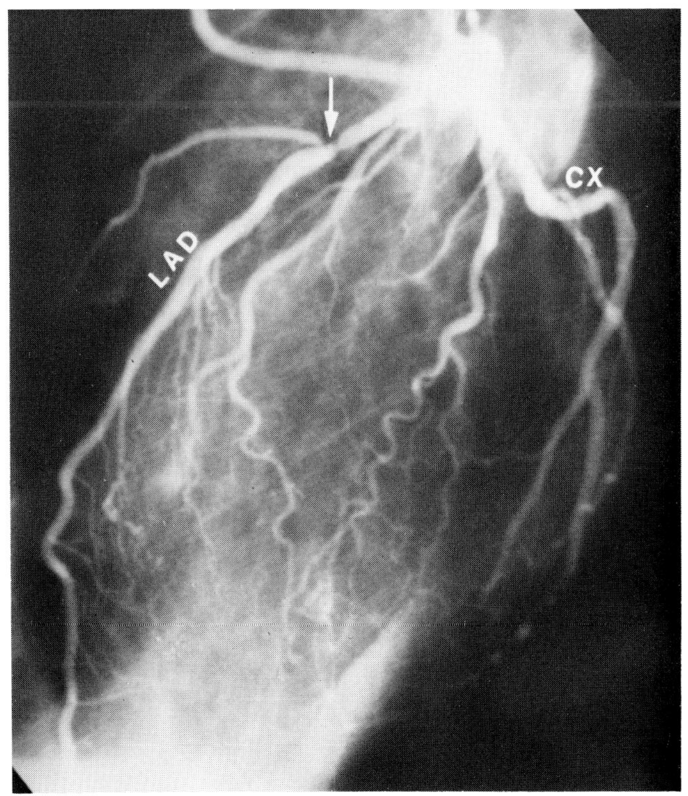

FIGURE 7.8

Figure 7.9:   Left coronary arteriogram; lateral projection. A severe (greater than 90%) stenosis (arrow) in the left anterior descending coronary artery (LAD) is seen before the first septal and diagonal arteries. The distal segment is size "A".

(Refer to pages 6 and 7 for grading of vessels.)

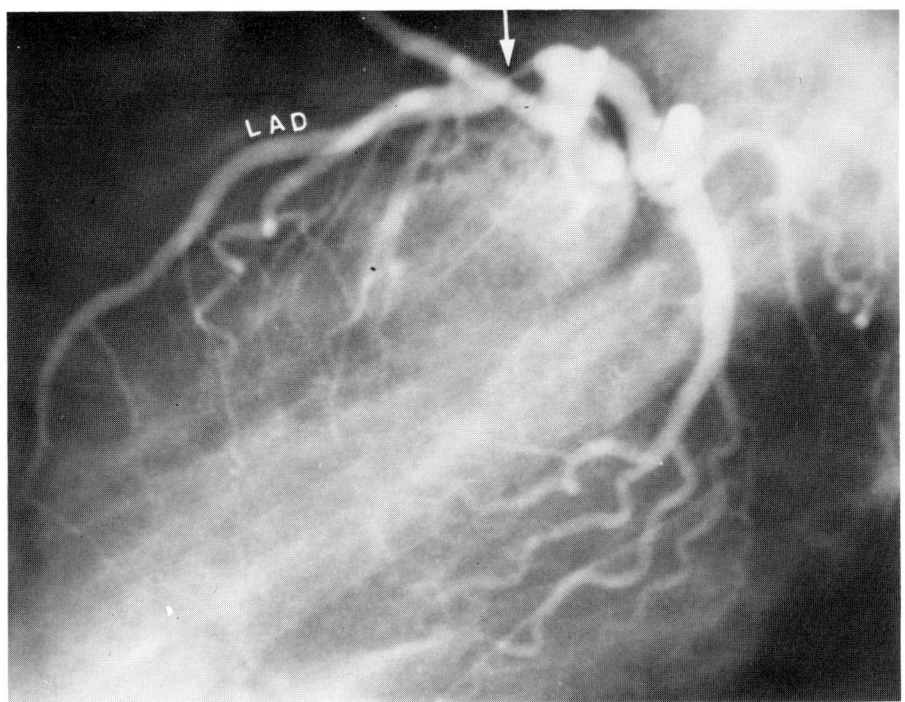

FIGURE 7.9

Figure 7.10:   Left coronary arteriogram; lateral projection.

A. A severe (greater than 90%) stenosis (arrow) is seen in the left anterior descending artery (LAD) after the origin of the first septal artery. There is a 50-70% stenosis following the first diagonal branch. The distal vessel is size "A".

CX = left circumflex artery. LM = left marginal branch of circumflex artery.

B. Diagrammatic representation of **A**.

(Refer to pages 6 and 7 for grading of vessels.)

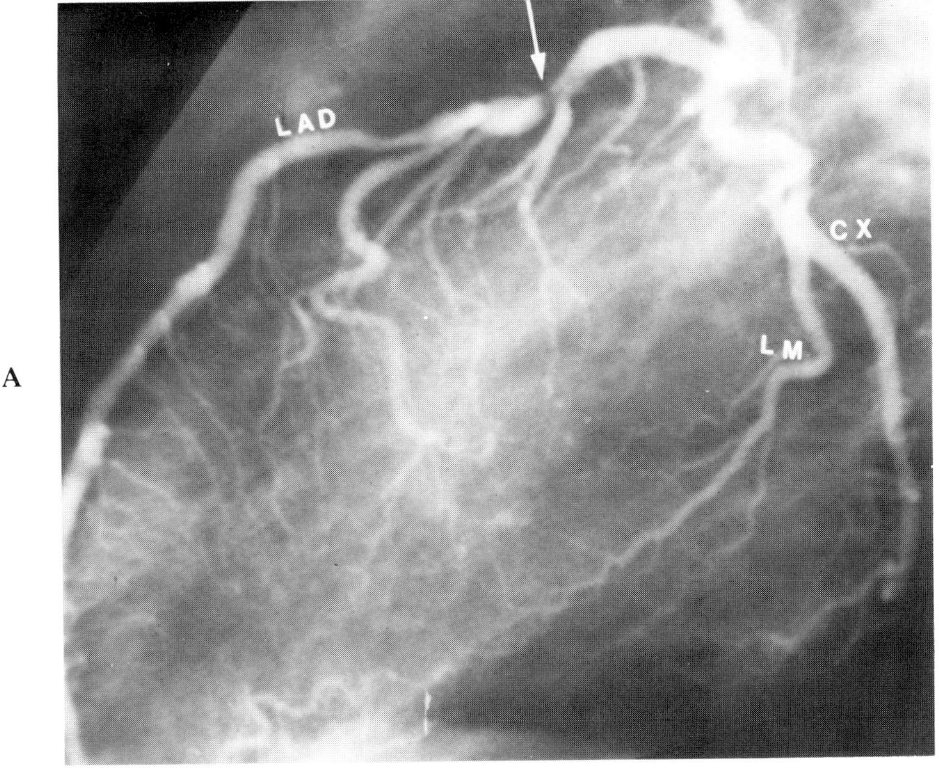

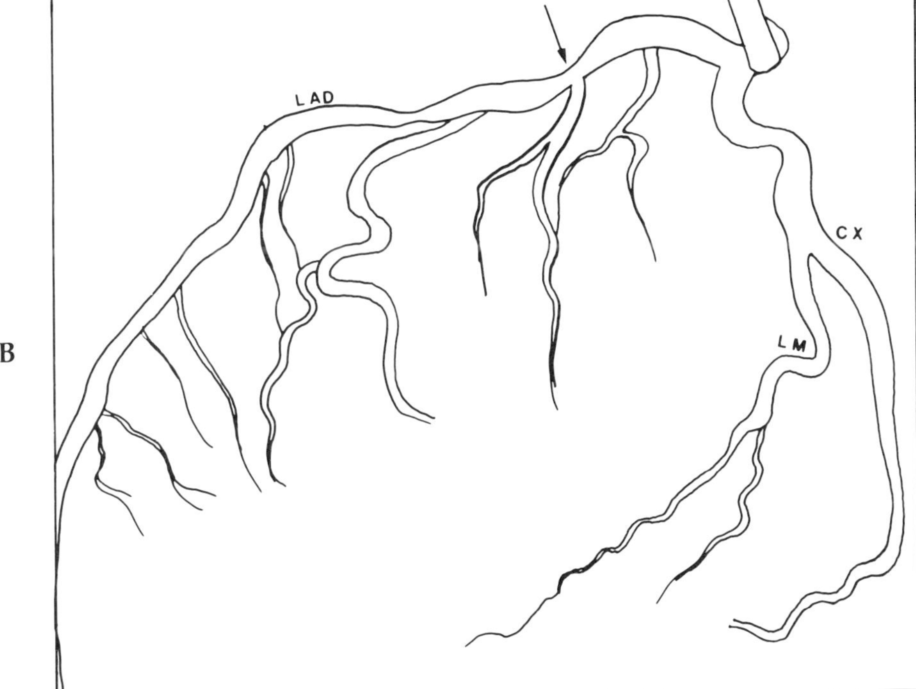

FIGURE 7.10

Figure 7.11:   Left coronary arteriogram; lateral projection. Two stenoses (arrows) in the left anterior descending artery (LAD) are present after the origin of the first diagonal (D) artery but before and after the second diagonal (D) branch. The proximal lesion is 70-90% stenotic and the distal lesion involves 50-70% of the arterial diameter. The distal LAD is size "A".

CX = left circumflex artery. S = septal branch of the left anterior descending artery.

(Refer to pages 6 and 7 for grading of vessels.)

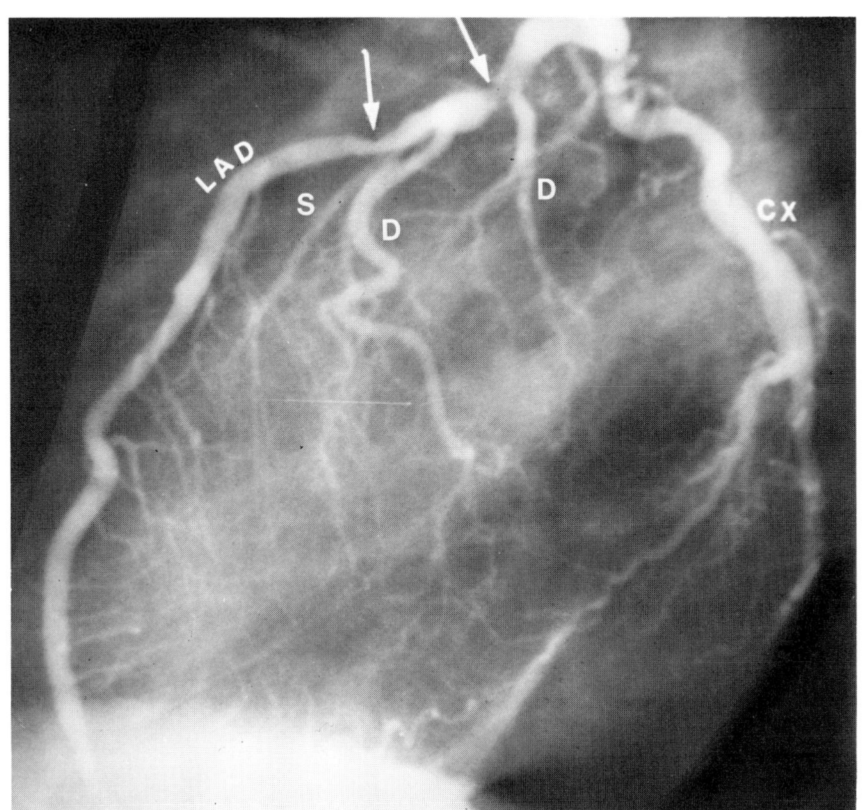

FIGURE 7.11

Figure 7.12:   Left coronary arteriogram; lateral projection.

A. A long stenotic segment in the proximal one-third of the left anterior descending coronary artery (LAD) is seen. The radiolucent strip (between the arrows) suggests a plaque.

D = diagonal branch of left anterior descending. CX = left circumflex artery. LM = left marginal branch of left circumflex artery.

B. Diagrammatic representation of **A**.

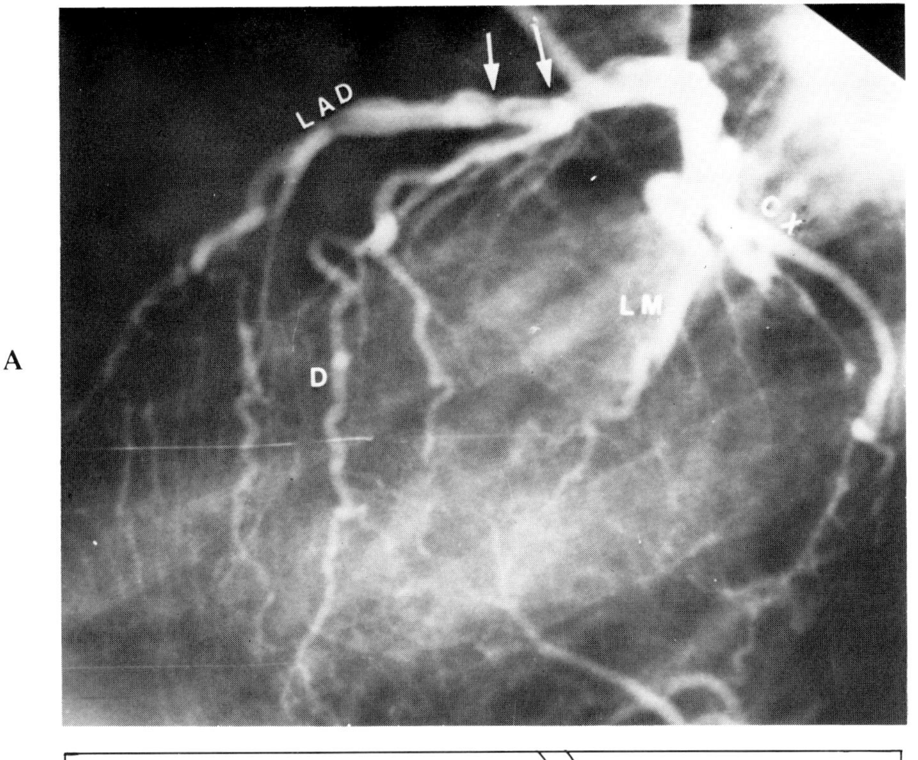

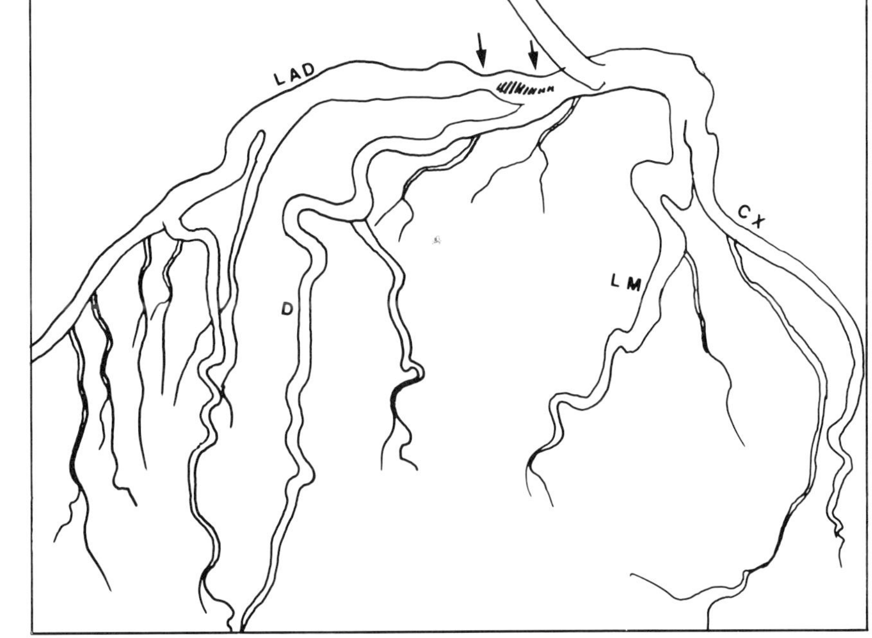

FIGURE 7.12

Figure 7.13:   Left coronary arteriogram; lateral projection.

A. Two stenoses (arrows) in the left anterior descending artery (LAD) are present, before and after the first septal branch. The distal segment of the left anterior descending is size "B". Both lesions compromise 50-70% of the arterial diameter.

CX = left circumflex artery.

B. Diagrammatic representation of **A.**

(Refer to pages 6 and 7 for grading of vessels.)

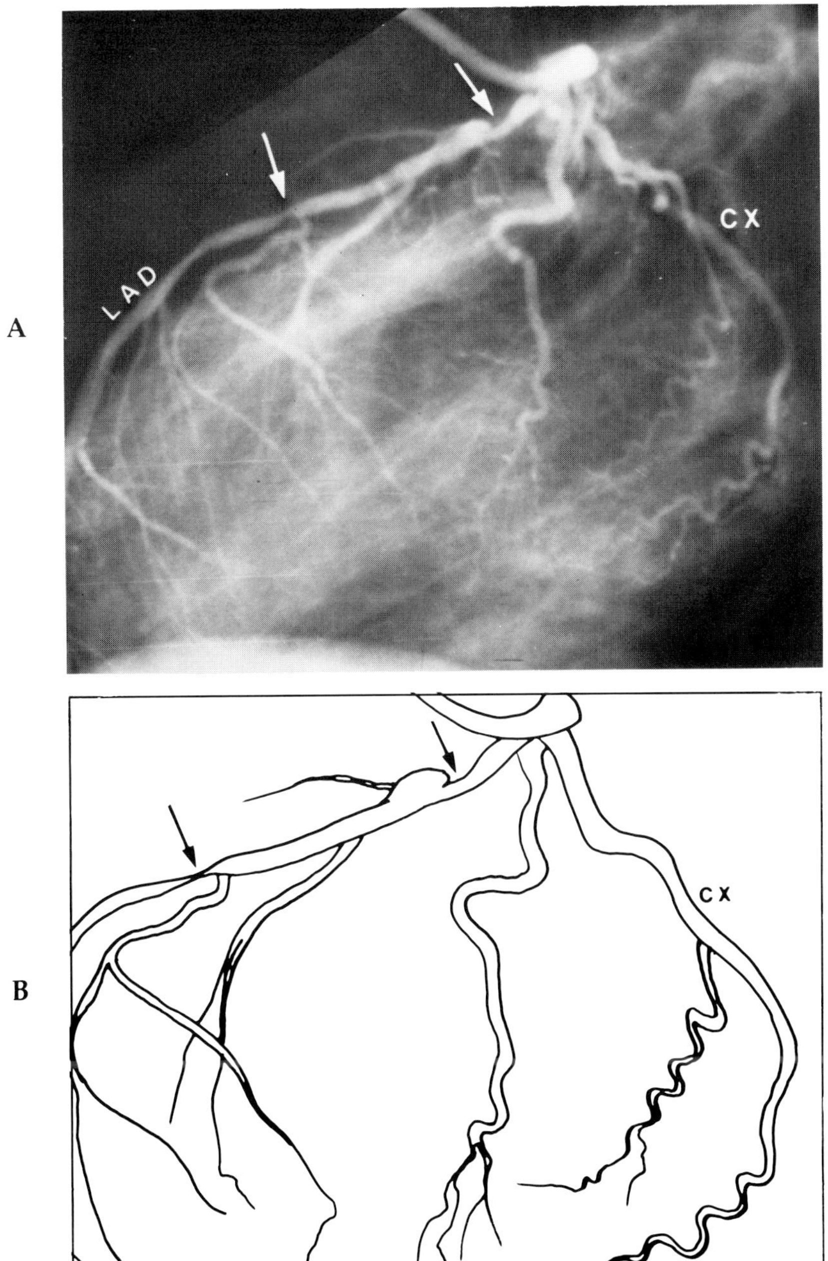

FIGURE 7.13

Figure 7.14:   Left coronary arteriogram; left anterior oblique projection.

A. Stenosis in the left anterior descending artery (LAD), just after the origin of the first septal artery (arrow). In this projection the severity of this lesion is not well appreciated. A filling defect representing a plaque is noted in the left circumflex artery (CX) proximal to the first left marginal artery.

B. Diagrammatic representation of **A.**

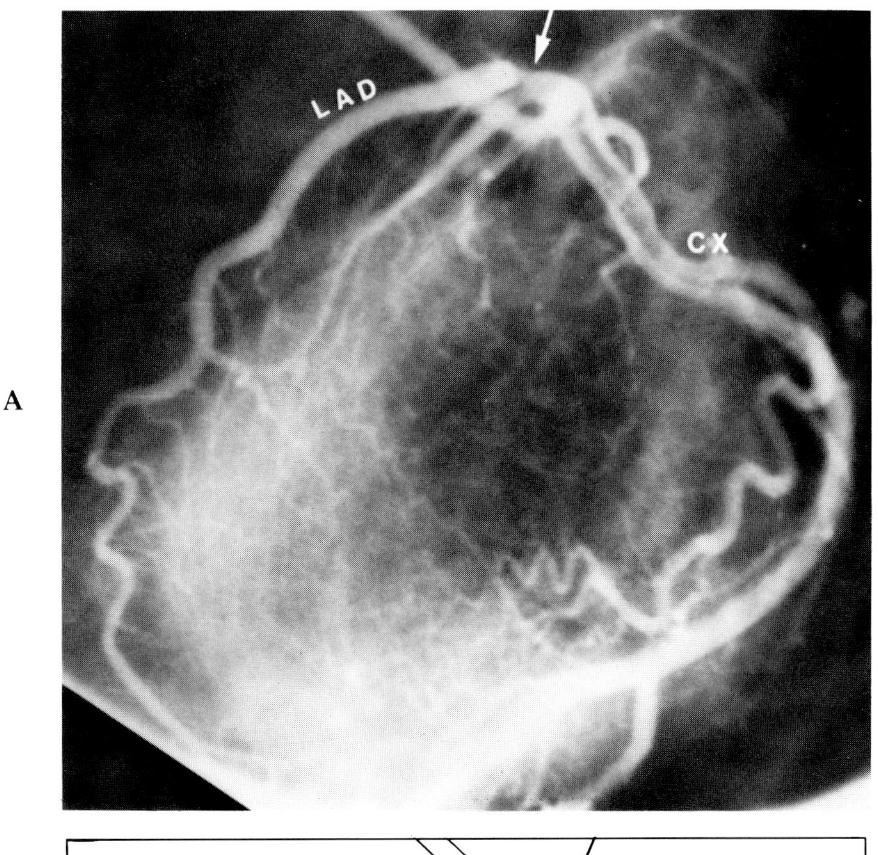

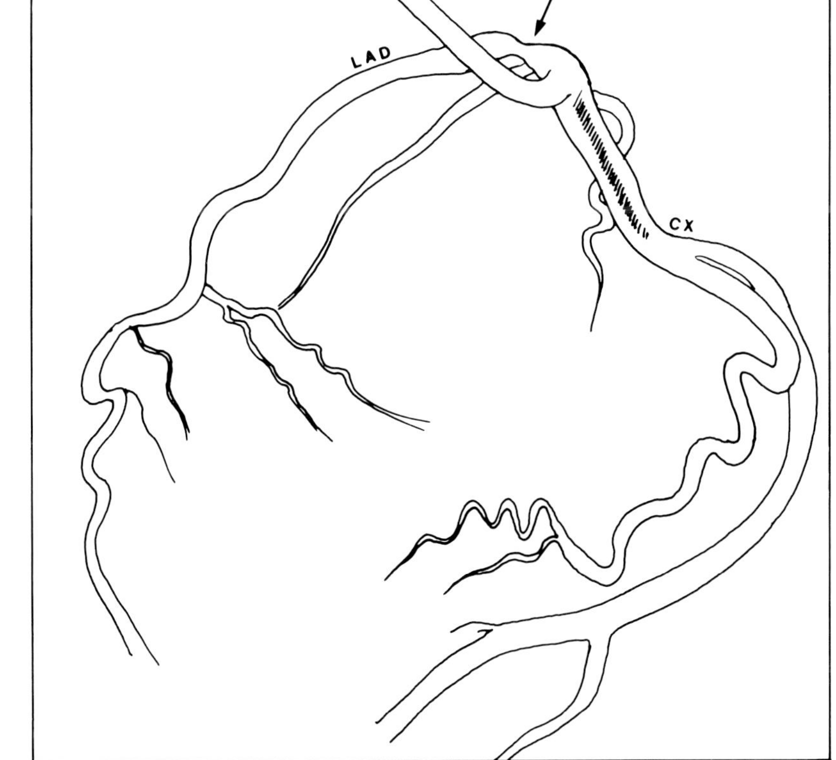

FIGURE 7.14

Figure 7.15:   Left coronary arteriogram; lateral projection. A severe (greater than 90%) stenosis is present in the proximal left anterior descending (LAD) after the origin of the first diagonal (D) branch which also has two lesions of greater than 90% stenosis. The left circumflex artery (CX) has a 70-90% lesion (arrow) after the first diagonal branch.

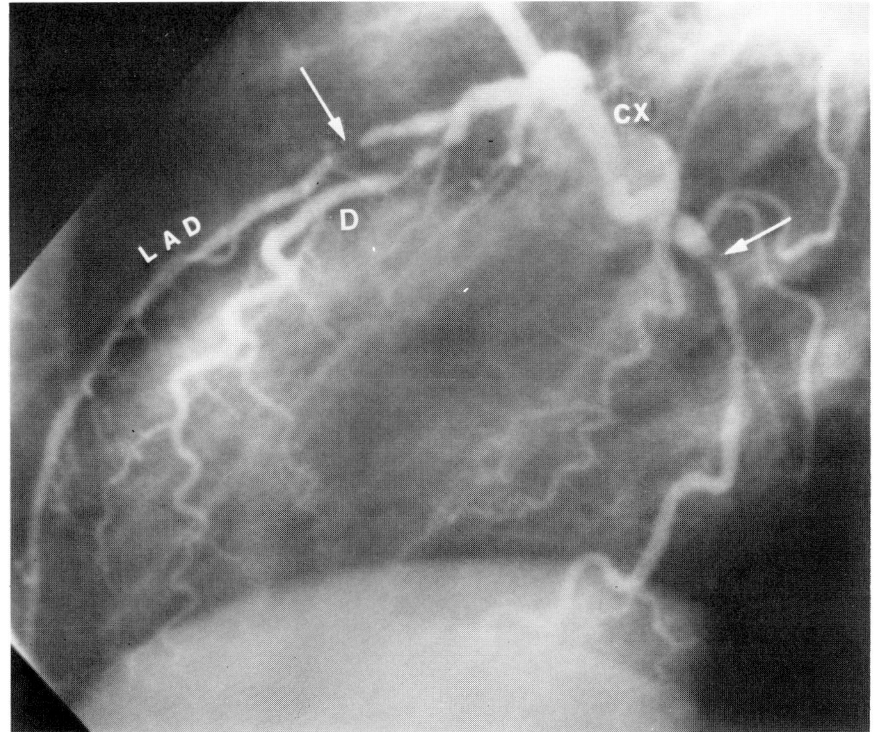

FIGURE 7.15

Figure 7.16:   Left coronary arteriogram; lateral projection.

A. Occlusion of the left anterior descending artery (between left upper arrows). The distal segment (LAD) is almost totally opacified by collateral channels over the left ventricular free wall originating from diagonal (D) and marginal (LM) branches. A stenosis is present in the circumflex artery (arrow on right).

S = septal branches of left anterior descending artery.

B. Diagrammatic representation of **A**.

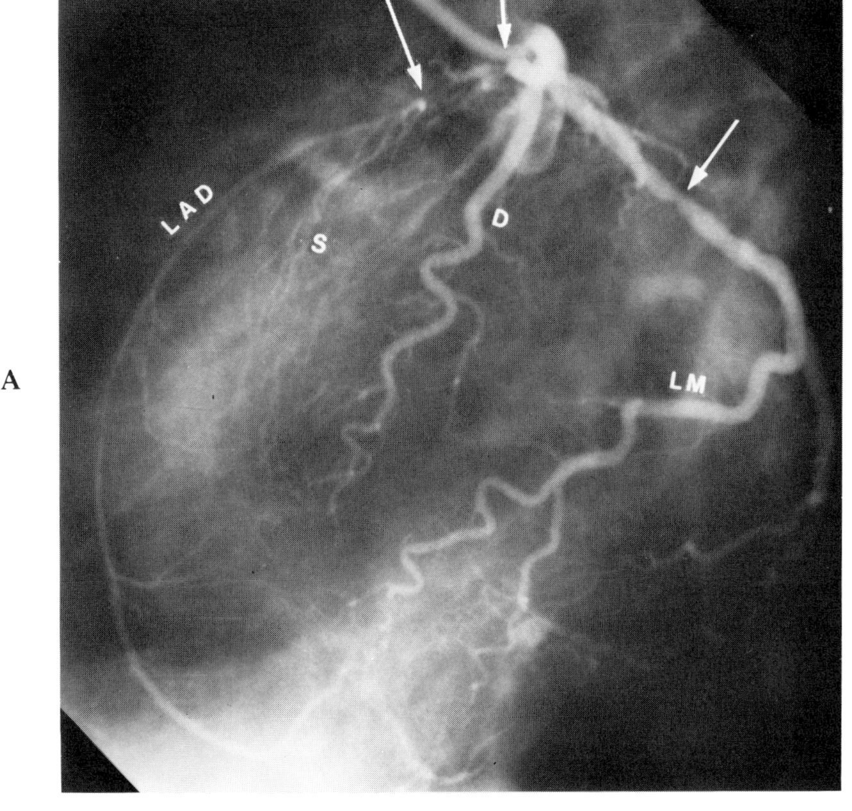

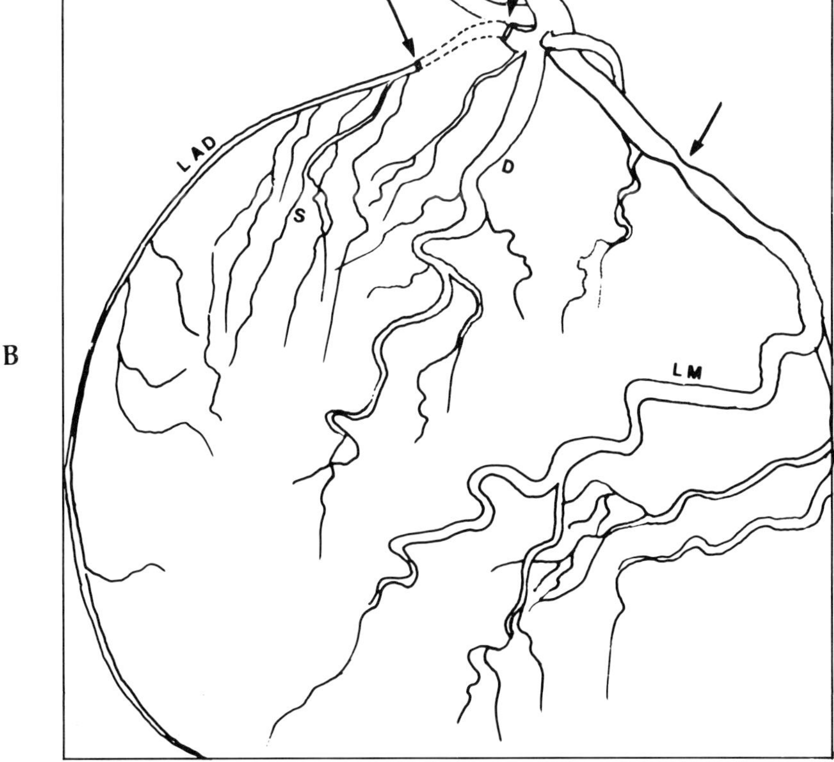

FIGURE 7.16

Figure 7.17:   Left coronary arteriogram; right anterior oblique projection.

A. There is a total occlusion of the left anterior descending artery at its origin (arrow). The distal segment of the left anterior descending artery is not visualized.

B. In a later stage of this arteriogram, an enlarged diagonal (D) branch of the left anterior descending artery fills in retrograde fashion, but the left anterior descending artery does not fill. The circumflex artery (CX) is normal, but the left marginal (LM) has a less than 50% stenosis proximally as seen in **A**. The system is left dominant as the posterior descending (PD) artery originates from the left circumflex (CX) artery.

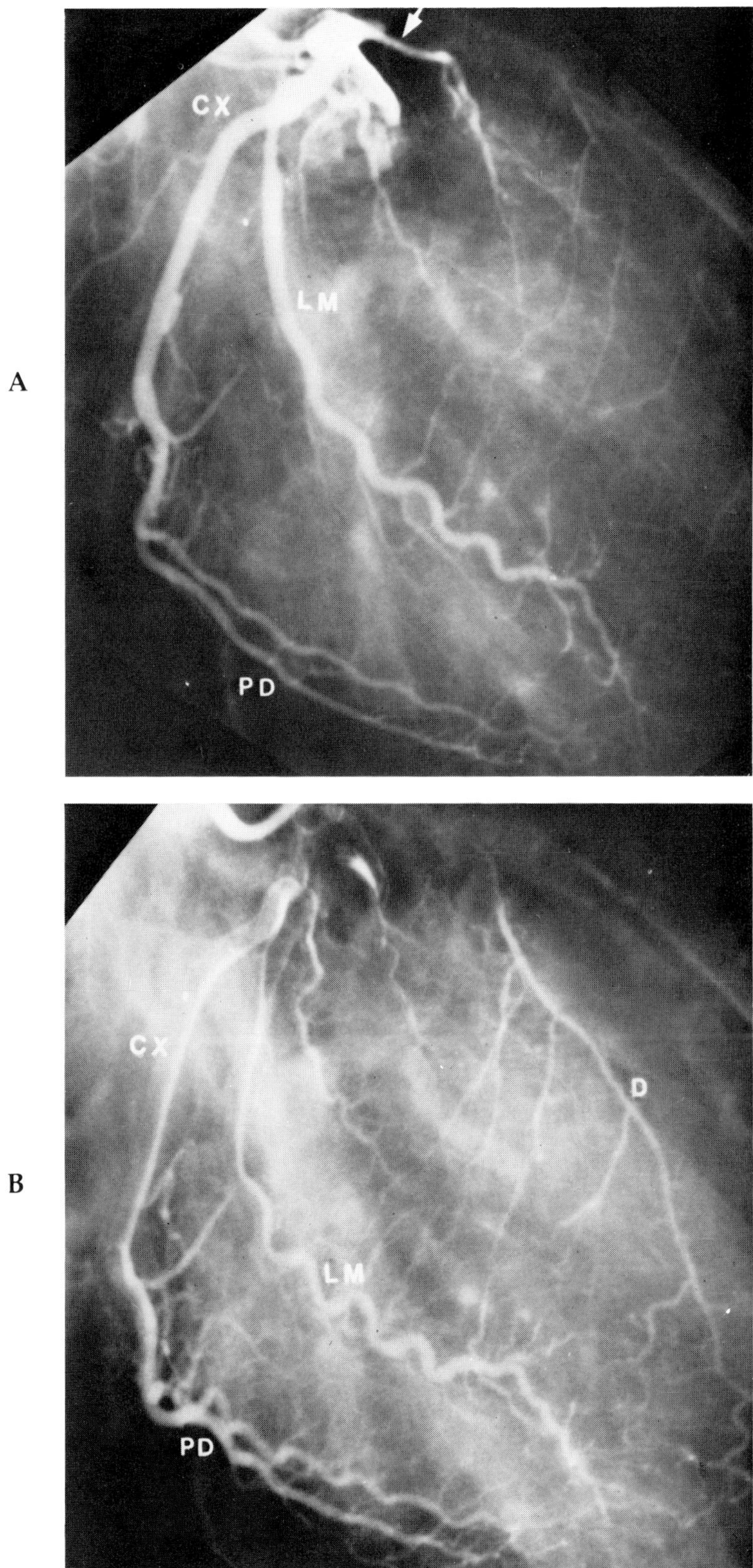

FIGURE 7.17

Figure 7.18:   Left coronary arteriogram; left anterior oblique projection. Complete occlusion of the left anterior descending artery (pointer). The circumflex artery (CX) is the only directly visualized vessel. A small diagonal branch of the left anterior descending artery (D), is opacified by collaterals from the left marginal artery.

Figure 7.19:   Left coronary arteriogram; left anterior oblique projection. Occlusion of the left anterior descending artery (LAD) in the proximal one-third (arrow), immediately after the origin of the first diagonal branch (D). The distal segment of the left anterior descending artery is poorly visualized (size "C" vessel) through collateral channels over the left ventricular free wall. The circumflex (CX) has irregularities in its wall. The left marginal branch of the circumflex (LM) is normal.

(Refer to pages 6 and 7 for grading of vessels.)

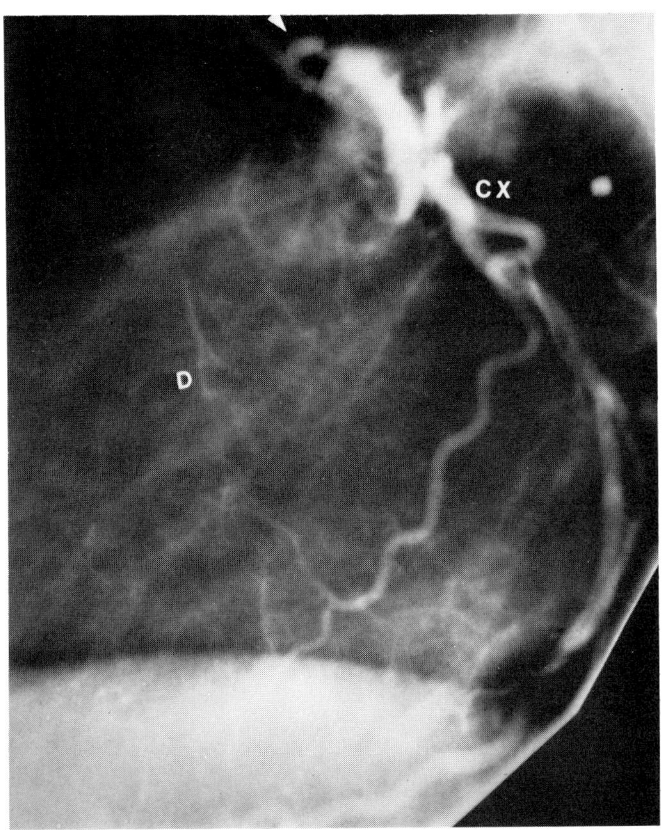

FIGURE 7.18

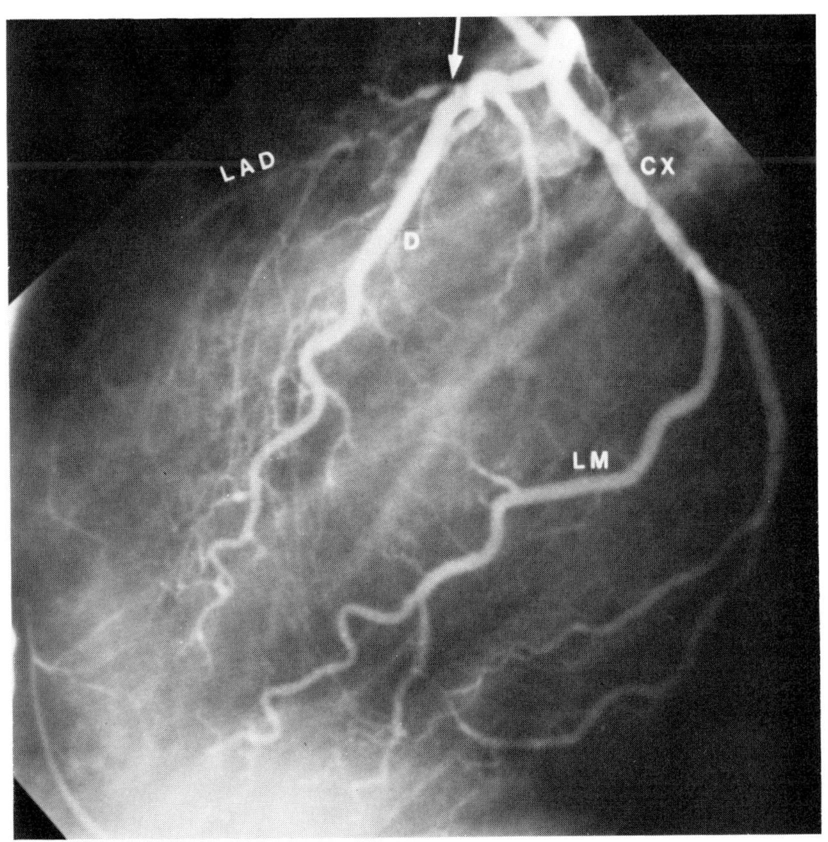

FIGURE 7.19

Figure 7.20:   Left coronary arteriogram; right anterior oblique projection. A 20 mm. segment of the left anterior descending is occluded (between vertical arrows). The distal vessel is opacified as a size "C" vessel. Notice the enlargement of the first septal branch (S). The left circumflex artery (CX, horizontal arrows) is also enlarged.

LM = left marginal branch of the left circumflex artery.

(Refer to pages 6 and 7 for grading of vessels.)

Figure 7.21:   Left coronary arteriogram; right anterior oblique projection. There is total occlusion of the left anterior descending artery in the proximal one-third before the first septal artery. The upper arrow points to the site of occlusion which in this projection is overlapped by a diagonal vessel. The distal one-third of the left anterior descending artery is opacified from the point of the lower arrow by collateral flow from the left marginal (LM) artery. The large LM artery is a major channel for the supply of blood to the left ventricle in this patient. The segment of the left anterior descending artery between the arrows is probably occluded.

LCA = left main coronary artery. CX = left circumflex artery. PDA = posterior descending branch of right coronary artery (at pointer).

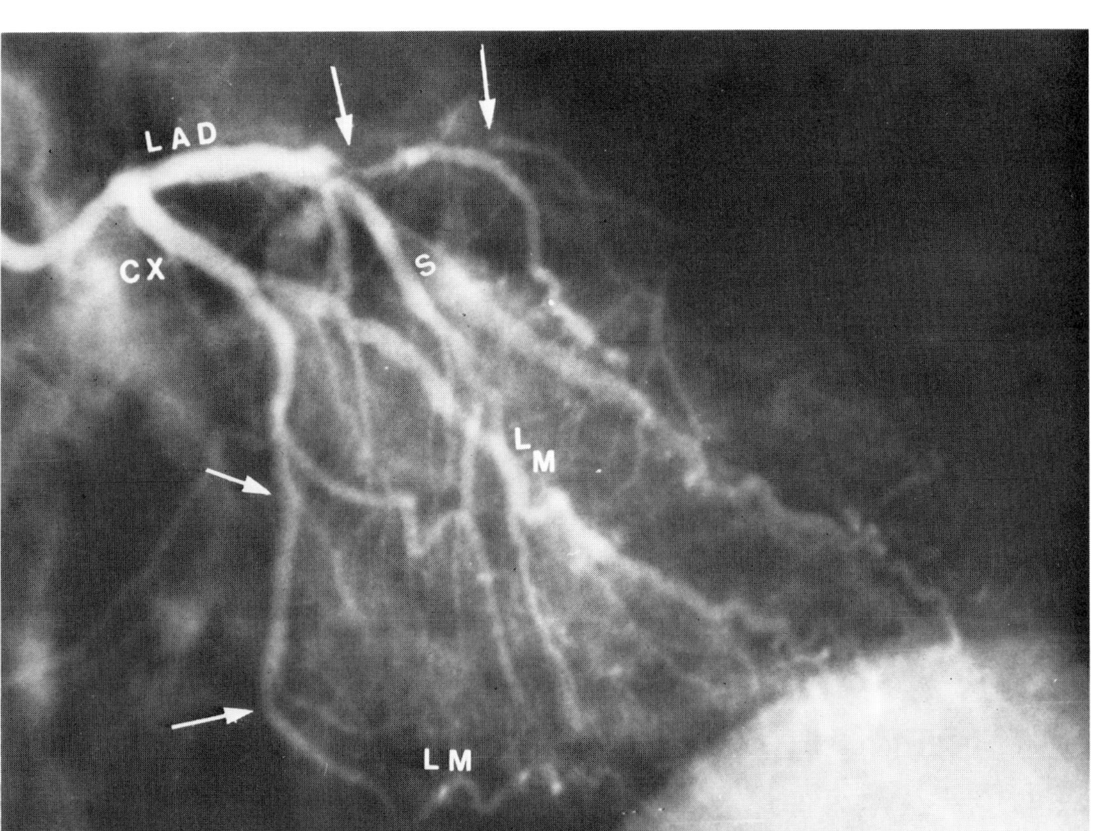

FIGURE 7.20

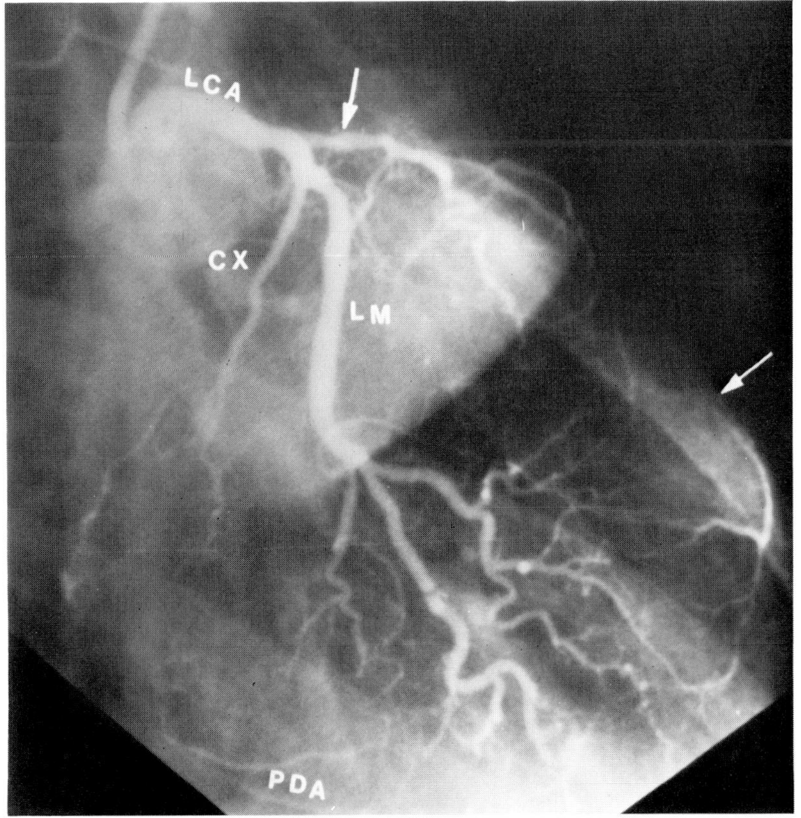

FIGURE 7.21

Figure 7.22:   Right coronary arteriogram; right anterior oblique projection. Two examples of retrograde filling of the left anterior descending artery (LAD) from the right coronary artery (RCA, arrows on lower left) provide indirect evidence for complete occlusion of the left anterior descending artery (arrow on right).

A. The septal (S) and epicardial vessels constitute the collateral channels.

B. There is a direct communication at the apex (lower right arrow) between the posterior descending (PDA) and left anterior descending (LAD) arteries. Septal collaterals are also present.

RM = right marginal branch of right coronary artery.

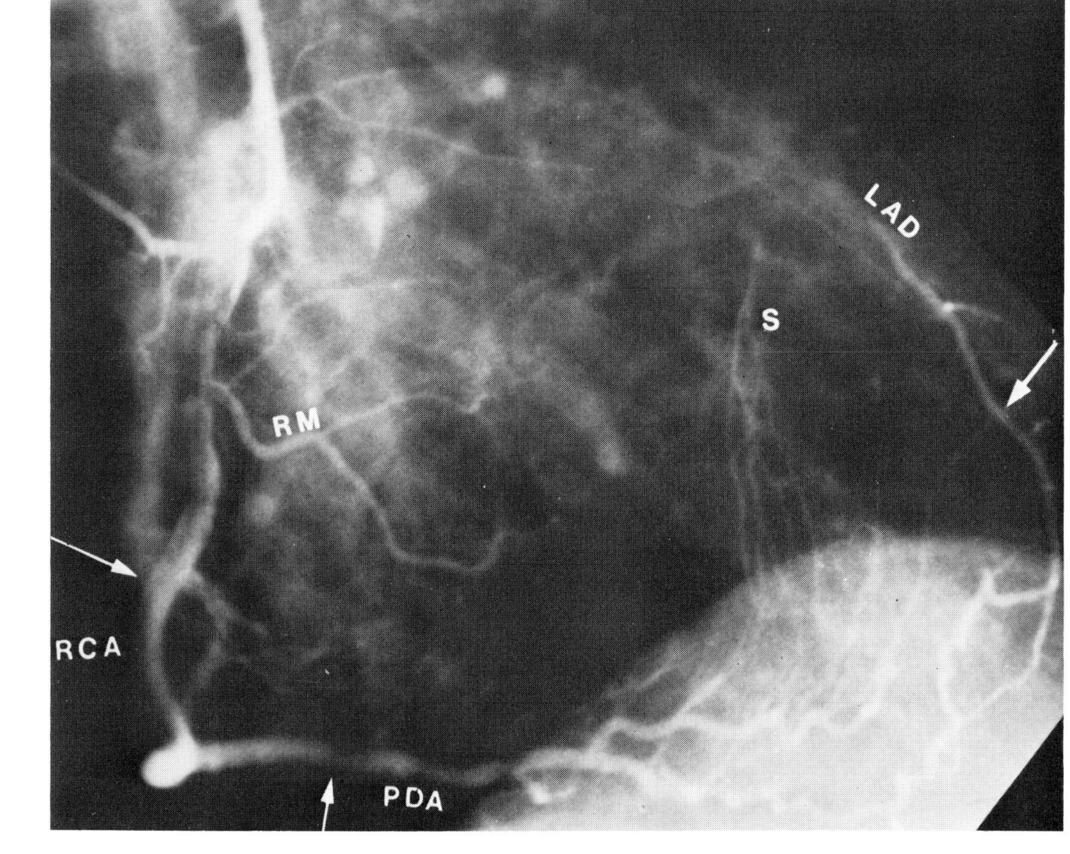

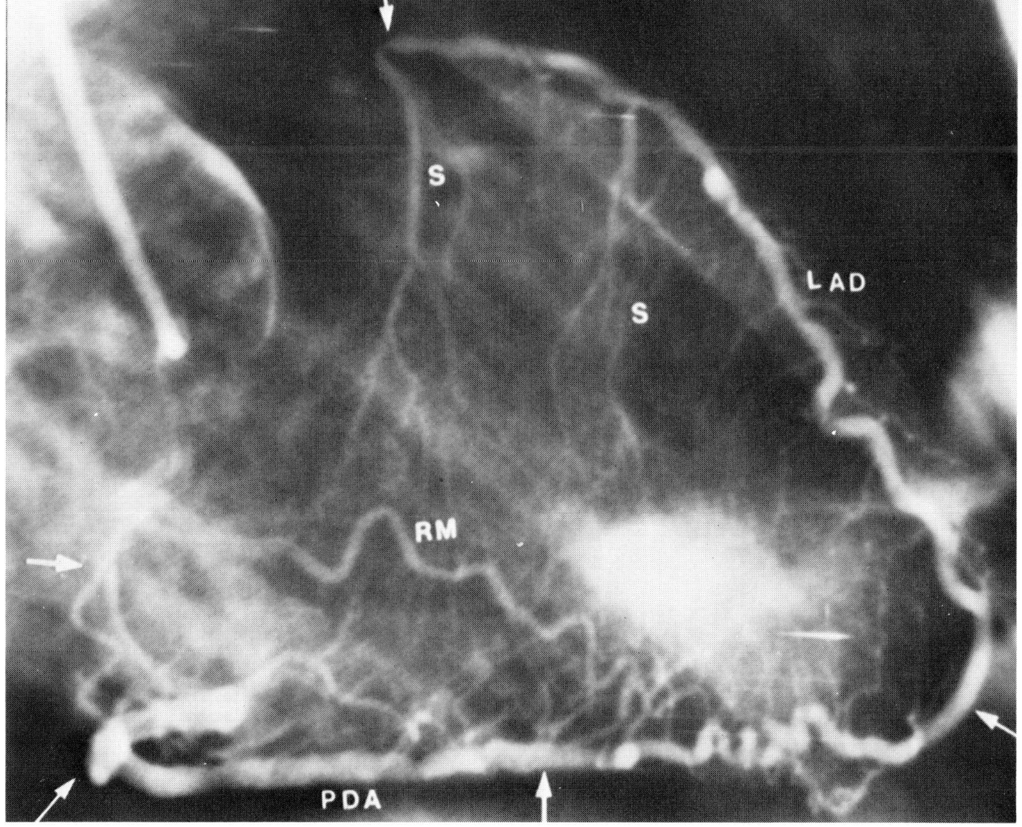

FIGURE 7.22

Figure 7.23:   Left coronary arteriogram; lateral projection.

A. Occlusion of the left anterior descending (LAD, arrow) in the middle one-third after the origin of the first septal artery (S). The distal LAD is faintly opacified by collateral channels originating in left marginal branches (LM), and is size "C".

D = diagonal branch of left anterior descending artery. CX = left circumflex artery.

B. Diagrammatic representation of **A**.

(Refer to pages 6 and 7 for grading of vessels.)

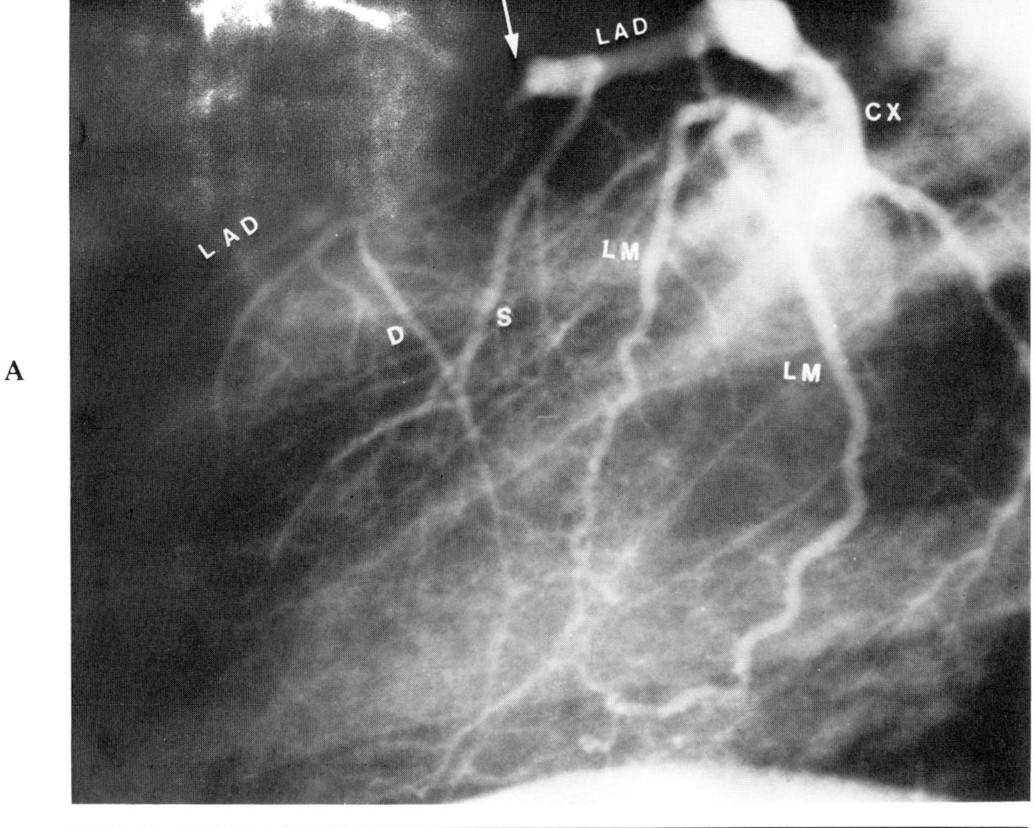

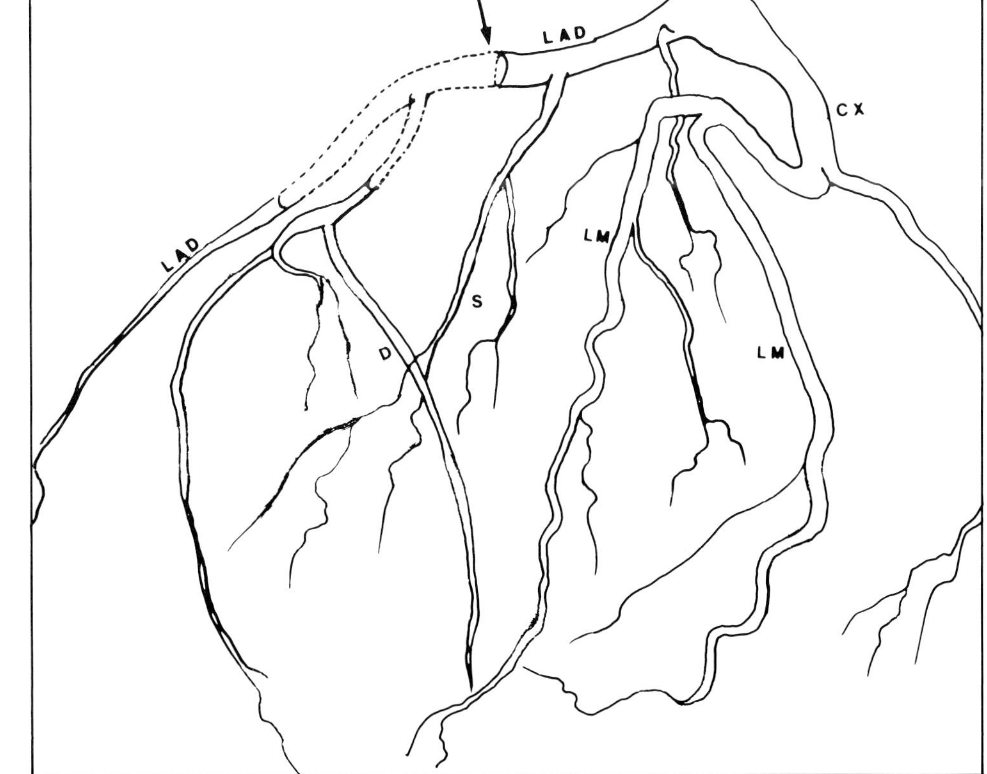

FIGURE 7.23

Figure 7.24: Left coronary arteriogram; lateral projection. The left anterior descending artery (LAD) is small, but the first septal artery (S) is quite large. A mild (less than 50%) stenosis in the left circumflex (CX) artery (arrow) is easily appreciated and is located before the marginal(LM)arteries. The left marginal arteries are size "A".

(Refer to pages 6 and 7 for grading of vessels.)

Figure 7.25: Left coronary arteriogram; right anterior oblique projection. Complete occlusion of the circumflex artery (CX, arrow), proximal to the origin of the left marginal artery. There is no filling of the distal circumflex artery or left marginal branch.

LAD = left anterior descending artery. S = septal branches of left anterior descending artery. D = diagonal branch of left anterior descending artery. PD = posterior descending artery, a continuation of the left anterior descending artery after it wraps around the apex.

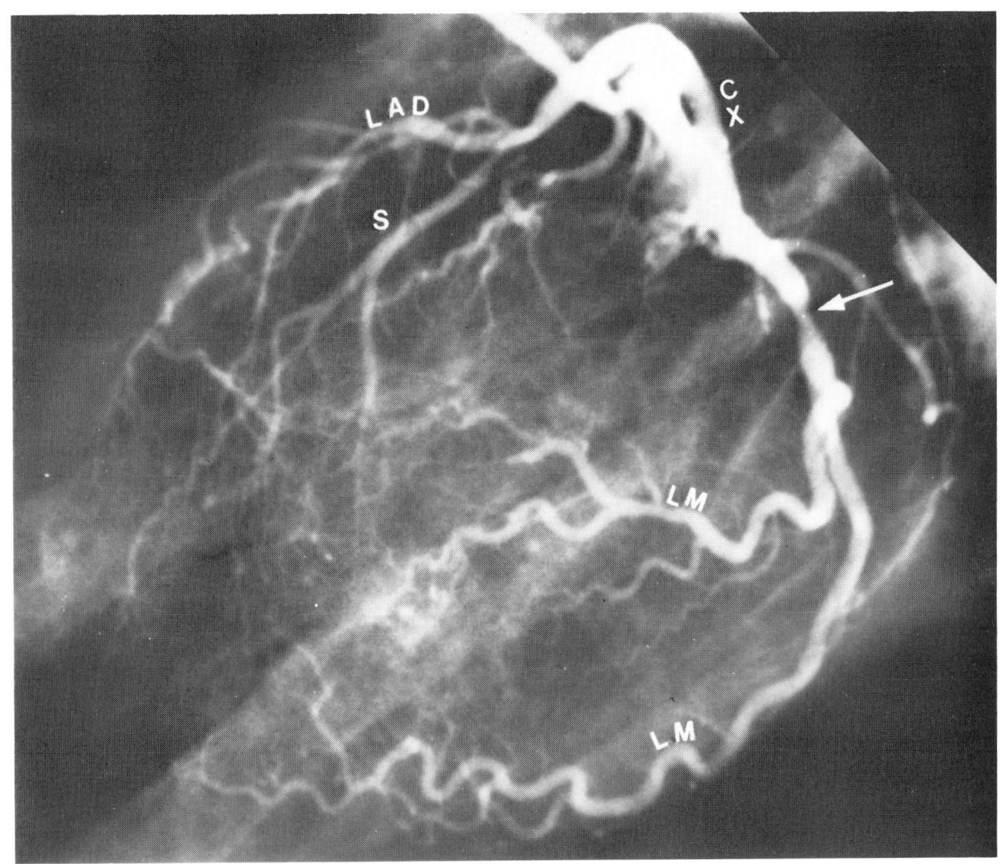

FIGURE 7.24

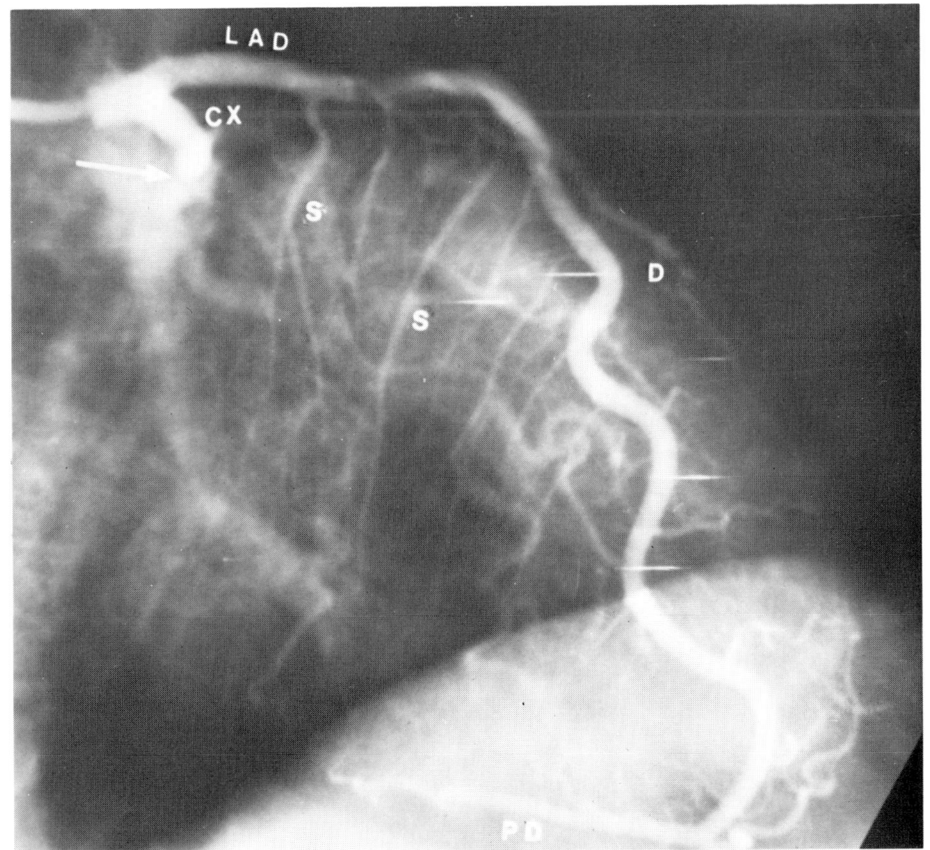

FIGURE 7.25

Figure 7.26:   Left coronary arteriogram; right anterior oblique projection. Four different examples of stenosis in the circumflex artery are shown.

A. Stenosis in the proximal one-third (leftward arrow) of the circumflex artery (CX), just after the origin of a large single left marginal artery (LM). The left anterior descending artery is occluded quite early (rightward arrow).

B. This is a circumflex artery (CX) with two left marginal branches. There is a stenosis (upper-most horizontal arrow) in the proximal one-third of the circumflex artery immediately after the first marginal artery (LM). The second left marginal artery also has a 70 to 90% stenosis in its middle segment (lower horizontal arrow). The left anterior descending artery is occluded just after its onset (rightward vertical arrow).

C. An isolated stenosis is seen in the middle segment of the left circumflex artery (CX, horizontal arrow), between the origins of the first and second left marginal arteries (LM). The left anterior descending artery is occluded in its proximal one-third (rightward arrow).

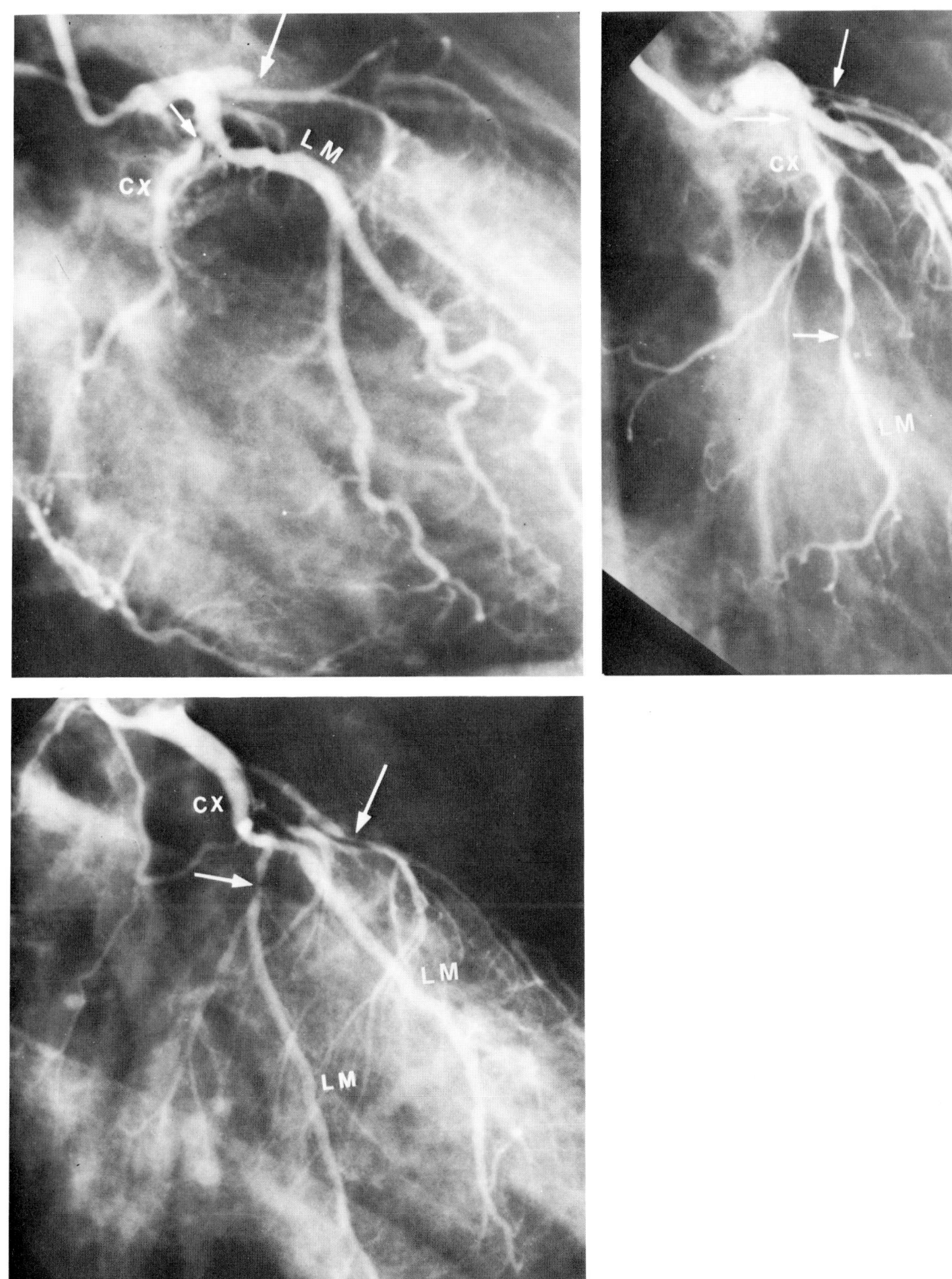

FIGURE 7.26

Figure 7.27:   Left coronary arteriogram; lateral projection. **A** in systole; **B** in diastole. Total occlusion of a segment of the circumflex artery (CX) is noted between the two rightward arrows. A bridging collateral vessel joins the proximal and distal segments of the circumflex artery and simulates continuity between these two segments. There are two lesions present in the left anterior descending artery (LAD, leftward arrows). Disease isolated to the left circumflex artery is unusual.

D = Diagonal branches of left anterior descending artery.

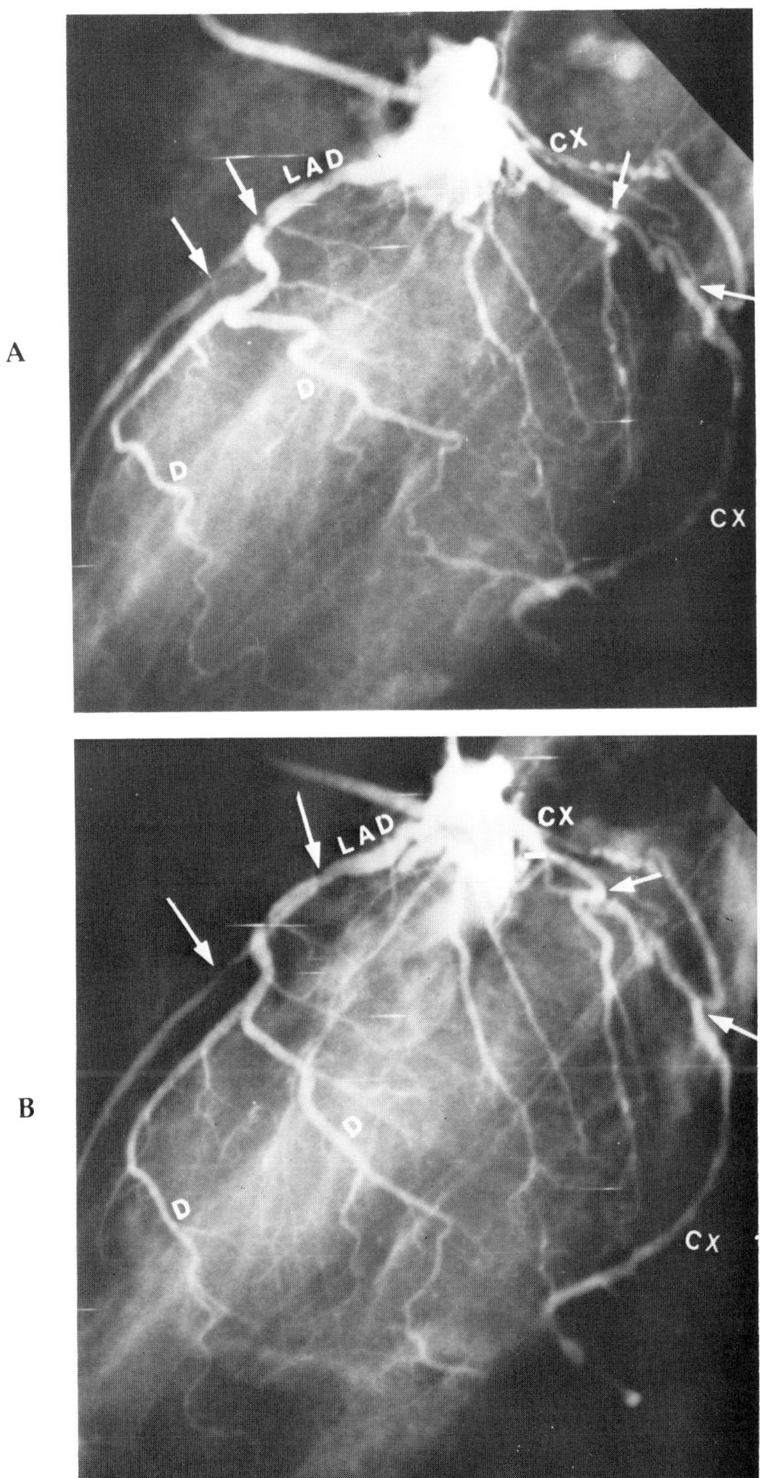

FIGURE 7.27

Figure 7.28:   Left coronary arteriogram; right anterior oblique projection. There is a long segment of 70-90% stenosis (between left-sided horizontal arrows) in the middle segment of the left circumflex artery (CX). The system is left dominant. Moderate proximal stenosis is followed by a 70-90% stenosis in the middle one-third of the left anterior descending (LAD) artery (between right-sided horizontal arrows). In addition there is a severe (70-90%) lesion in the left main coronary artery (upper vertical arrow). Such extensive disease in a left dominant system which is responsible for most if not all of the blood flow to the left ventricle presents a most critical clinical situation.

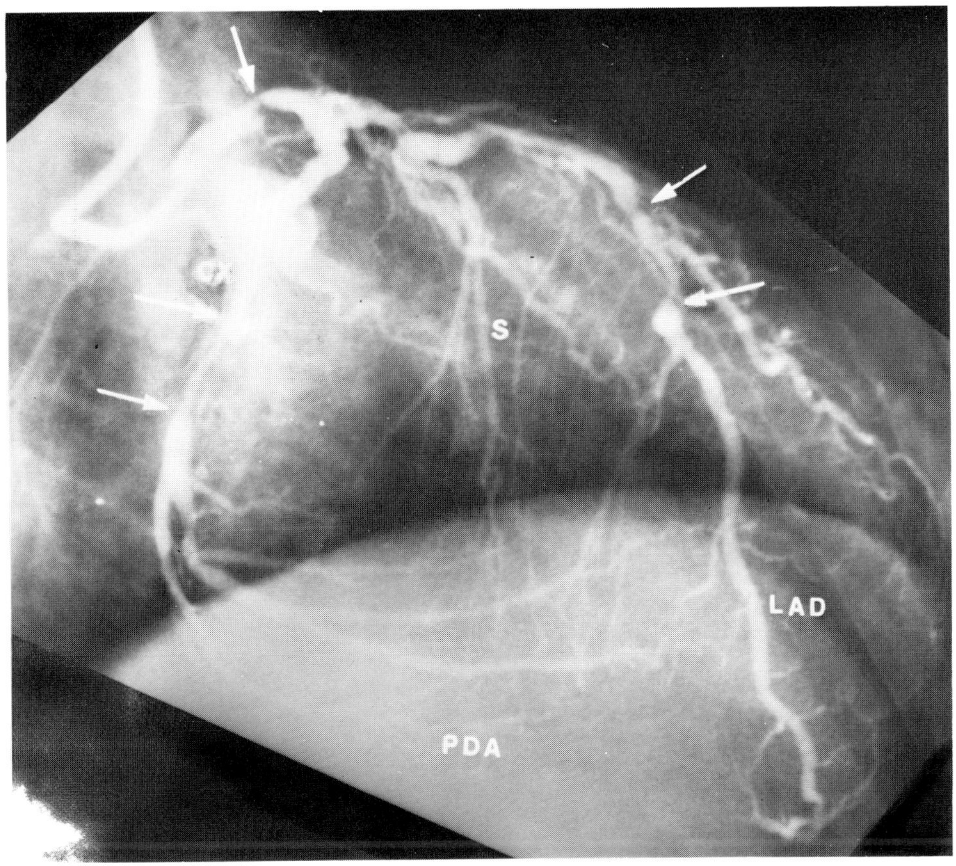

FIGURE 7.28

Figure 7.29:   **A**. Left coronary arteriogram; right anterior oblique projection. Severe (70-90%) stenosis in the left marginal artery (arrows) is present.

C. Left coronary arteriogram; left anterior oblique projection. The same lesion demonstrated in **A** is seen in this projection. The left marginal artery (arrows) is very well separated from the circumflex artery (CX) in this projection.

LAD = left anterior descending artery.

B. Diagrammatic representation of **A**.

D. Diagrammatic representation of **C**.

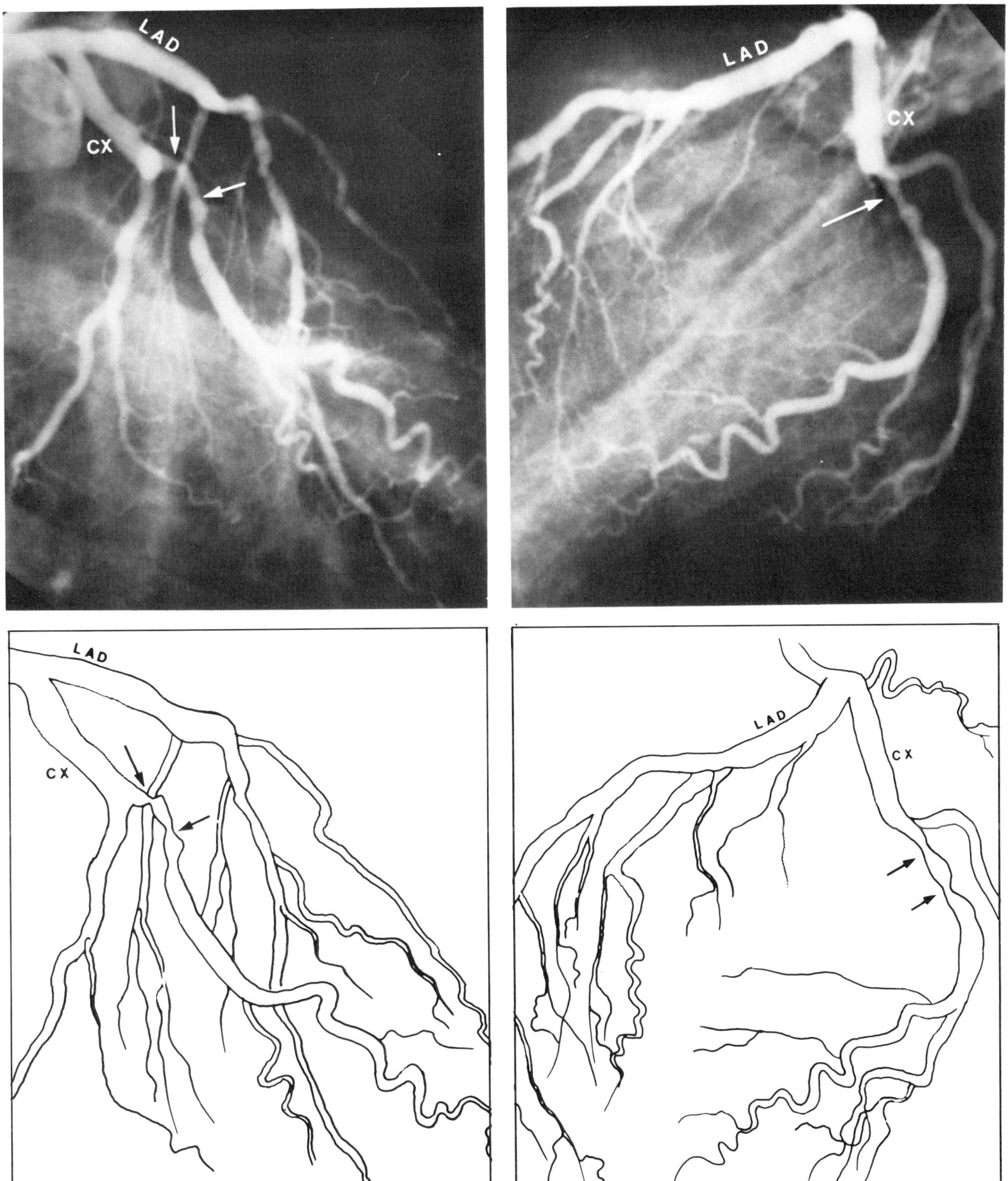

FIGURE 7.29

Chapter 8

Obstructive Disease of the Right Coronary Artery

Isolated disease in the right coronary artery has been reported to occur in 10% of patients with angiographically documented coronary artery disease.[1] Most frequently atherosclerotic lesions in the right coronary artery are associated with disease in other vessels. Complete arterial occlusion is encountered very frequently in the right coronary artery (Figures 8.1-8.4).

Although lesions may be found at any location in the proximal right coronary artery (Figures 8.5-8.8) or its major branches, the posterior descending (Figure 8.9) and distal right (Figure 8.10) coronary arteries, it is imperative to detect significant stenosis proximal to the crux and at the crux of the heart. This information is important because anastomosis of a saphenous vein bypass graft with the right coronary artery is frequently placed at the crux or in the posterior descending artery. When the right coronary artery is totally occluded proximally collateral filling of the posterior descending and distal right coronary arteries must be carefully sought. When present, collateral filling may occur from the left coronary artery (Figure 8.1 B) or via intracoronary collateral channels (Figure 8.3 C, D).

Catheterization of the right coronary artery in the presence of a severe ostial or proximal stenosis may be quite difficult. In this situation the arterial pressure frequently drops precipitously necessitating prompt withdrawal of the catheter from the right coronary artery. In these instances we have found it advantageous to place the patient in position for obtaining the desired projection prior to entering the coronary ostium. Successful catheterization of the ostium is heralded by the arterial pressure drop, and at that instant two or three milliliters of contrast material should be injected and the catheter immediately withdrawn. Filming should be continued in order to obtain adequate visualization of the artery and any collateral flow.

Reference

1.   Proudfit, W.L., Shirey, E.K., and Sones, F.M. Jr.: Distribution of arterial lesions demonstrated by selective cinecoronary arteriography. *Circulation,* **36**:54-62, 1967.

Figure 8.1: **A.** Right coronary arteriogram; right anterior oblique projection. Total occlusion of the right coronary artery (RCA) in the middle one-third (arrow), immediately following the origin of the right marginal branch (RM).

B. Left coronary arteriogram; lateral projection; same patient as in **A.** The posterior descending (PDA) and distal right coronary artery (DRCA) are visualized via collateral channels from the left coronary artery and are size "B".

LAD = left anterior descending artery. D = diagonal branch of left anterior descending artery. LM = left marginal branch of circumflex artery. CX = left circumflex artery. S = septal branches of left anterior descending coronary artery.

(Refer to pages 6 and 7 for grading of vessels.)

Figure 8.2: Right coronary arteriogram; right anterior oblique projection. Two examples of total occlusion of the right coronary artery (RCA) in its middle portion (arrow). In **A,** additional stenoses are seen in the proximal portion of the right coronary artery and in its right marginal branch (RM, pointers).

PDA = posterior descending branch of right coronary artery. SN = sinus node artery, here arising from the right coronary artery.

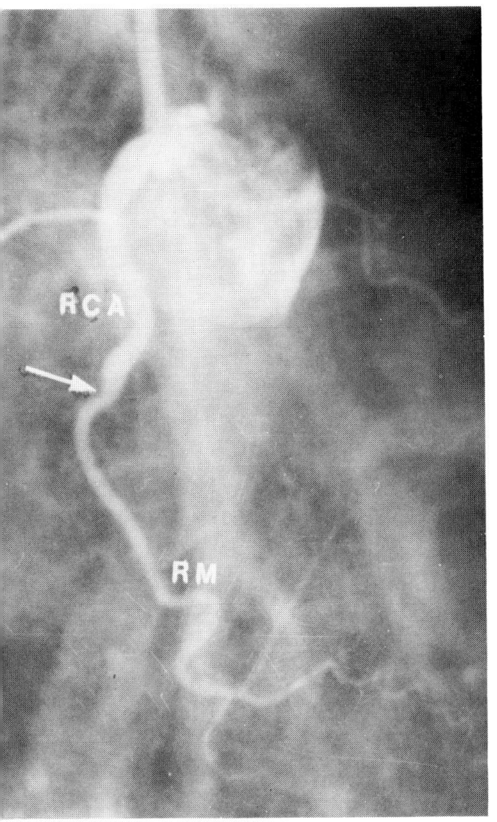

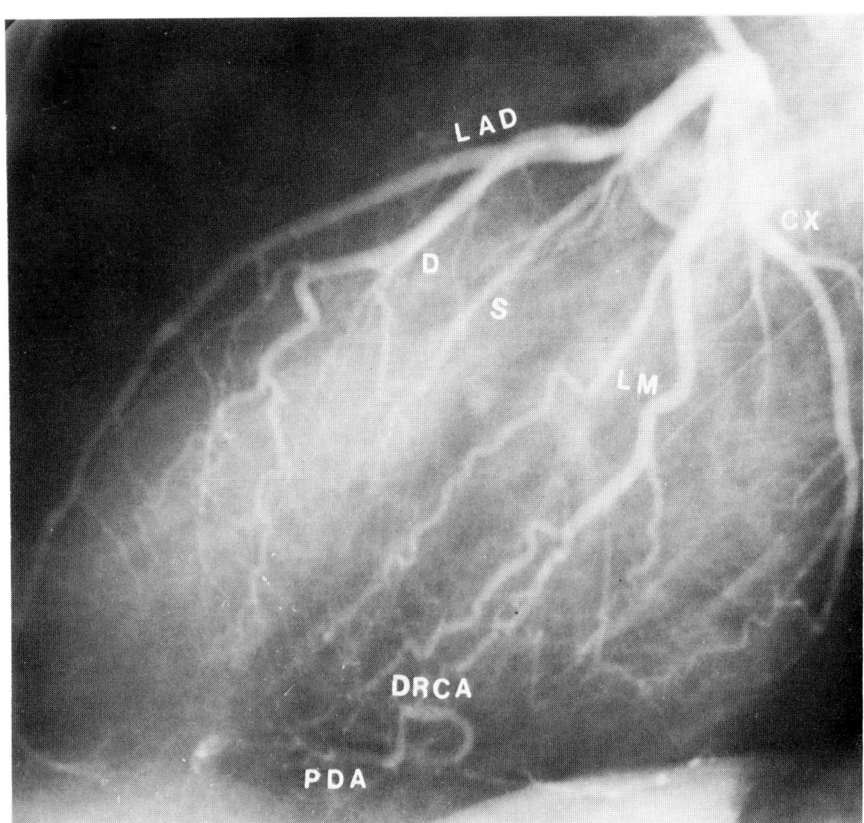

FIGURE 8.1

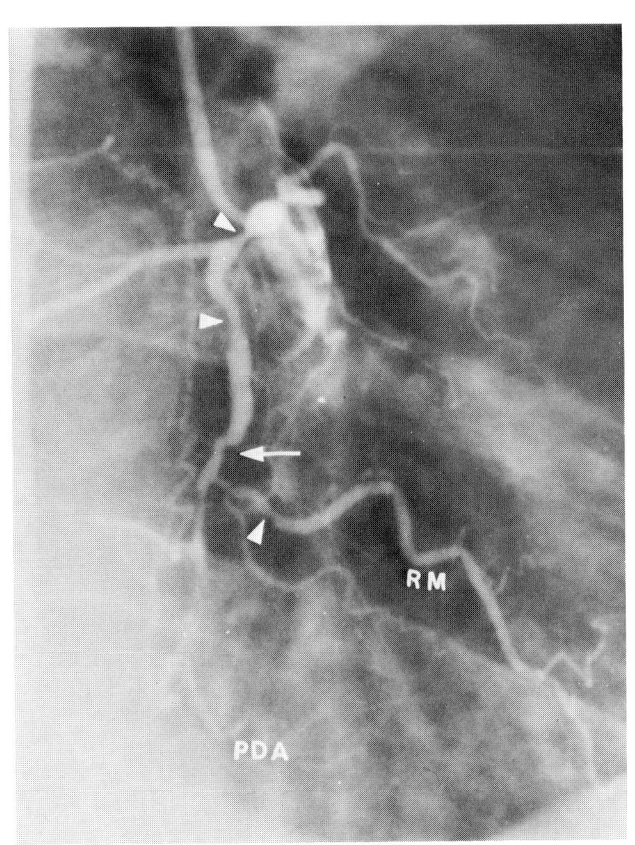

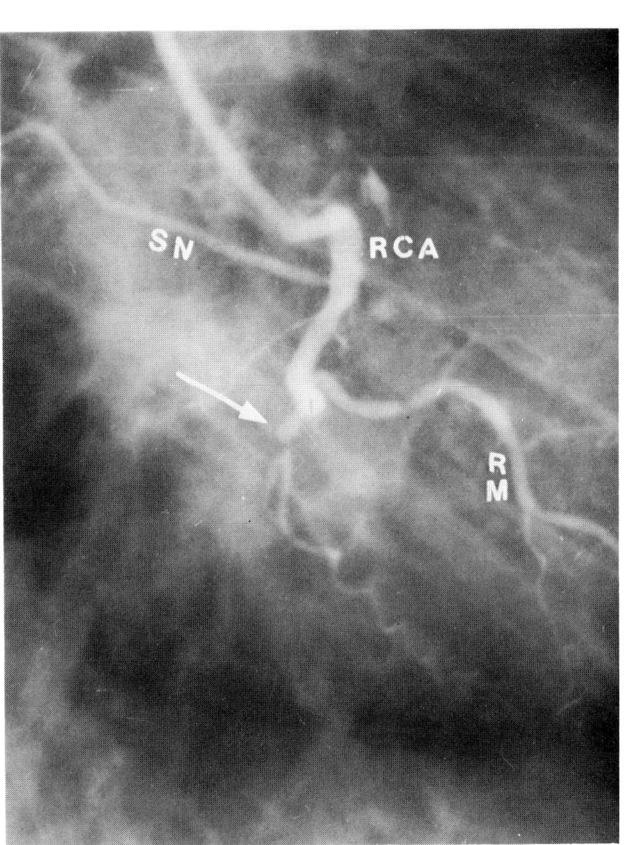

FIGURE 8.2

Figure 8.3:   Right coronary arteriogram; left anterior oblique projection.

A and **B**: Two examples of total occlusion of the right coronary artery (RCA) in the proximal portion (arrow). There is no distal opacification.

C and **D**: Two examples of total occlusion of the right coronary artery in its middle portion. In **C** an intracoronary collateral channel is seen bridging the obstructed segment (between arrows). In **D** collateral circulation between the proximal (arrow) and distal (pointers) segments via epicardial channels originates from the right marginal artery (RM).

C = conus branch of right coronary artery.

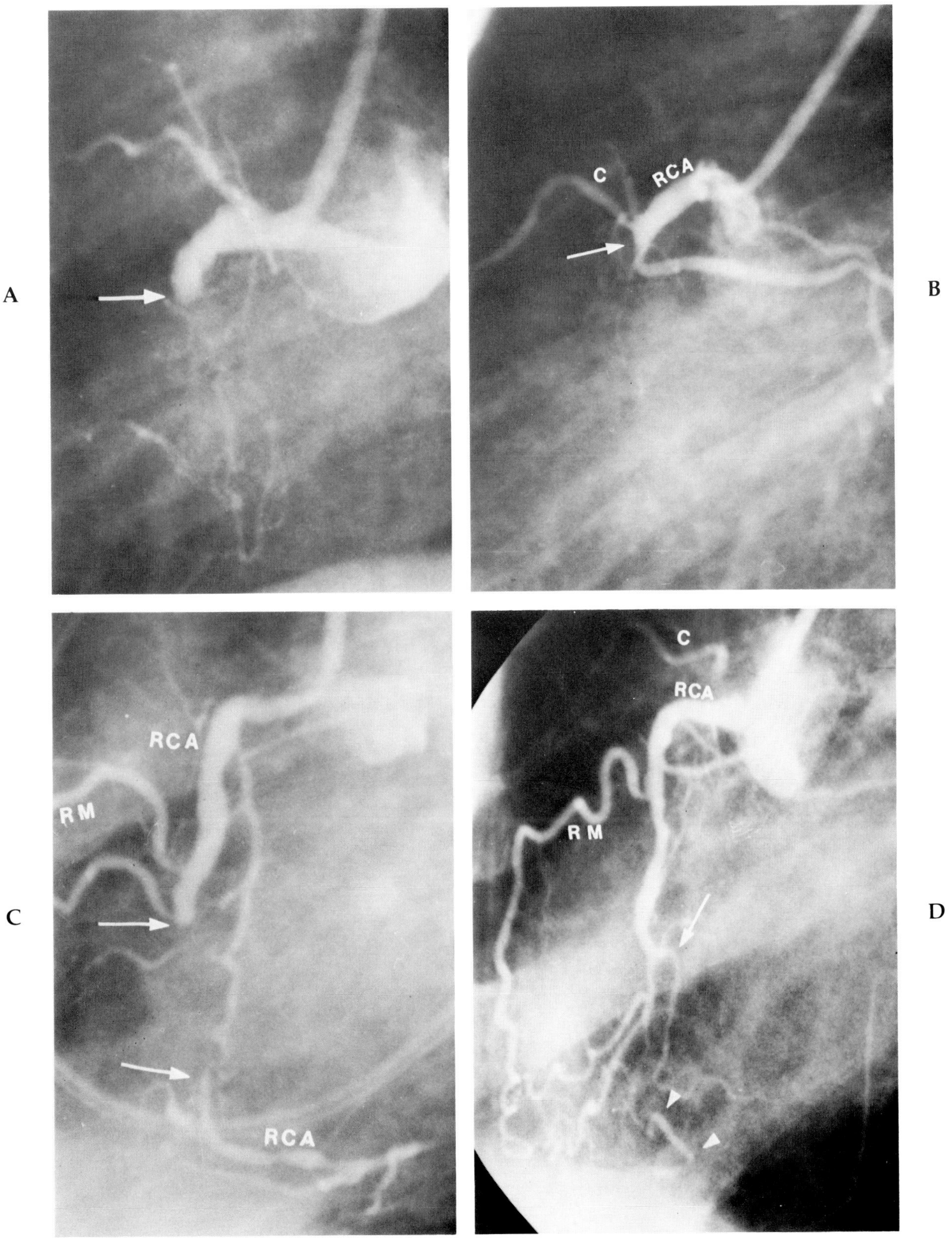

FIGURE 8.3

Figure 8.4:   Right coronary arteriogram; lateral projection.

A. There is total occlusion in the proximal segment of the right coronary artery (RCA) after the origin of the conus (C), sinus node (SN) and right marginal (RM) arteries (arrow). There is no distal opacification.

B. Diagrammatic representation of **A**.

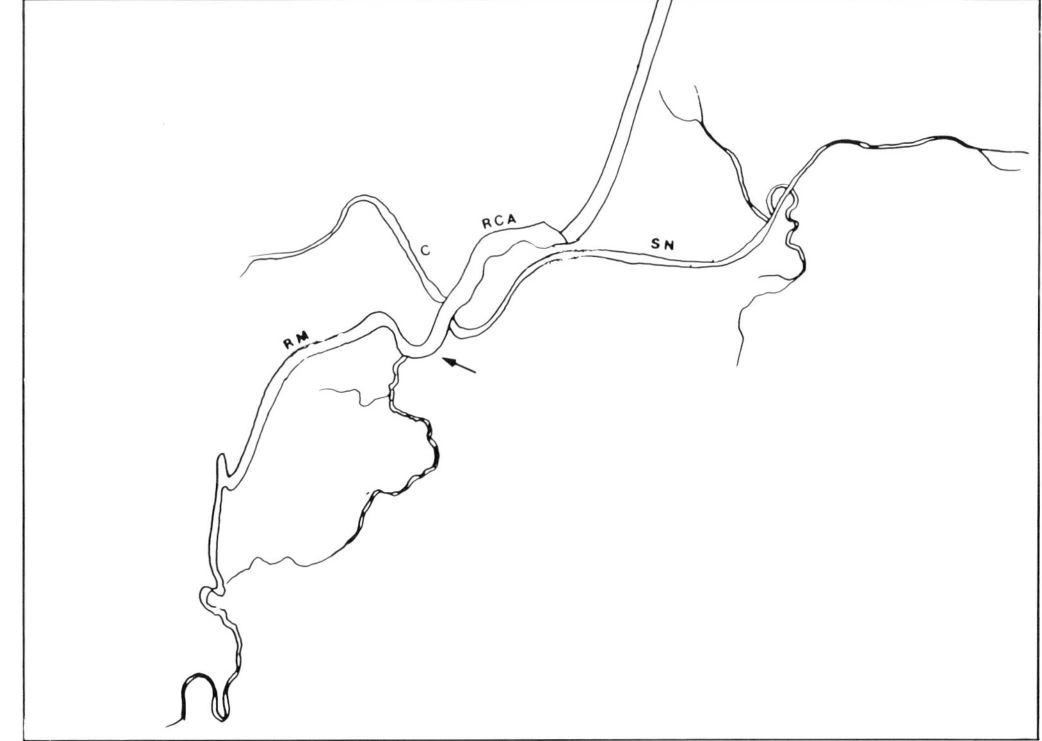

FIGURE 8.4

Figure 8.5:   Right coronary arteriogram; lateral projection. Two minor filling defects (pointers) in the mid-portion of the right coronary artery (RCA). These lesions represent an early stage of atherosclerotic coronary artery disease.

RM = right marginal branch of right coronary artery. PDA = posterior descending branch of right coronary artery. AV = atrioventricular node artery. DRCA = distal right coronary artery.

Figure 8.6:   Right coronary arteriogram; **A**. Right anterior oblique projection. **B**. Left anterior oblique projection. Severe, circumscribed (greater than 90%) isolated stenosis in the middle portion of the right coronary artery (RCA). The posterior descending coronary artery (PDA) is size "A".

RM = right marginal branch of right coronary artery. DRCA = distal right coronary artery.

(Refer to pages 6 and 7 for grading of vessels.)

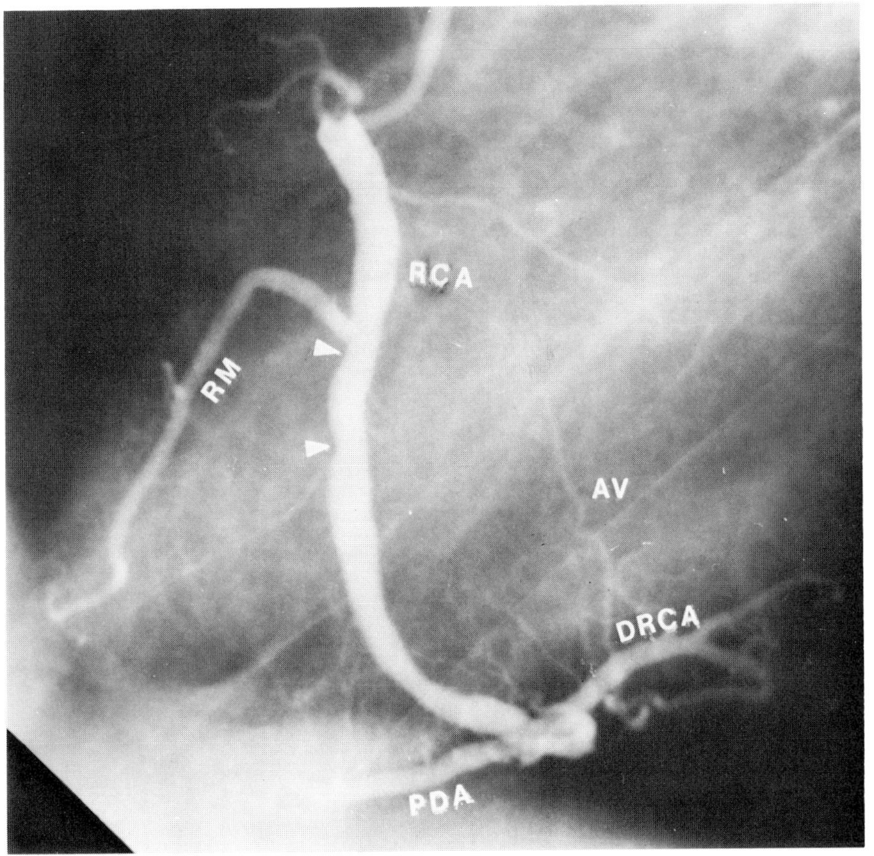

FIGURE 8.5

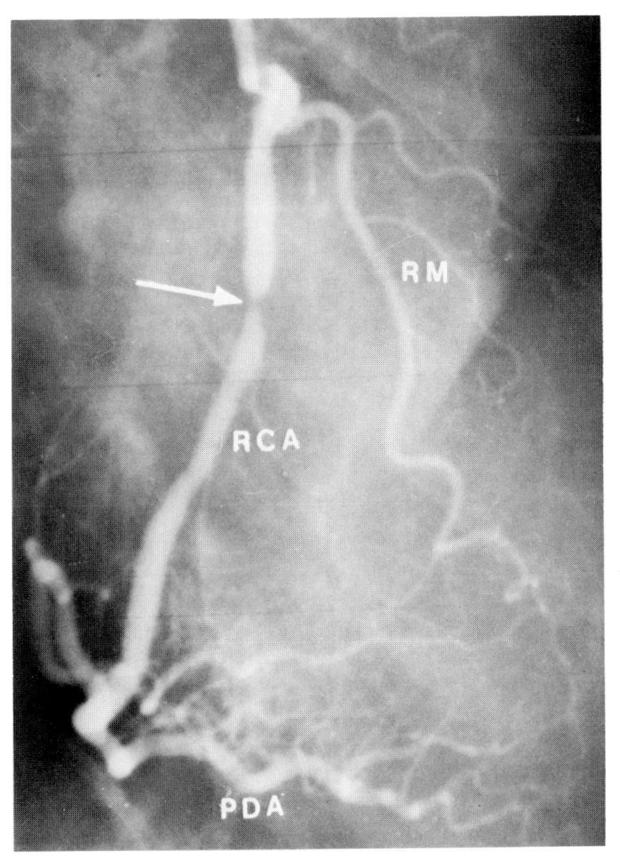

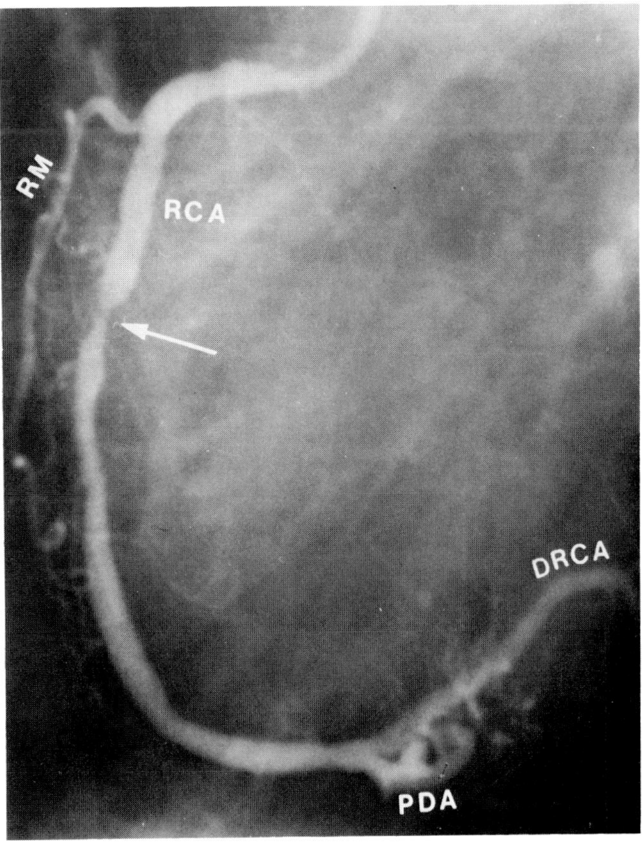

A   **FIGURE 8.6**   B

Figure 8.7:   Right coronary arteriogram; lateral projection. Two examples of severe (70-90%) stenosis (arrows) in the distal portion of the right coronary artery(RCA)just prior to the crux. The posterior descending artery (PDA) and the distal right coronary artery (DRCA) are size "B" vessels. In **A**, a lesion is also seen in the proximal portion of the right coronary artery.

C = conus artery. SN = sinus node artery.

(Refer to pages 6 and 7 for grading of vessels.)

Figure 8.8:   Right coronary arteriogram; **A**. Right anterior oblique projection; **B**. Left anterior oblique projection. Diffuse disease in the entire right coronary artery is demonstrated. Arrows locate very severe stenotic lesions. The posterior descending (PDA) and distal right coronary arteries (DRCA) are size "B".

C = conus artery. SN = sinus node artery.

(Refer to pages 6 and 7 for grading of vessels.)

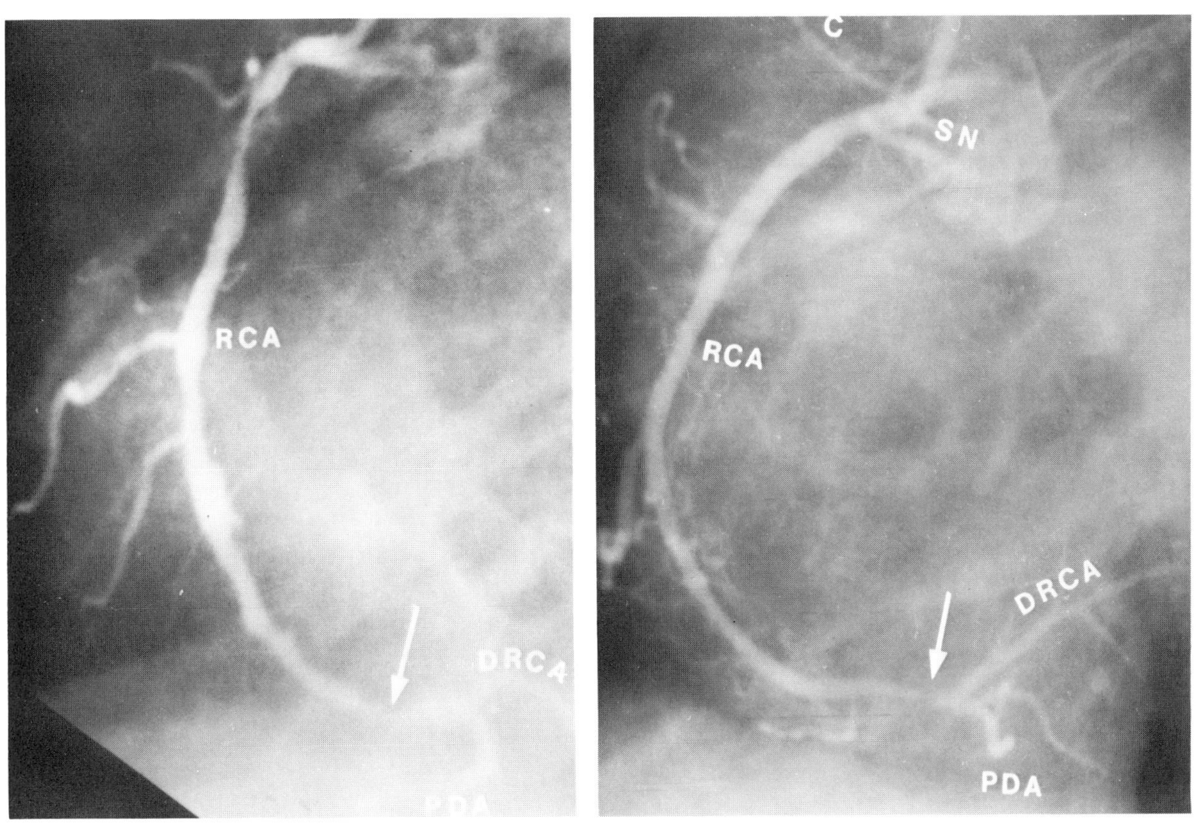

A   **FIGURE 8.7**   B

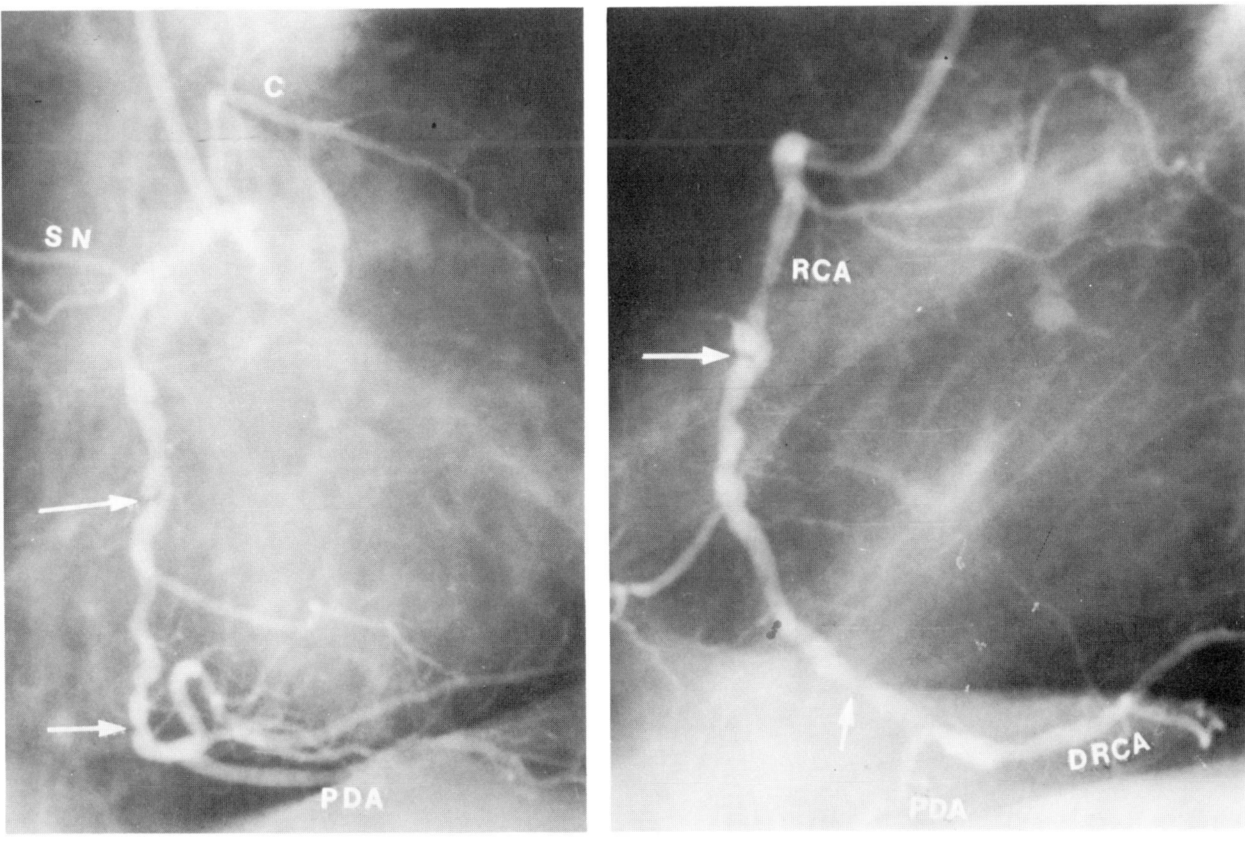

A   **FIGURE 8.8**   B

Figure 8.9:   Right coronary arteriogram; right anterior oblique projection. A severe (greater than 90%) stenosis (arrow) is seen at the origin of the posterior descending coronary artery (PDA). The distal posterior descending coronary artery is size "A".

RM = right marginal branch of right coronary artery. RCA = right coronary artery.

(Refer to pages 6 and 7 for grading of vessels.)

Figure 8.10:   Right coronary arteriogram; lateral projection. A severe (greater than 90%) stenosis (lower arrow) is demonstrated in a left ventricular branch of the distal right coronary artery (DRCA).

A. Several mild stenoses are seen in the middle portion of the right coronary artery (pointers).

B. A moderately severe (50-70%) stenosis is present in the mid-portion of the right coronary artery (RCA, upper-arrow).

AV = atrioventricular node artery. PDA = posterior descending branch of right coronary artery.

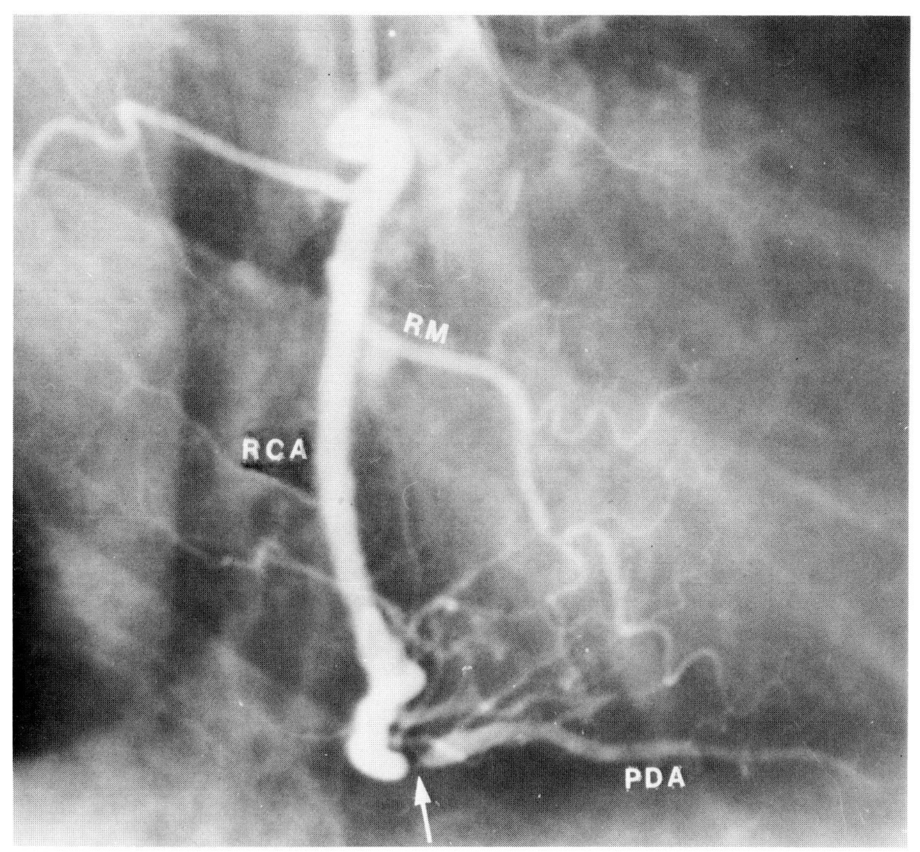

FIGURE 8.9

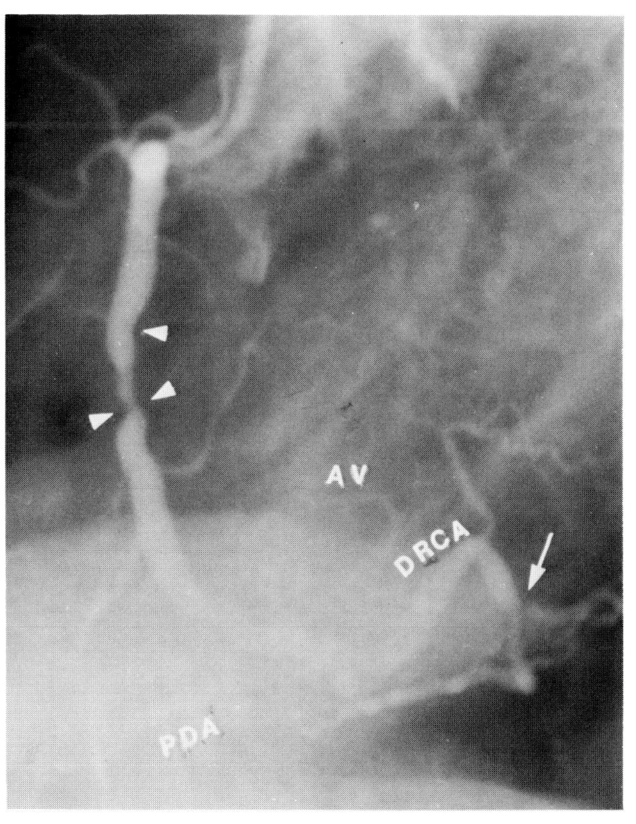

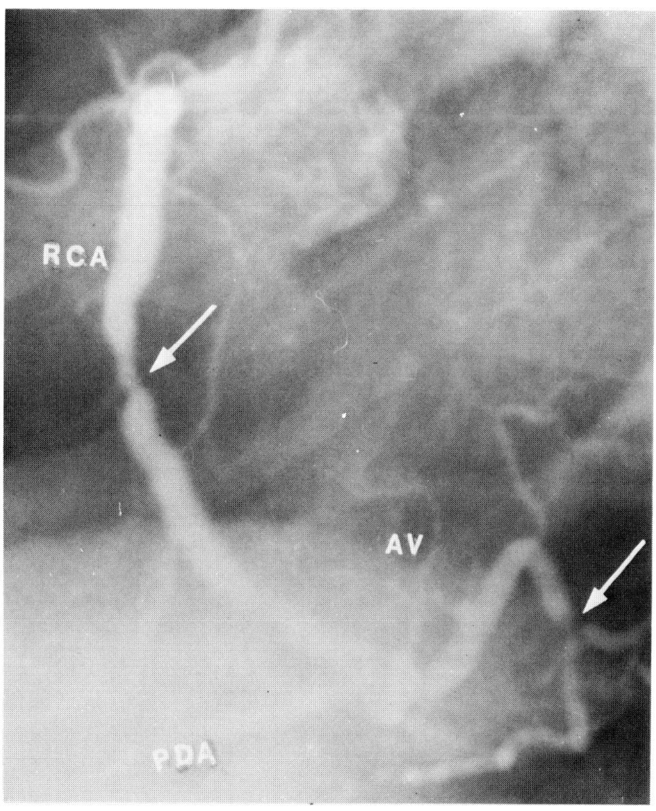

A   **FIGURE 8.10**   B

Chapter 9

Multiple Vessel Disease

When data from a large series of patients undergoing coronary arteriography are analyzed, the majority of patients are found to have multiple vessel disease. Twenty-five to thirty-five percent of patients with coronary artery disease have two vessel disease (Figures 9.1-9.5) and 23-40% of patients are found to have three vessel disease (Figure 9.6).[1,2] Various combinations of two vessel involvement occur, but disease in the left anterior descending and right coronary arteries is the most common two vessel combination. (Figures 9.2-9.5).

Information is now available that patient survival and left ventricular function are inversely proportional to the number of coronary arteries involved. While myocardial revascularization is performed primarily for relief of severe angina pectoris, saphenous vein bypass grafts are increasingly being employed in hopes of improving patient survival and preserving left ventricular function.

Thus, since most of the patients coming to coronary arteriography have involvement of multiple coronary arteries, it is imperative that adequate and complete examination by arteriography be performed. This chapter will illustrate various combinations of coronary lesions.

References

1.   Proudfit, W.L., Shirey, E.K., and Sones, F.M. Jr.: Distribution of arterial lesions demonstrated by selective cinecoronary arteriography. *Circulation,* **36**:54-62, 1967.
2.   Jochem, W., Soto, B., Karp, R.B., Russell, R.O. Jr., Holt, J.H., and Barcia, A.: Radiographic anatomy of the coronary collateral circulation. *American Journal of Roentgenology, Radium Therapy and Nuclear Medicine,* **116**:50-61, 1972.

Figure 9.1:   Left coronary arteriogram:

A. Left anterior oblique projection. There is total occlusion of the left anterior descending and circumflex (CX, arrow) arteries. The left marginal artery (LM) is a large vessel and provides epicardial collateral (pointers) circulation to a large diagonal (D) branch of the left anterior descending artery. The occlusion of the circumflex is present after the second left ventricular marginal artery. A left marginal artery is also opacified in retrograde fashion to the point of occlusion (arrow).

B. Right coronary arteriogram, right anterior oblique projection, same patient as in **A.** The left anterior descending coronary artery (LAD) is now visualized as a size "B" vessel following opacification via a well developed septal collateral network (S) from the posterior descending artery (PDA).

(Refer to pages 6 and 7 for grading of vessels.)

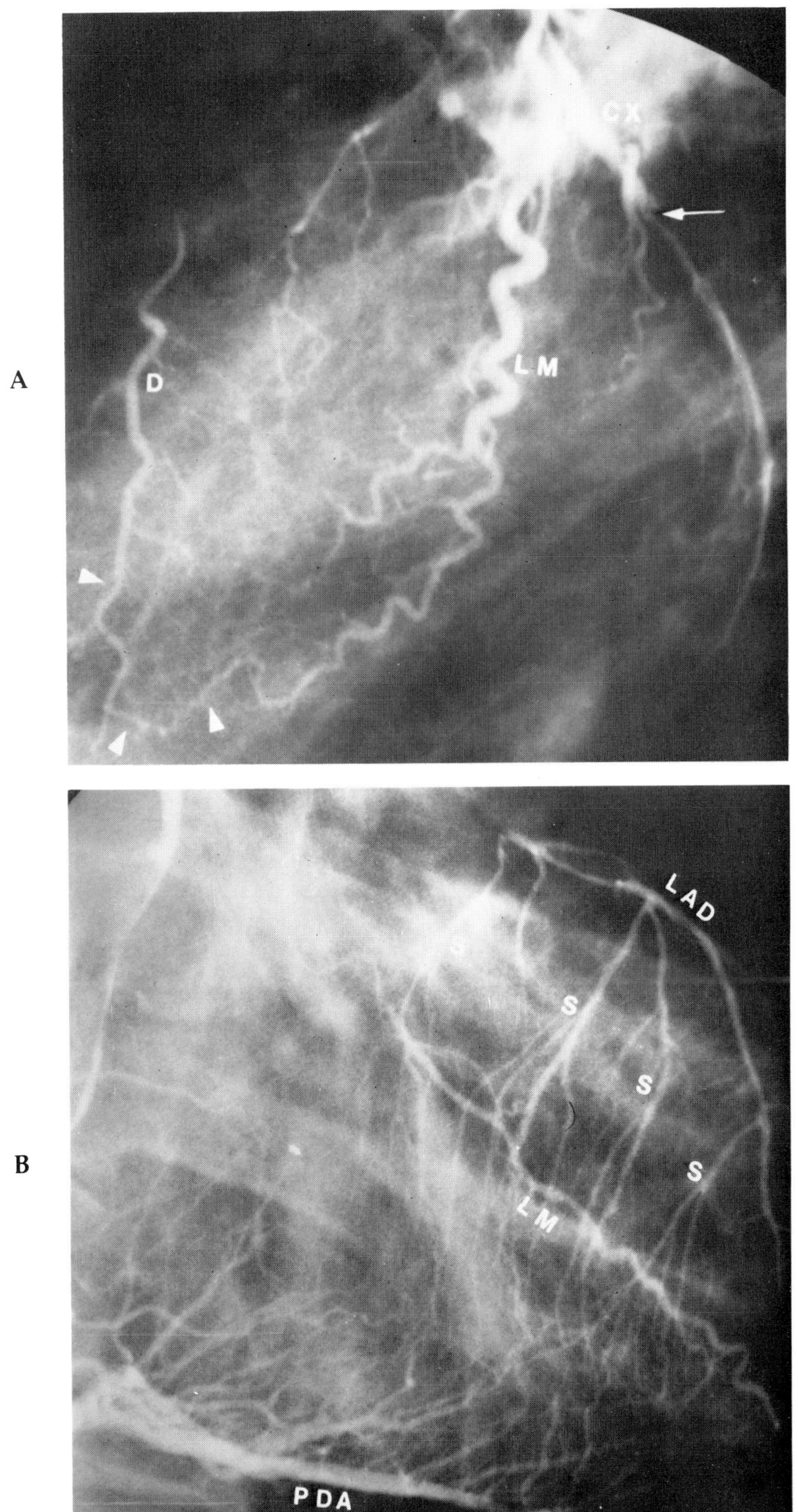

FIGURE 9.1

Figure 9.2:   An example of two vessel disease with occlusion of left anterior descending (LAD) and right coronary arteries (RCA):

A. Left coronary arteriogram; lateral projection. Total occlusion of the left anterior descending (LAD, arrow) immediately following origin of first small diagonal branch. The left circumflex (CX, between pointers) originates from its own ostium.

B. Right coronary arteriogram; left anterior oblique projection. Total occlusion of the right coronary artery (RCA) immediately following origin of the conus (C) and right marginal (RM) vessels. Several collateral channels (pointers) join the right coronary artery with the left anterior descending (LAD) and a diagonal (D) branch of the left anterior descending artery.

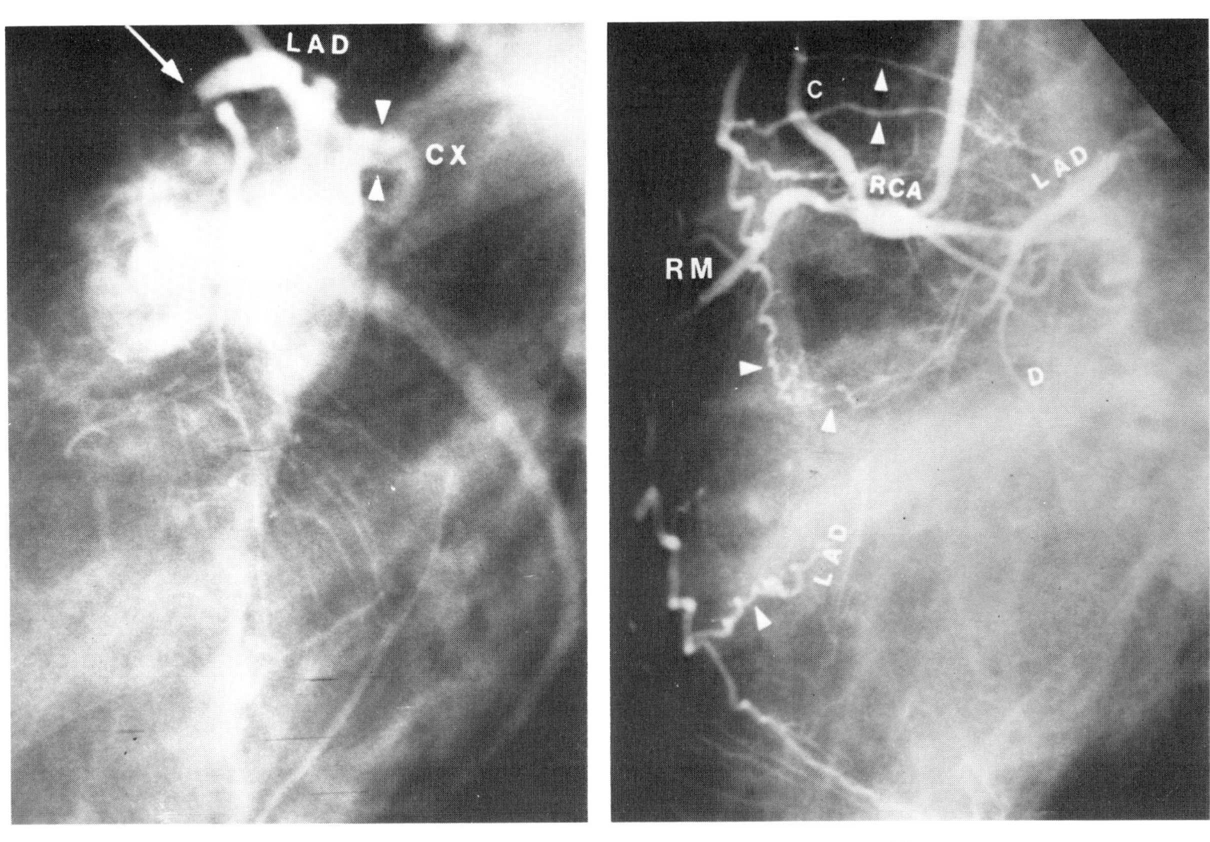

FIGURE 9.2

Figure 9.3:   Right coronary arteriogram; left anterior oblique projection. Same patient as in Figure 9.2 showing successive stages of opacification of the left anterior descending (LAD) via collateral channels from the occluded right coronary artery (RCA). Pointers indicate collateral circulation:

A. Segmental opacification of the LAD.

C = Conus artery. D = diagonal branch of left anterior descending.

B. Almost complete opacification of the LAD.

C. Opacification of entire vessel without complete filling.

S = septal collateral branches.

D. Complete filling of LAD to a size "B" vessel.

(Refer to pages 6 and 7 for grading of vessels.)

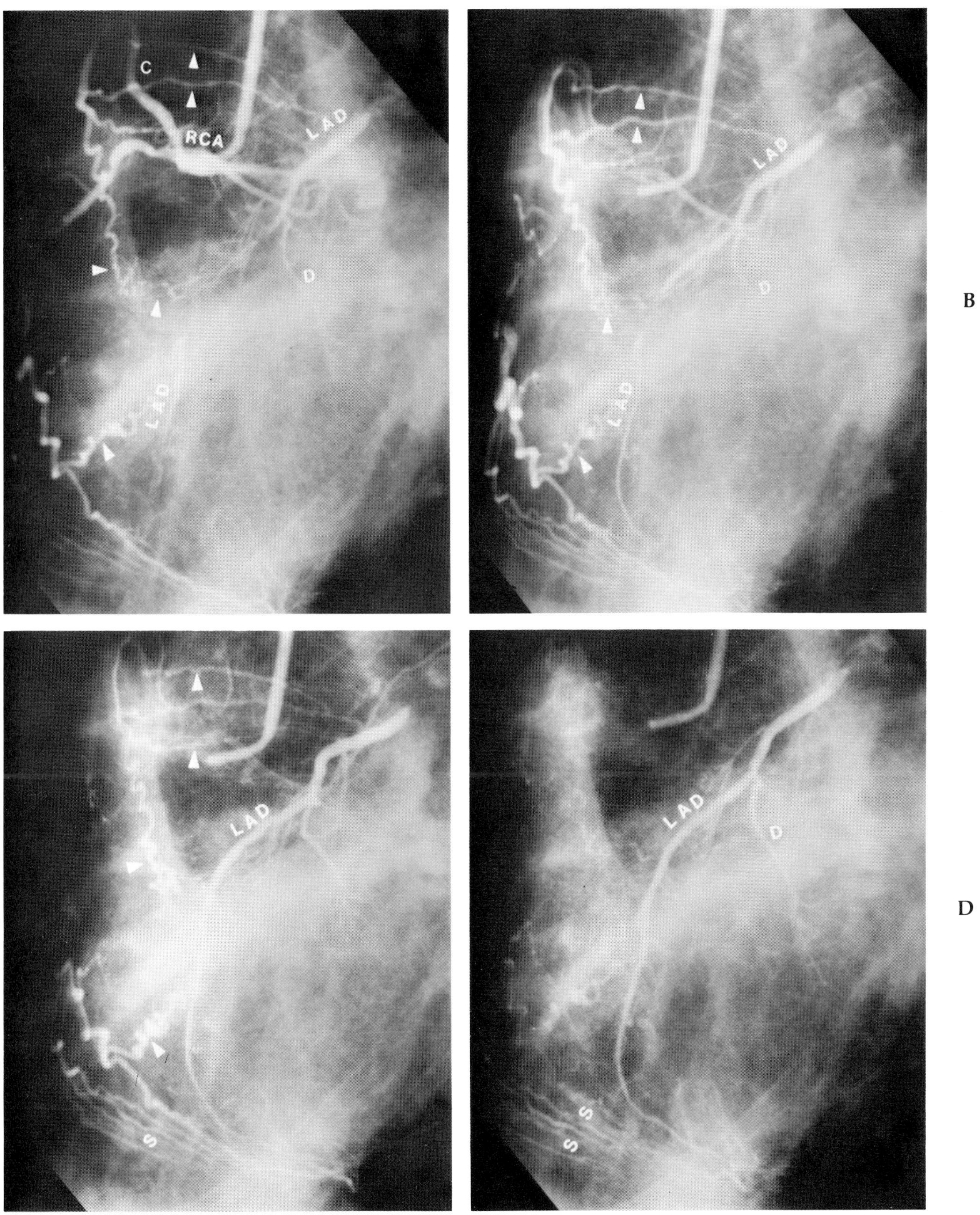

FIGURE 9.3

Figure 9.4:   **A** and **B**. Left coronary arteriogram; right anterior oblique projection. The left anterior descending artery (LAD) is occluded after the first septal branch (between the arrows) but is seen again in the middle one-third as a size "C" vessel. A ramus medianus is present between the LAD and the left circumflex artery (CX) and is occluded (arrow in **A** and pointer in **B**). It fills distally as a size "C" vessel. A diagonal (D) branch of the LAD fills in its distal one-half. A tortuous collateral channel (leftward pointers in **B**) fills the posterior descending artery (PDA) which in this patient is a branch of the right coronary artery. Two left marginal (LM) branches arise from the CX.

(Refer to pages 6 and 7 for grading of vessels.)

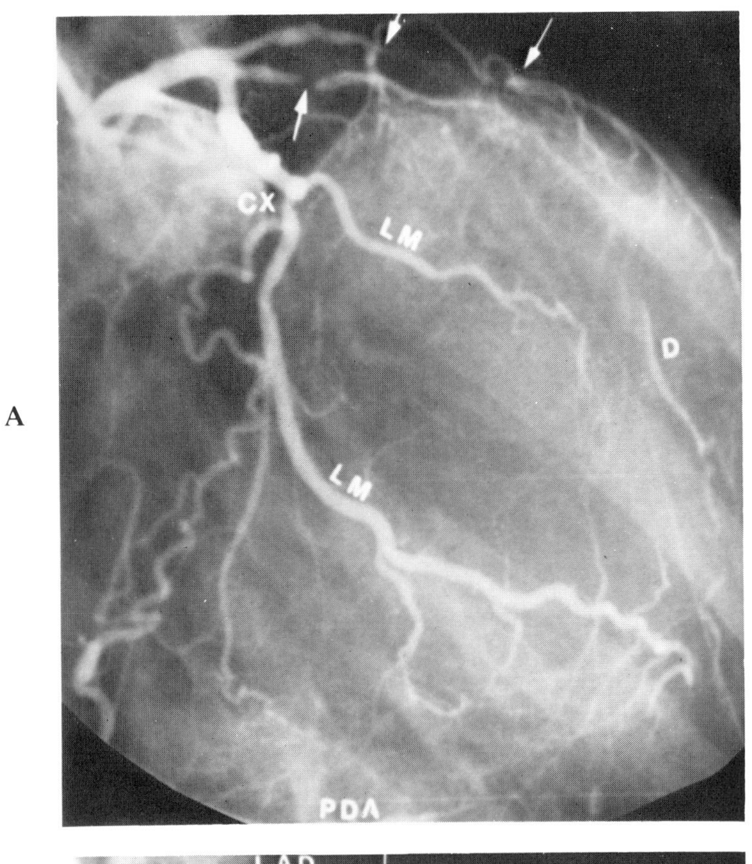

A

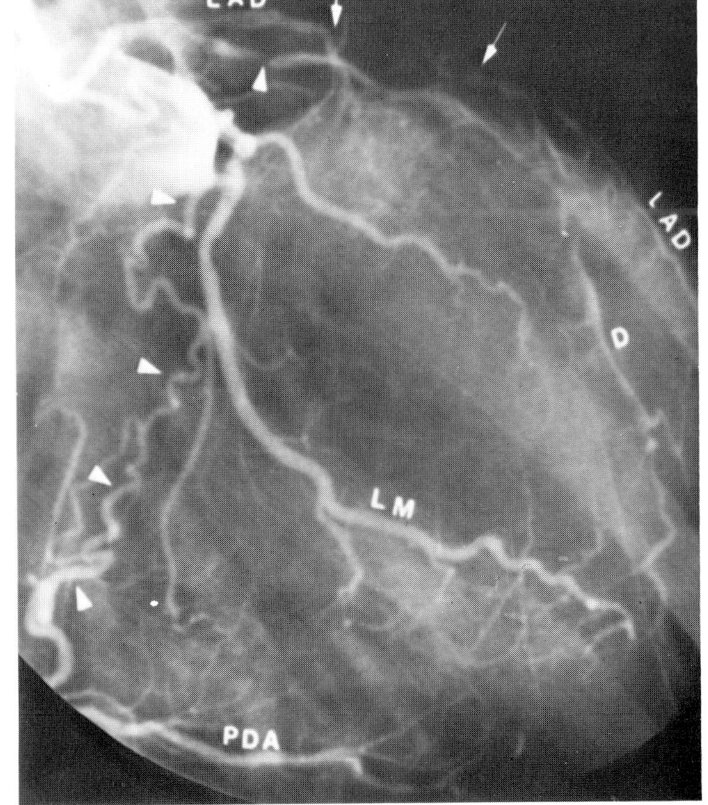

B

FIGURE 9.4

Figure 9.4:   C and **D**. Right coronary arteriogram; left anterior oblique projection. The right coronary artery (RCA) is occluded in the proximal one-third after the right marginal (RM) branch. Segments of the RCA refill by intracoronary collateral vessels (arrows). **C**. Early phase; **D**. Later phase. In **D** the middle one-third of the LAD and a septal (S) branch of the LAD are opacified from the RCA injection.

(Refer to pages 6 and 7 for grading of vessels.)

C

D

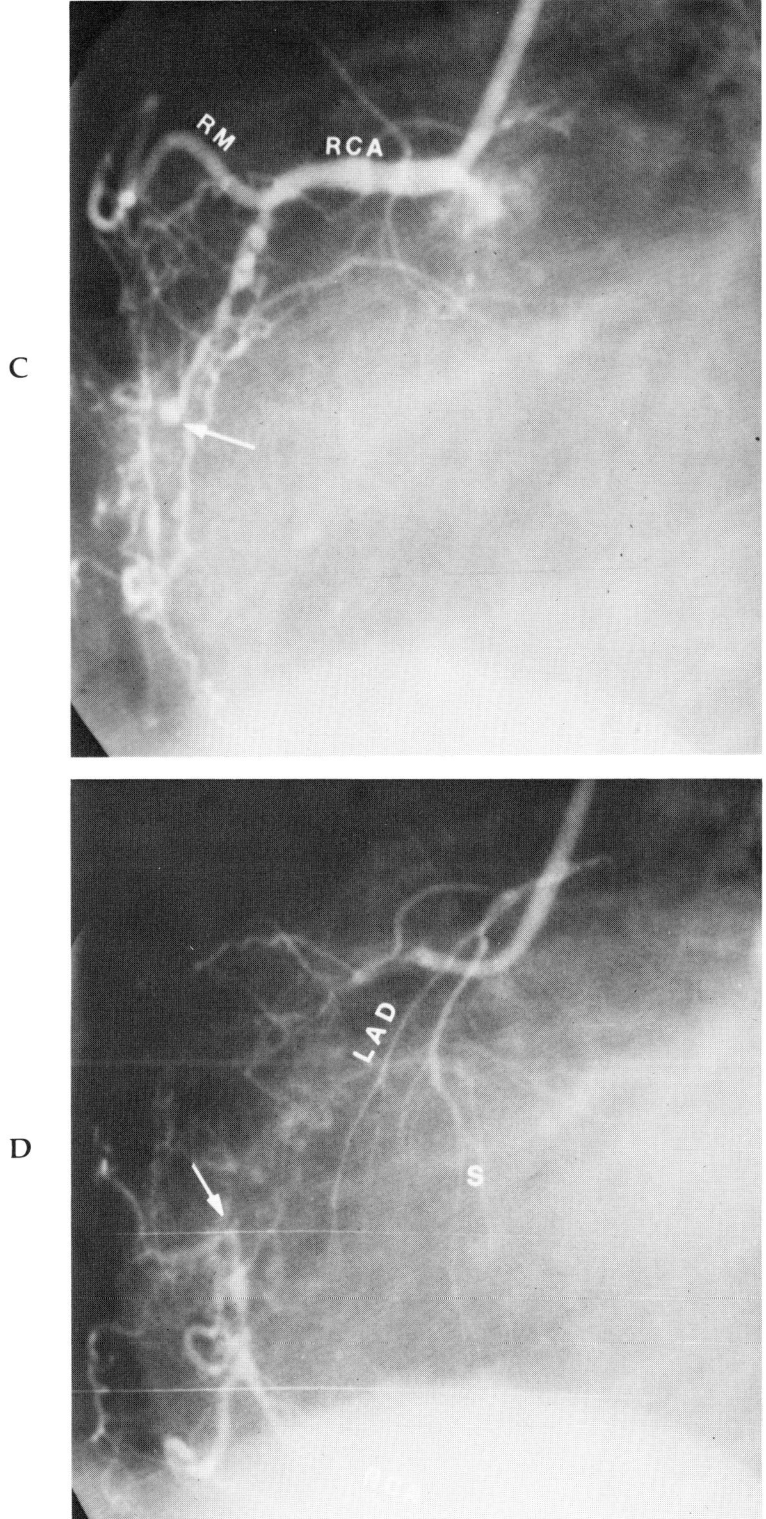

FIGURE 9.4

Figure 9.5:   Left coronary arteriogram; right anterior oblique projection. There is a 50-70% stenosis at the distal end of the left main coronary artery (LCA). The left anterior descending (LAD) is occluded after the first septal (S) and first diagonal (D) arteries, between the arrows, and fills in its middle and distal one-thirds as a size "B" vessel. The dilated diagonal branch simulates the LAD between the arrows. The left circumflex artery (CX) gives rise to several tortuous channels after the origin of the left marginal (LM) to supply the posterior descending artery (PDA), a branch of the right coronary artery which in this patient was occluded proximally.

(Refer to pages 6 and 7 for grading of vessels.)

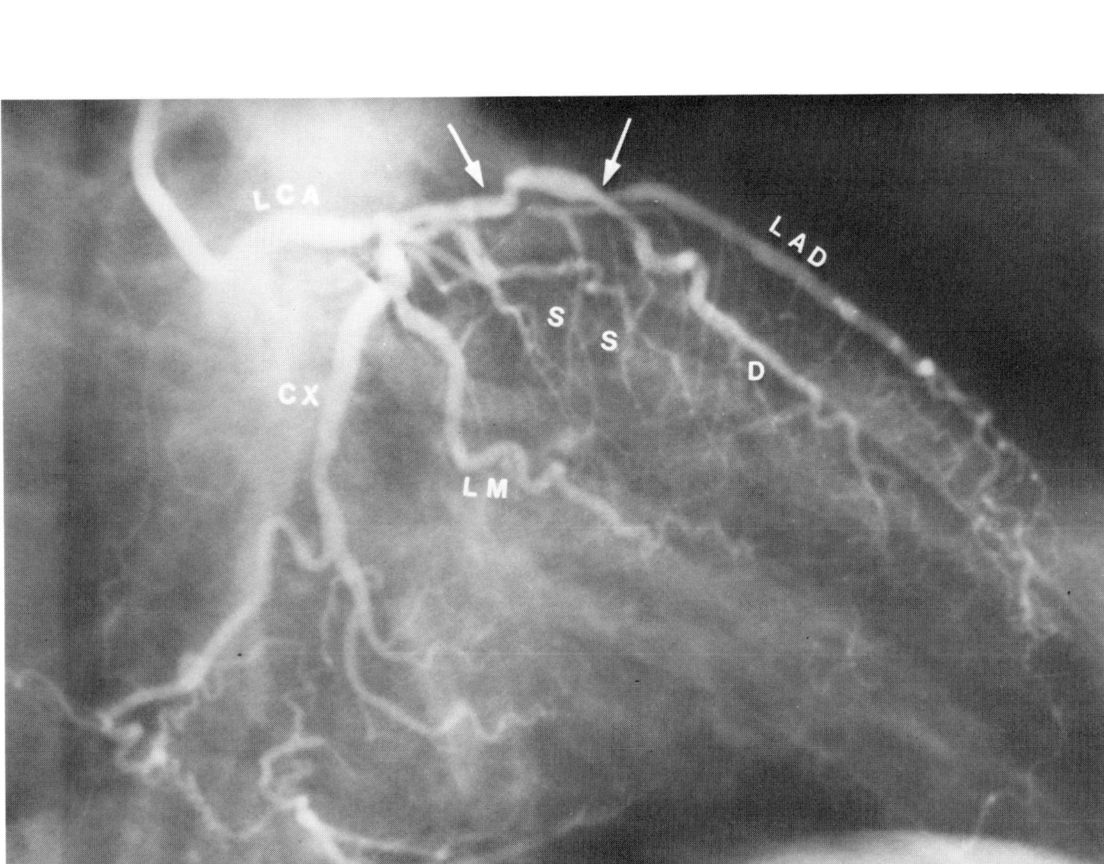

FIGURE 9.5

Figure 9.6:   Severe disease of the three major coronary arteries.

A. Right coronary arteriogram; right anterior oblique projection. There is total occlusion of the right coronary artery (RCA) in the middle segment just after the origin of a right marginal (RM) artery. The posterior descending artery (PDA) is partially opacified by intracoronary collaterals and is size "C". A collateral channel (pointers) proceeds toward the left anterior descending artery.

B. Left coronary arteriogram, lateral projection. There is total occlusion (upper arrow) of the left anterior descending artery (LAD) in the proximal one-third after the origin of the first diagonal artery (D). The left circumflex (CX) is also occluded (lower arrow) after the origin of the left marginal (LM) artery.

(Refer to pages 6 and 7 for grading of vessels.)

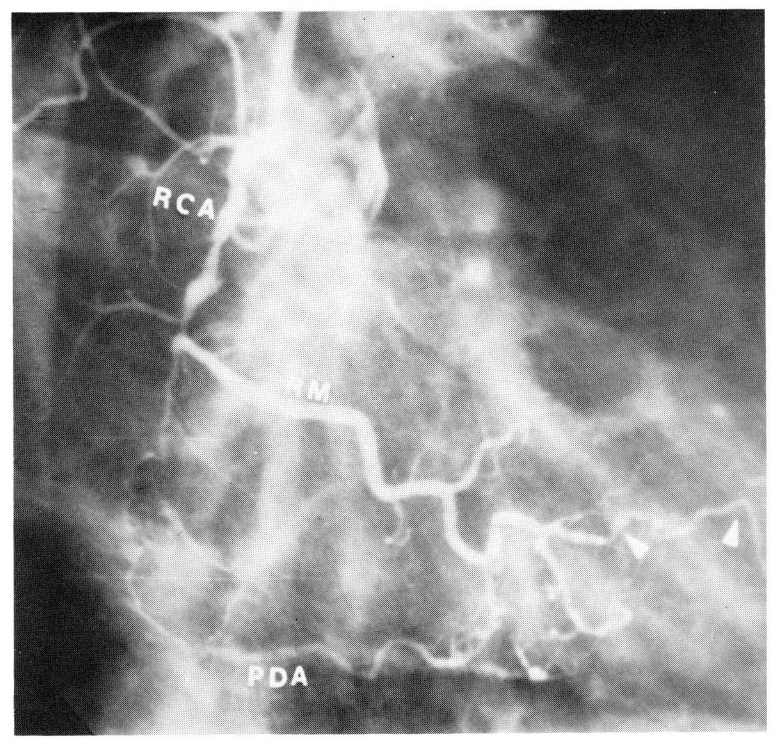

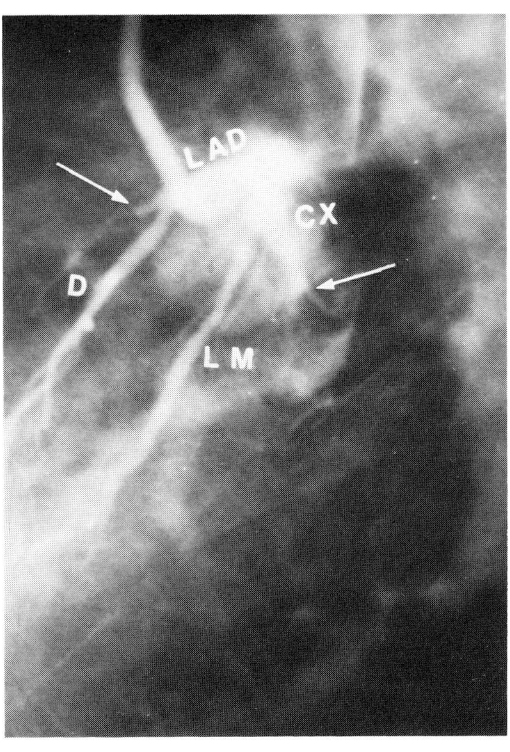

A   **FIGURE 9.6**   B

Chapter 10

Collateral Circulation

The radiographic and post-mortem anatomy of the coronary circulation has been extensively examined and the published investigations reviewed.[1,2] While there is not yet a universal classification of coronary collateral circulation, the system followed in this chapter is based upon a frequency distribution from a study of 100 consecutive coronary arteriograms in patients with coronary artery disease[1] (Figure 10.1).

Collateral Circulation To The Left Anterior Descending Artery

Collateral flow to a diseased left anterior descending artery may occur: 1—via septal collaterals from the posterior descending artery (Figures 10.2-10.6); 2—through anastomoses over the apex by epicardial branches from the posterior descending artery; 3—through anastomoses from a left marginal branch of the circumflex artery to diagonal branches of the left anterior descending (Figures 10.2 A, 10.6 C); 4—via anastomotic channels from the conus artery or Vieussen's circle (Figures 10.3, 10.7); 5—through anastomoses from the right marginal branch of the right coronary artery (Figure 10.3); 6—via diagonal branches which function as anastomoses to the post-stenotic segment (Figure 10.8); 7—through intracoronary collateral channels which bridge the stenotic segment; and less commonly, 8—through the atrioventicular node artery to a septal branch of the left anterior descending artery (Figure 10.3 E).

Collateral Circulation To The Left Circumflex Artery

Collateral flow to a stenotic or occluded left circumflex artery may course: 1—through anastomoses from any atrial branch as the left atrial circumflex artery or sinus node artery (when it arises from the left) to the distal circumflex artery (Figures 10.9, 10.10); 2—through anastomoses from the right coronary artery through the sinus node artery when it arises from the right coronary artery (Figures 10.11, 10.12); 3—via diagonal branches of the left anterior descending to the circumflex artery (Figure 10.13); 4—via intracoronary collateral circulation bridging the occlusion; or 5—through a left marginal branch to the post-stenotic segment (Figure 10.14).

Collateral Circulation To The Right Coronary Artery

Collateral circulation to a diseased right coronary artery may occur: 1 — via septal collateral from the left anterior descending to the posterior descending artery (Figures 10.9, 10.15-10.17); 2 — via apical anastomoses from the left anterior descending to the posterior descending artery (Figures 10.16, 10.18); 3 — through the left circumflex to the distal right coronary artery in the atrioventricular sulcus; 4 — through the left atrial circumflex to the distal right coronary artery (Figures 10.16, 10.17, 10.19); 5 — through right marginal branches over the free wall of the right ventricle to post-stenotic segments of right coronary artery and its posterior descending branch (Figures 10.7, 10.11, 10.12, 10.20); 6 — via the left marginal branch of the circumflex artery coursing near the apex to the posterior descending artery (Figure 10.14); 7 — through the sinus node artery or other atrial arteries to the right coronary artery or right marginal branch beyond an occlusion (Figures 10.21, 10.22); 8 — via the arteria anastomotica auricularis magna, or Kugel's artery, to the atrioventricular node artery and distal right coronary artery (Figure 10.23); 9 — bridging intracoronary anastomoses across an occlusion (Figures 10.12, 10.23); 10 — less commonly, the left anterior descending artery provides collateral channels to a left ventricular branch of the distal right coronary artery (Figures 10.13, 10.18); and 11 — the left anterior descending may also provide flow to the right coronary artery by collateral channels over the anterior surface of the right ventricle (Figure 10.24).

References

1. Jochem, W., Soto, B., Karp, R.B., Russell, R.O. Jr., Holt, J.H., and Barcia, A.: Radiographic anatomy of the coronary collateral circulation. *American Journal of Roentgenology, Radium Therapy and Nuclear Medicine,* **116**:50-61, 1972.
2. James, T.N.: The delivery and distribution of coronary collateral circulation. *Chest,* **58**:183-203, 1970.

Figure 10.1:   Anastomoses of the coronary arteries in order of frequency.

I. Left Anterior Descending Artery: 1. Septal anastomoses; 2. Anastomoses over the apex; 3. Left Marginal anastomoses to the LAD; 4. Vieussen's circle; 5. Right marginal anastomoses to the LAD; 6. Intracoronary anastomoses.

II. Right Coronary Artery: 1. Septal anastomoses; 2. Apical anastomoses; 3. Left circumflex anastomoses with distal RC; 4. Atrial circumflex anastomoses with distal RC; 5. Right marginal anastomoses with posterior descending; 6. Left marginal anastomoses with distal RC; 7. Sinus node artery anastomoses with distal RC; 8. Kugel's artery; 9. Conus artery anastomoses with the right marginal branches; 10. Intracoronary anastomoses across occlusion.

III. Left Circumflex Artery: 1. Anastomoses from the left atrial circumflex to the circumflex; 2. Anastomoses from the right coronary artery to the left circumflex; 3. Anastomoses from a diagonal branch of the LAD to a marginal branch of the left circumflex; 4. Intracoronary anastomoses bridging the occlusion.

KEY: Cx = left circumflex artery; RC = right coronary artery; AVN = atrioventricular node artery; LAD = left anterior descending artery; LM = left marginal artery of the obtuse angle; RM = right marginal artery of the acute angle; SN = sinus node artery; CA = conus artery.

(From Jochem, W., Soto, B., Karp, R.B., Russell, R.O., Jr., Holt, J.H., and Barcia, A.: Radiographic anatomy of the coronary collateral circulation. *American Journal of Roentgenology, Radium Therapy and Nuclear Medicine,* **46**:50-61, 1972. Reproduced with permission.)

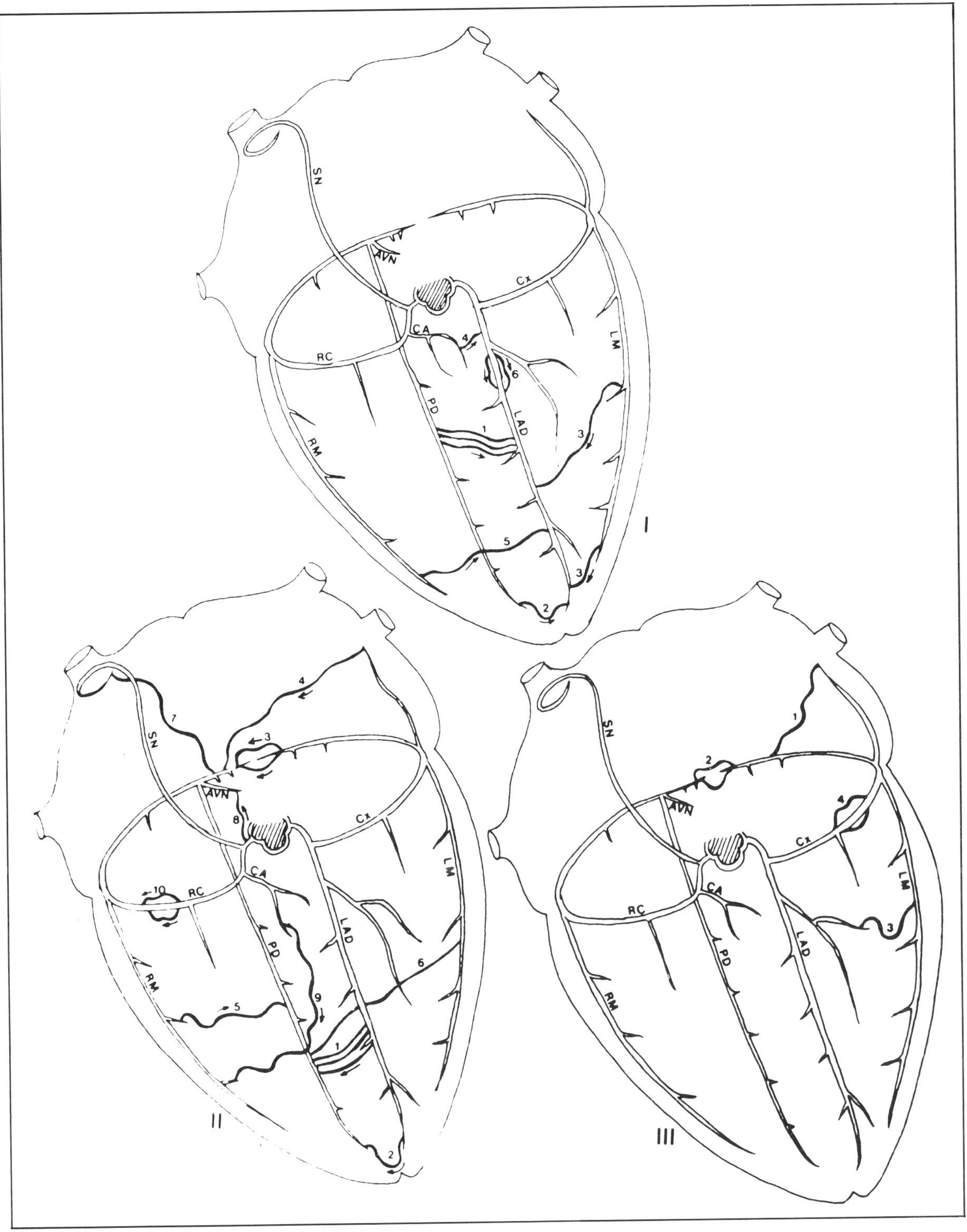

FIGURE 10.1

Figure 10.2:   Left coronary arteriogram.

A. Lateral projection. The left anterior descending is occluded at origin (arrow). The left circumflex (CX) is normal and gives rise to three left marginal (LM) branches. A diagonal (D) branch of the left anterior descending fills by collateral channels from the CX, but there is no opacification of the left anterior descending from the left injection.

B. The CX appears to be a direct extension of the left main coronary artery (LCA) because of the occlusion of the left anterior descending artery (arrow in **B**).

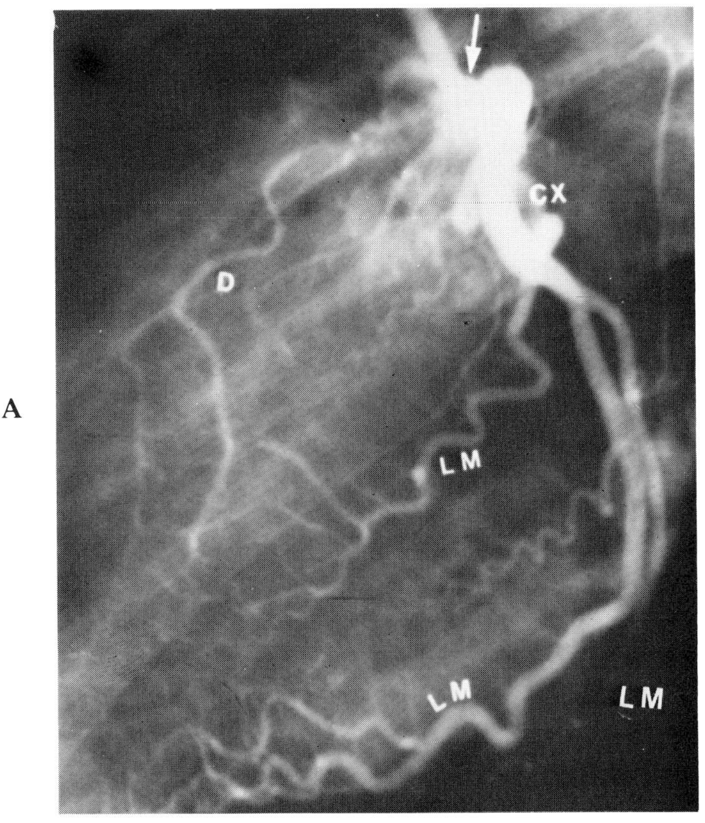

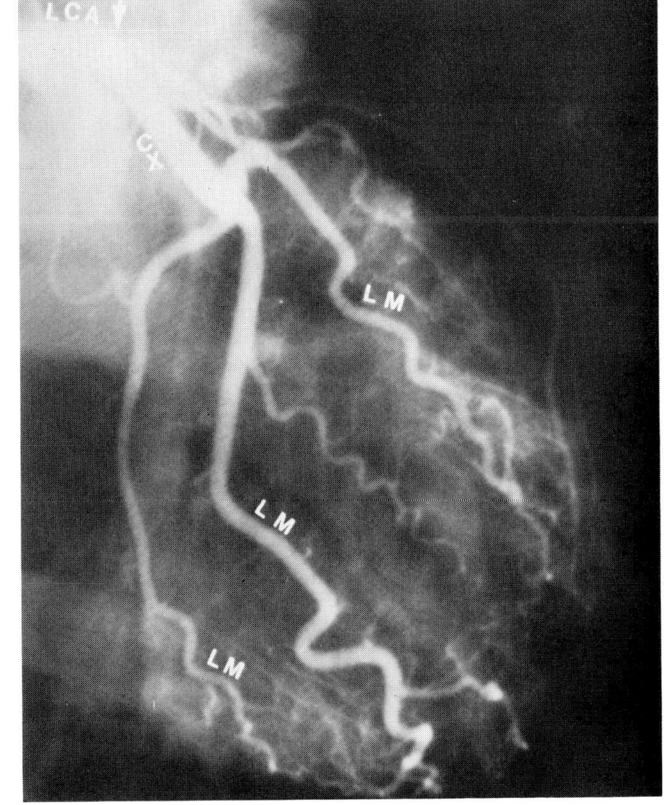

FIGURE 10.2

Figure 10.2:   C. Right coronary arteriogram; right anterior oblique projection, early stage of filling. The right coronary artery (RCA), and posterior descending artery (PDA) are normal. Large septal (S) branches of the PDA (lower group of S's) join septal branches of the left anterior descending (LAD) (upper group of S's).

D. Right coronary arteriogram; right anterior oblique projection, late stage of filling. Same arteriogram as in C. The left anterior descending (LAD) is now filled in its middle and distal trunk. This is a good demonstration of septal collateral flow from the PDA to an obstructed LAD.

C
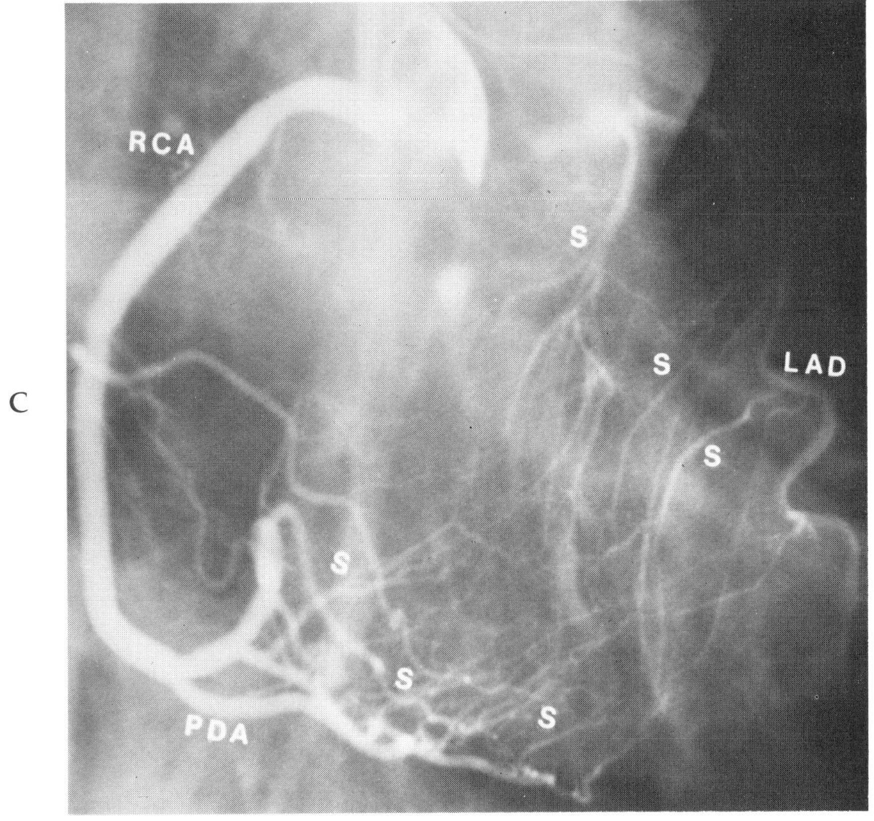

D
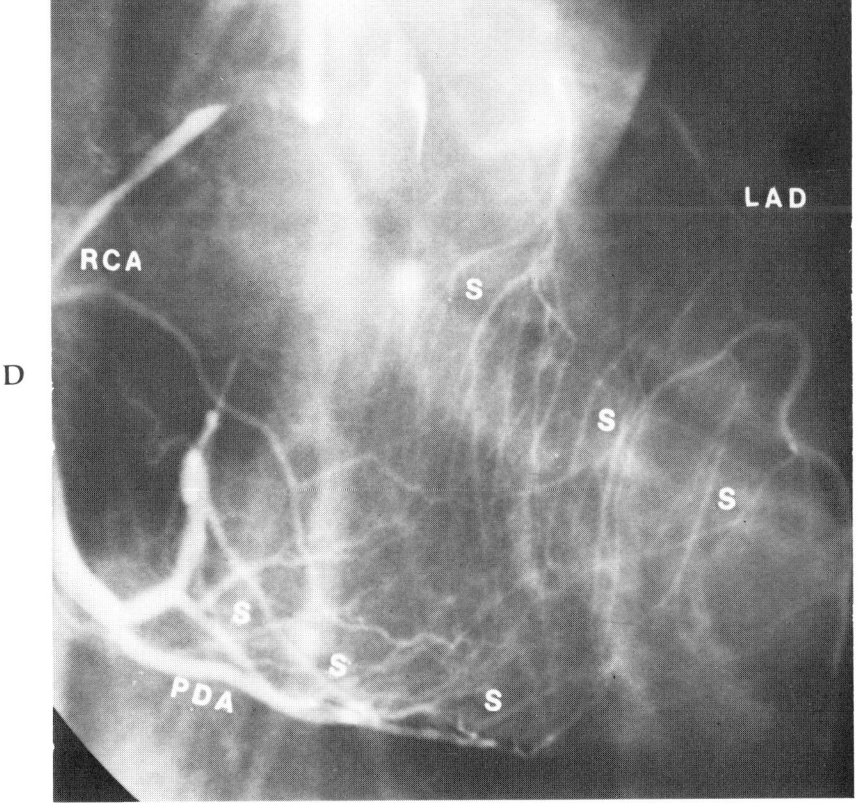

FIGURE 10.2

Figure 10.3:   Right coronary arteriogram; **A**. Left anterior oblique projection; **C** and **E**. Right anterior oblique projection. **A**, **C** and **E** are from the same patient.

A. The right coronary artery (RCA) has three occlusions (arrows) prior to the posterior descending artery (PDA). Three proximal branches of the RCA (pointers) function as collateral channels to fill a large septal (S) branch of the left anterior descending artery. These vessels comprise Vieussen's circle between proximal right coronary and left anterior descending arteries. Smaller septal branches (lower S's) are also seen. C, early and **E**, late stages of filling in right anterior oblique projection. Severe disease in RCA is indicated by the arrows in **C** and the left upper arrow in **E**. The conus (C) artery functions as a collateral channel to the large septal (S) branch of the LAD which is seen faintly in **C** and better in **E** (horizontal arrow). The right marginal (RM) branch is another source of collateral circulation to the LAD. The atrioventricular node artery also functions as a collateral channel (lower arrows in **E**) to the large septal branch (S) of the LAD.

B, **D** and **F**. Diagrammatic representations of **A**, **C** and **E**, respectively.

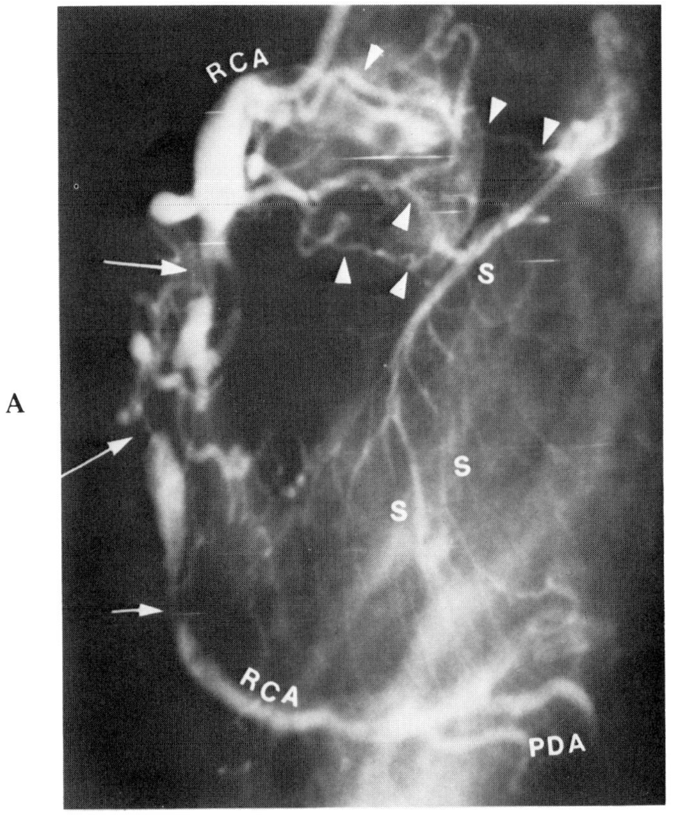

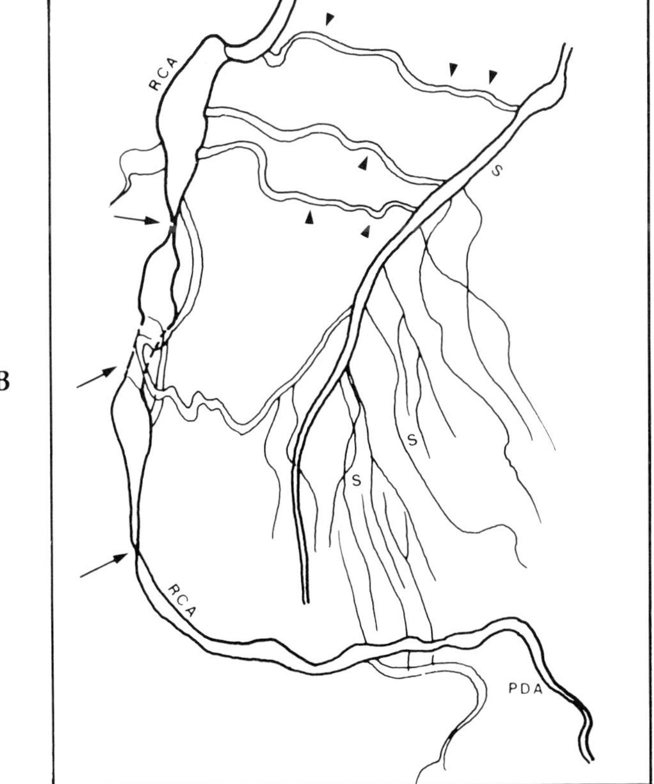

FIGURE 10.3

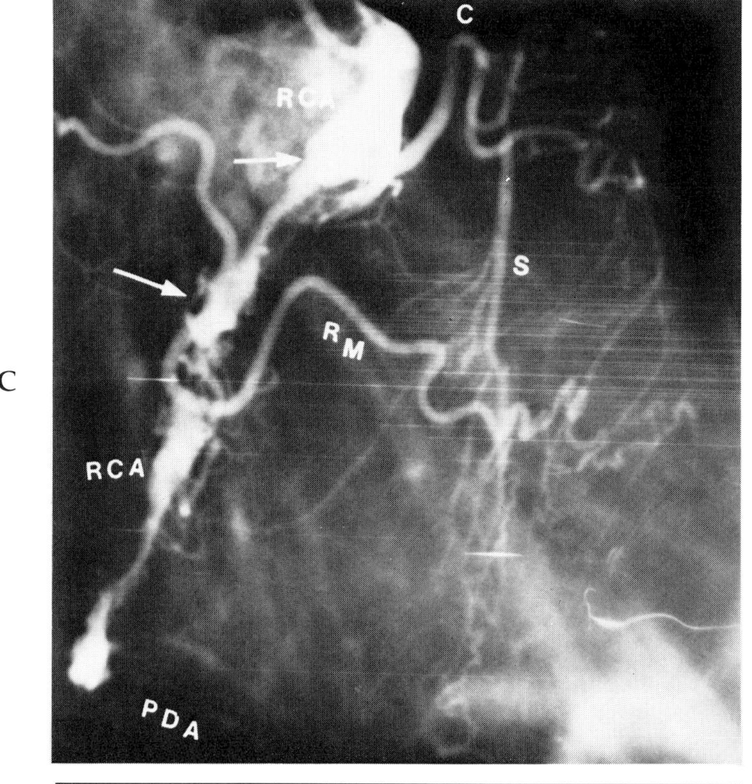

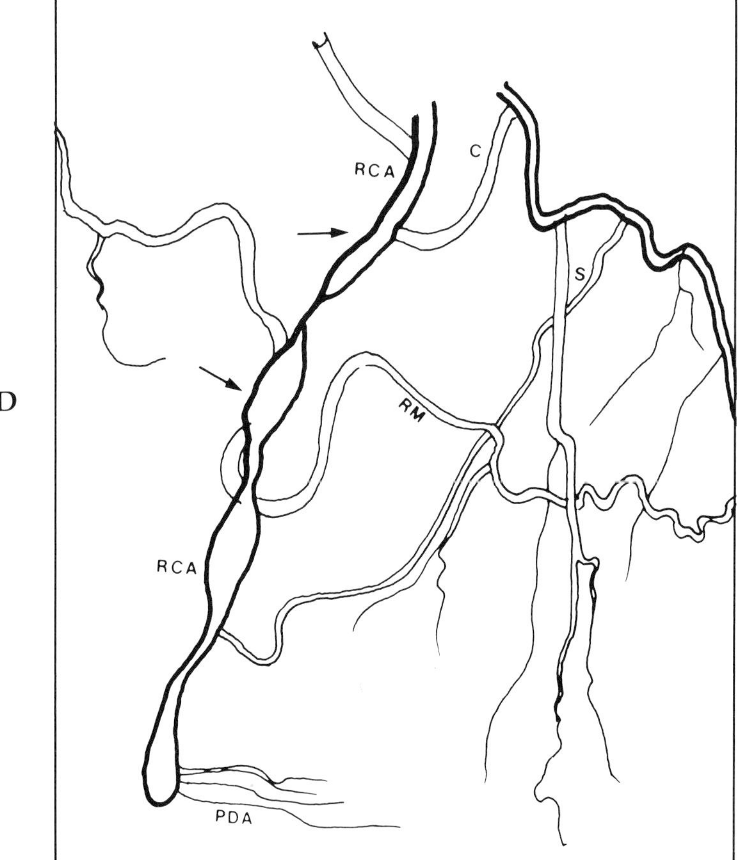

FIGURE 10.3

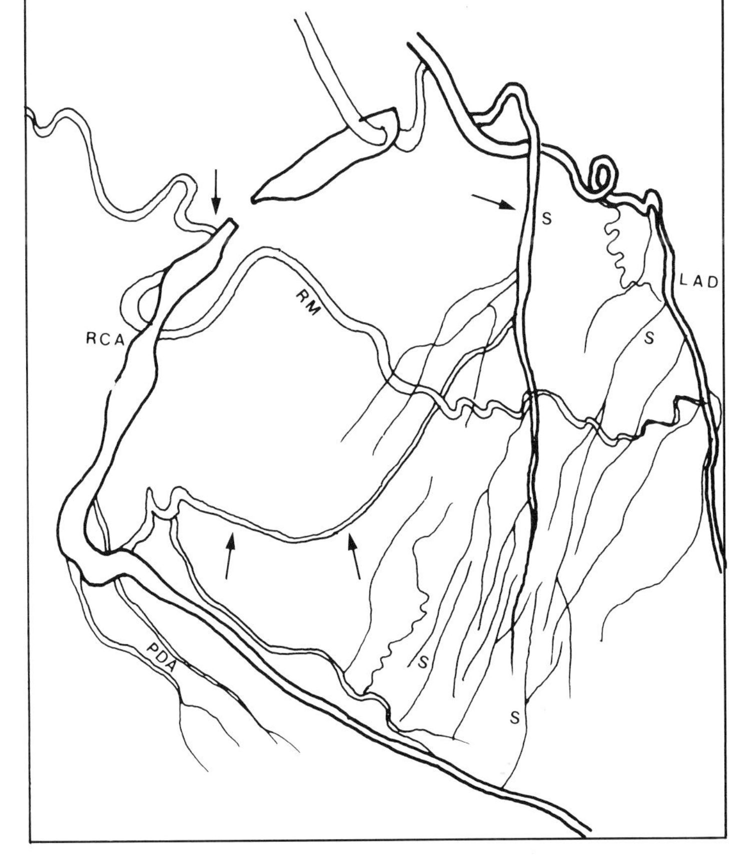

FIGURE 10.3

Figure 10.4:   Right coronary arteriogram; left anterior oblique projection. **A**, early, and **B**, late stages of filling: The right coronary artery (RCA), posterior descending artery (PDA) and the distal right coronary artery (DRCA) are normal. Septal (S) branches of the PDA are profuse and fill the septal (upper S) branch of the left anterior descending and the left anterior descending (LAD) itself. The atrioventricular node (AV) artery arises from the apex of the arch of the RCA at the crux.

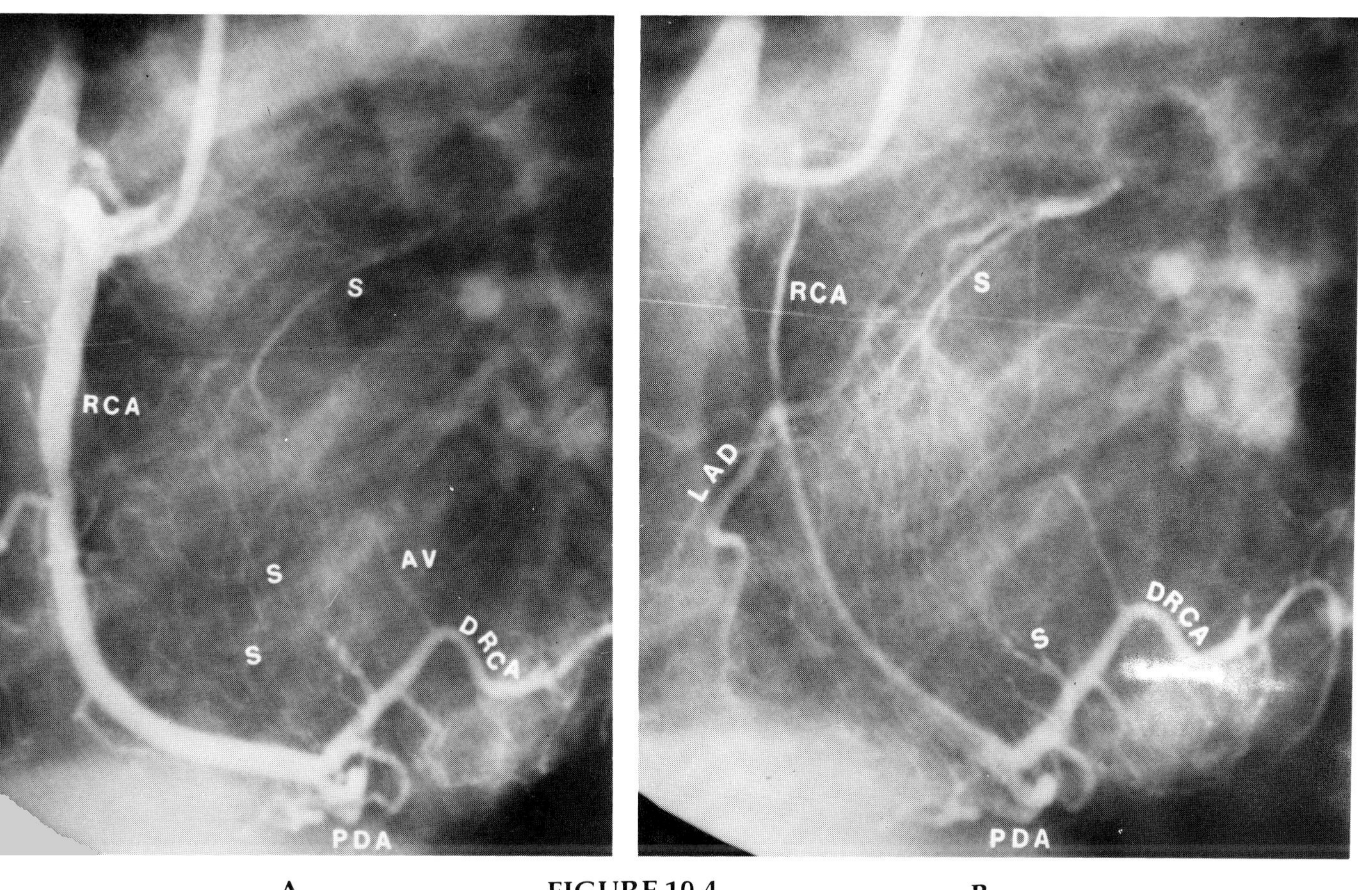

A   **FIGURE 10.4**   B

Figure 10.5:   Right coronary arteriogram; lateral projection. **A.** Early phase; **B.** Late phase. Following opacification of the right coronary artery (RCA), there is prompt visualization of the septal collaterals (lower S's) of the posterior descending coronary artery (PDA). These septal branches join the septal branches of the left anterior descending artery (LAD, upper S's). In **B**, filling of the main channel of the LAD is seen.

DRCA = distal right coronary artery.

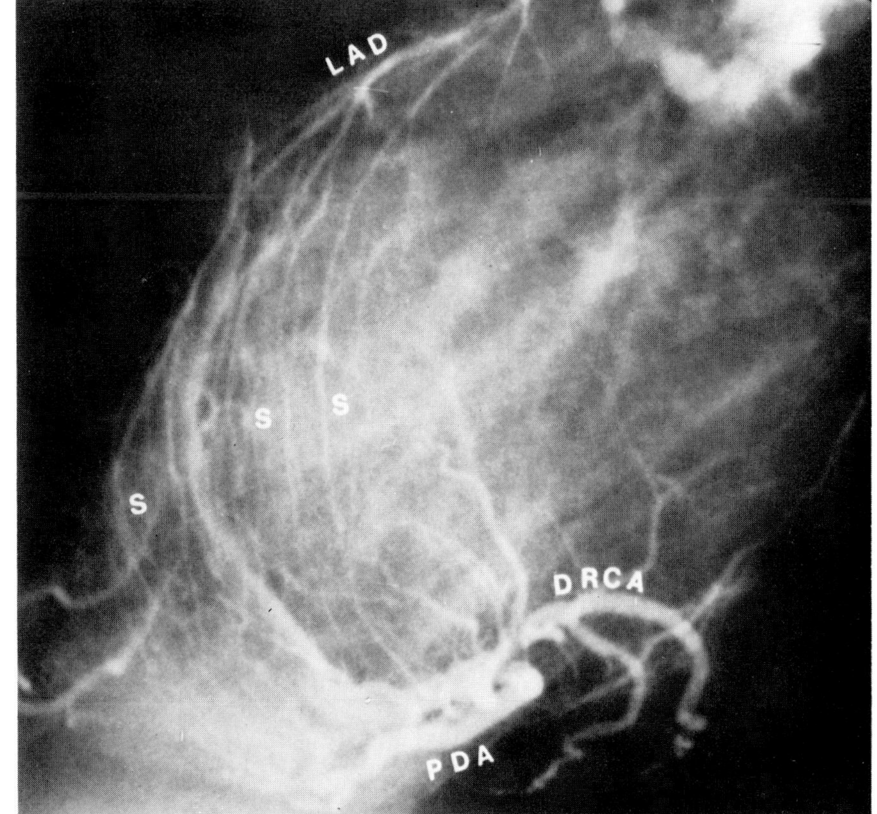

FIGURE 10.5

Figure 10.6:   **A.** Right coronary arteriogram; left anterior oblique projection. The right coronary artery (RCA) is unobstructed and the distal right coronary artery (DRCA) and posterior descending artery (PDA) are well filled. The latter is seen end-on. Prominent septal (S) branches from the PDA supply blood to the left anterior descending (LAD).

B. Right coronary arteriogram; right anterior oblique projection (same patient). The right coronary artery (RCA) and posterior descending artery (PDA), the latter now visualized in profile, are unobstructed and the prominent septal (S) branches supply small segments of the left anterior descending (LAD).

C. Left coronary arteriogram; left anterior oblique projection (same patient). The left circumflex (CX) is small after origin of the left marginal (LM) branch which has a 50-70% narrowing in its mid-course. The LM also supplies collateral circulation to the left anterior descending (LAD), primarily in its distal one-third. Although the LAD receives collateral blood from the right and left coronary arteries, it fills only sparsely and in segments.

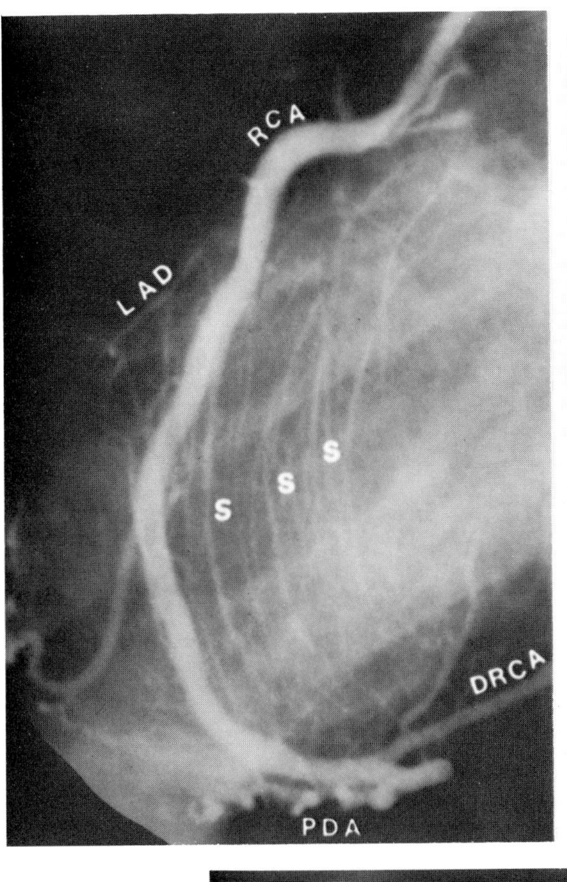

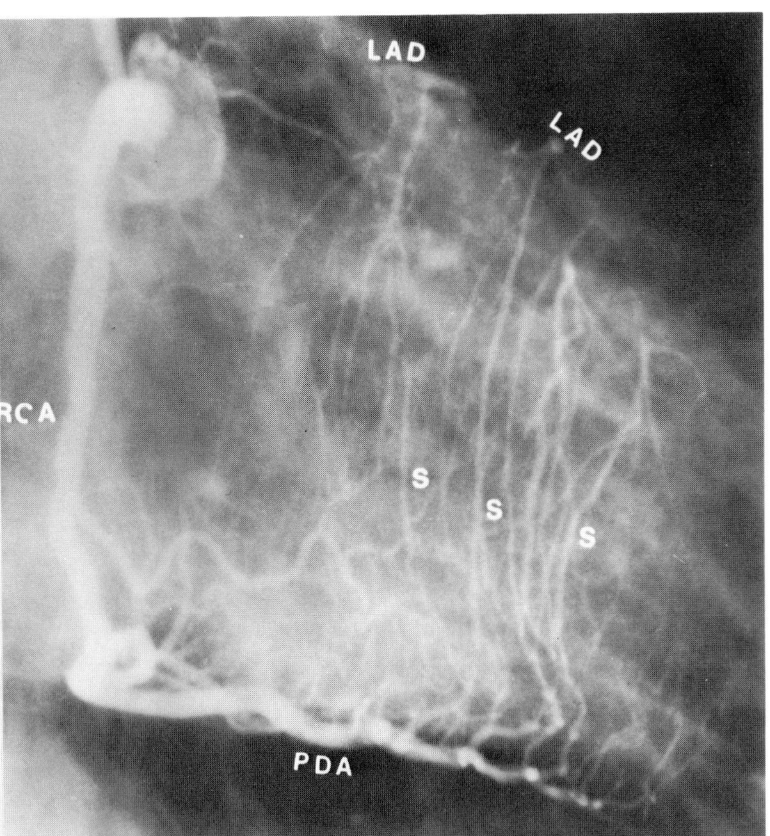

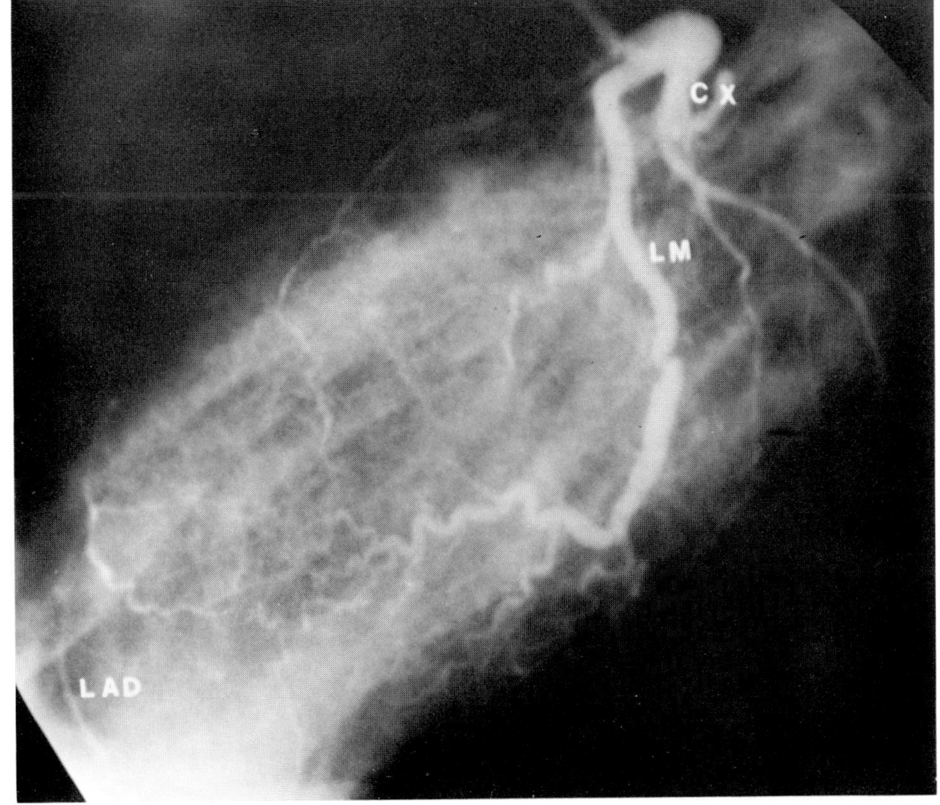

FIGURE 10.6

Figure 10.7:   Right coronary arteriogram; right anterior oblique projection.

A. The right coronary artery (RCA) is occluded after a very proximal origin of the right marginal (RM) branch. Note the collateral circulation between the two RM branches. These collaterals are present in the free wall of the right ventricle and are the source of blood supply to the distal one-third of the proximal portion of the RCA. The left anterior descending (LAD) fills primarily via the conus branch (C) of the RCA. The arrow indicates another source of collateral circulation through the sinus node artery.

B. Diagrammatic representation of A.

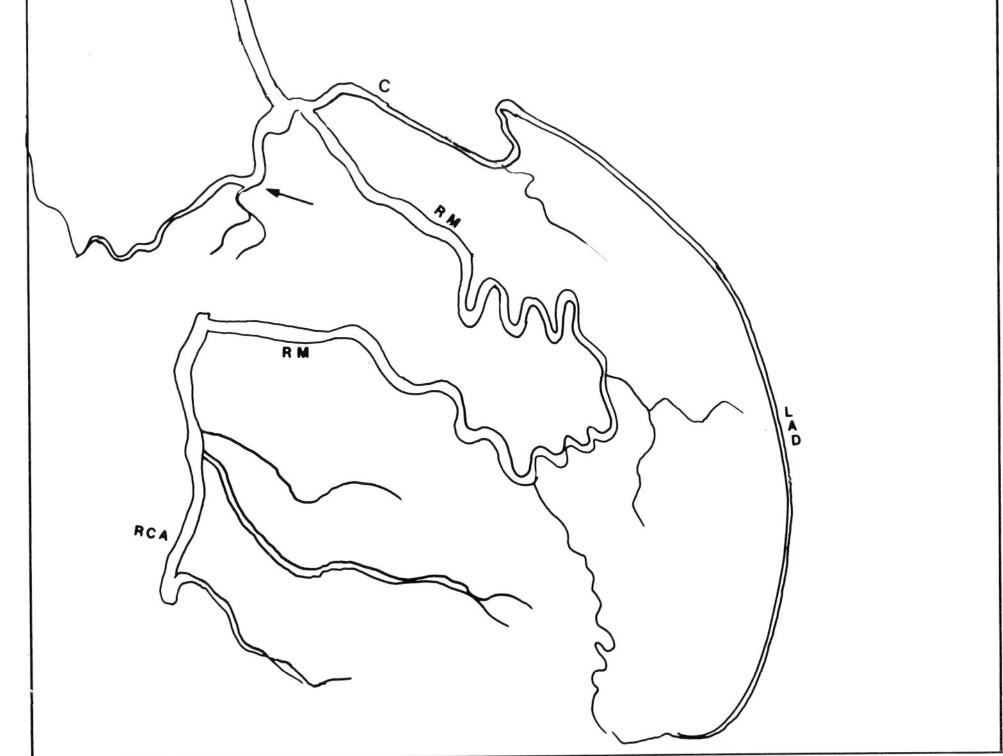

FIGURE 10.7

Figure 10.8:   Left coronary arteriogram; lateral projection. The occluded left anterior descending artery (LAD) fills distally
by well developed collateral flow through its two diagonal
branches (D). The left circumflex (CX) has a severe
stenosis (arrow).

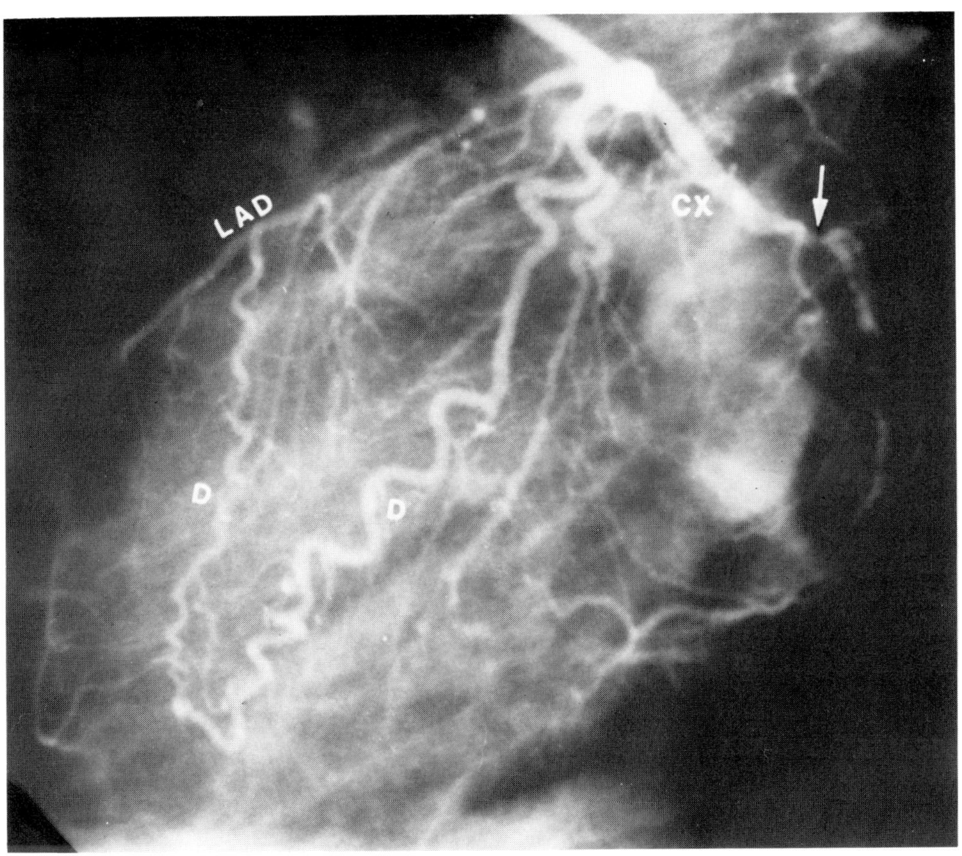

FIGURE 10.8

Figure 10.9:   Left coronary arteriogram: **A**. Lateral projection; **C**. Left anterior oblique projection in the same patient. Both projections demonstrate an occluded segment of left circumflex artery (CX) (between arrows in **C** and **D**) and filling beyond this occluded segment by collaterals (pointers) through an atrial branch originating from the proximal segment of the CX. In **A** the left anterior descending artery (LAD) has a moderately severe stenosis (arrow) after the origin of the first septal artery (S); other septal arteries (S) are seen in profusion in **A** and fill the posterior descending artery (PDA).

B. Diagrammatic representation of **A**.

D. Diagrammatic representation of **C**.

LM = left marginal branch of circumflex artery. D = diagonal branches of left anterior descending artery.

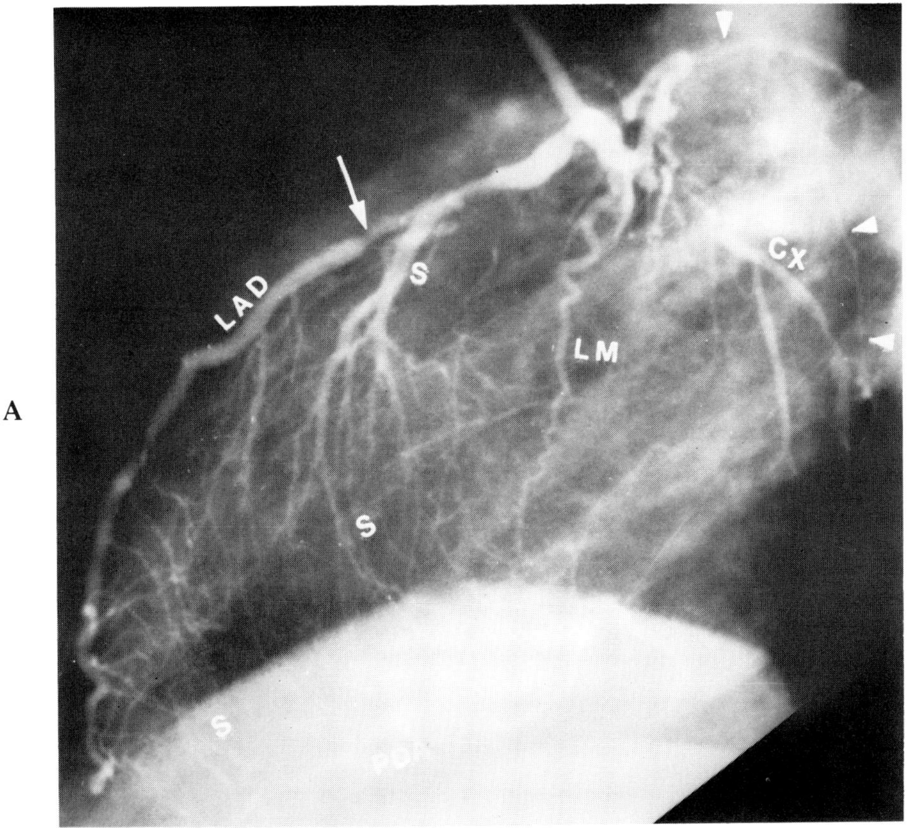

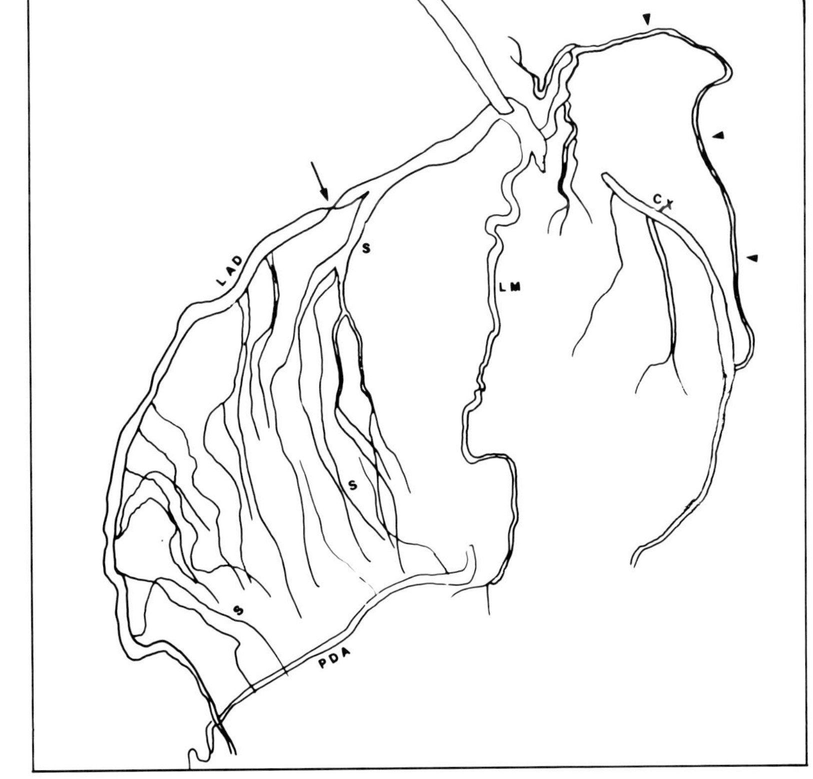

FIGURE 10.9

Figure 10.9:   C, D: See preceding page for legend.

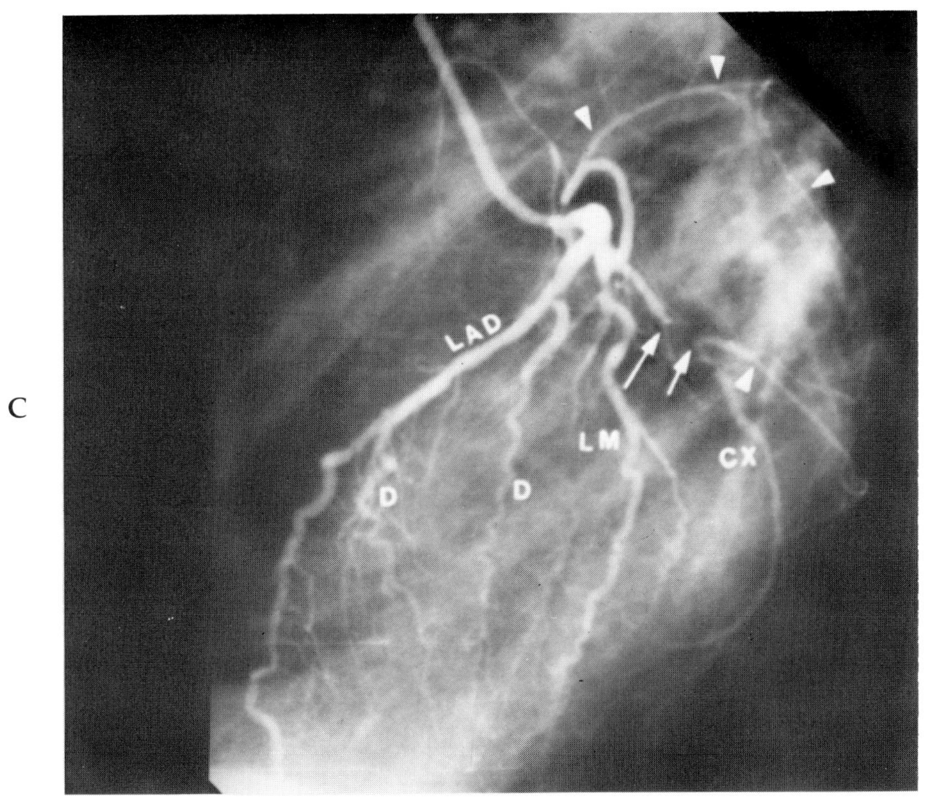

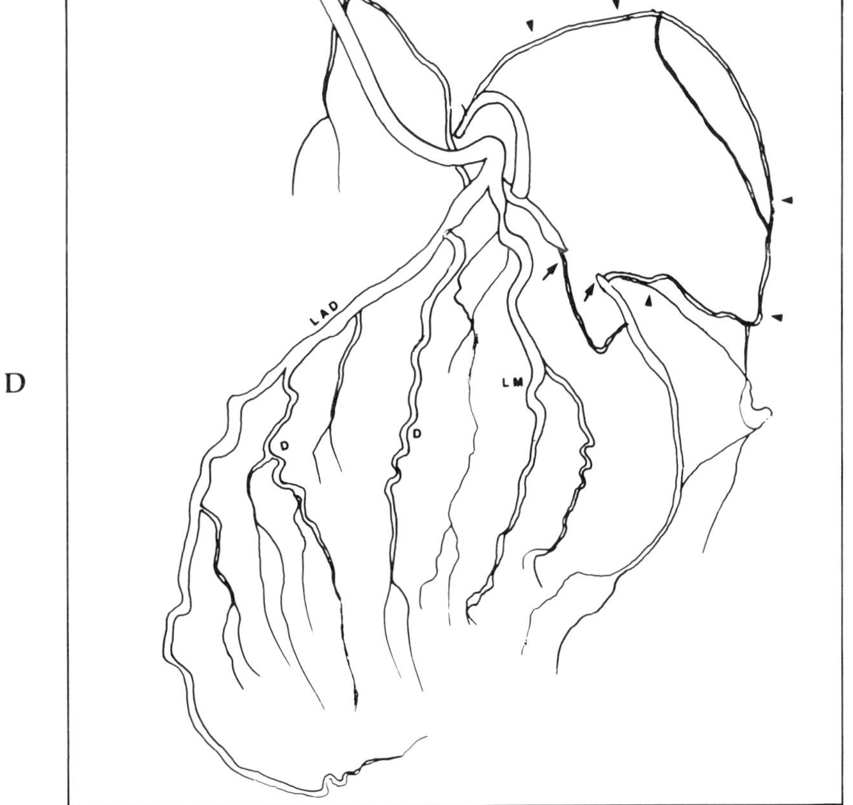

FIGURE 10.9

Figure 10.10: Left coronary arteriogram; lateral projection.

A. There is a total occlusion of the left circumflex artery (CX) just after the origin of the sinus node and left marginal (LM) arteries. Collateral flow through the sinus node artery and an additional collateral channel (pointers) provides filling of the distal left circumflex (CX) artery.

LAD = left anterior descending artery.

B. Diagrammatic representation of **A**.

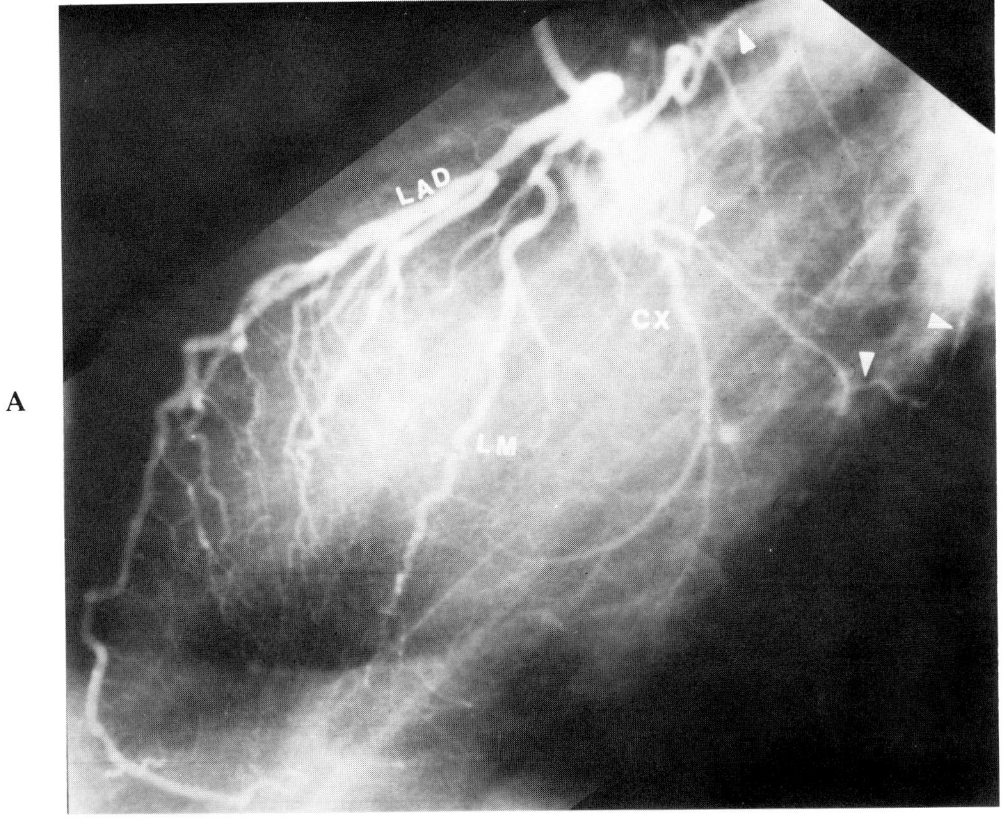

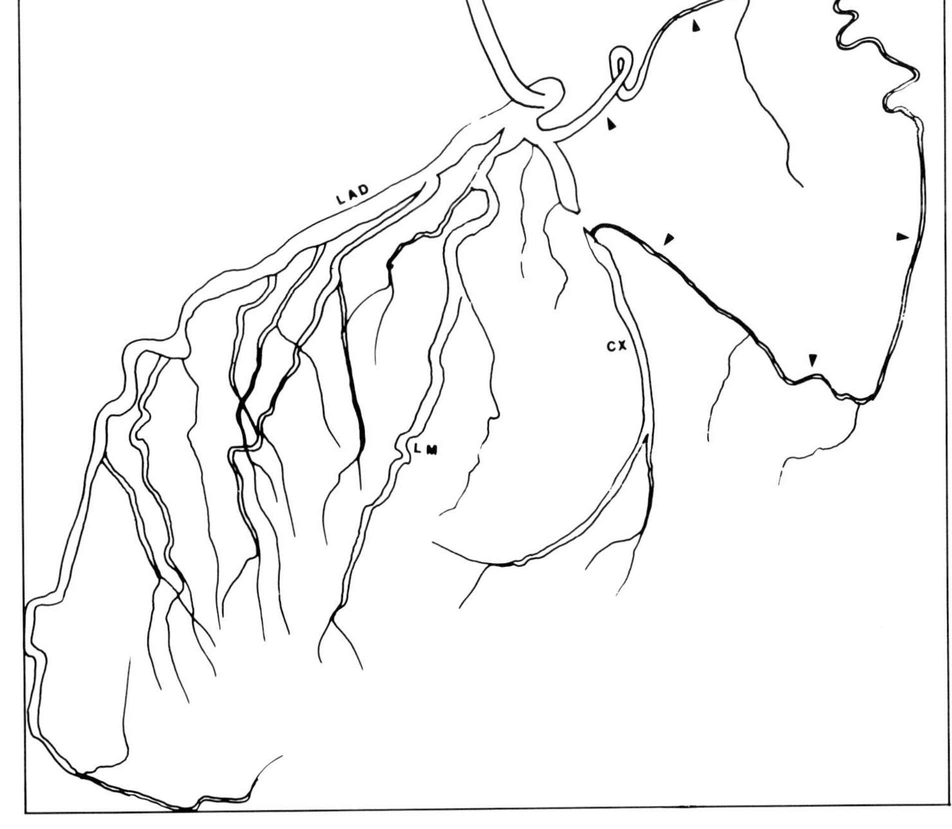

FIGURE 10.10

Figure 10.11: Right coronary arteriogram; left anterior oblique projection. The right coronary artery (RCA) is occluded at the left arrow. A net of collateral circulation is present in the right ventricular wall mainly via the right marginal artery (RM). The sinus node (SN) artery is an important source of collateral to the left circumflex (CX) artery (right arrows).

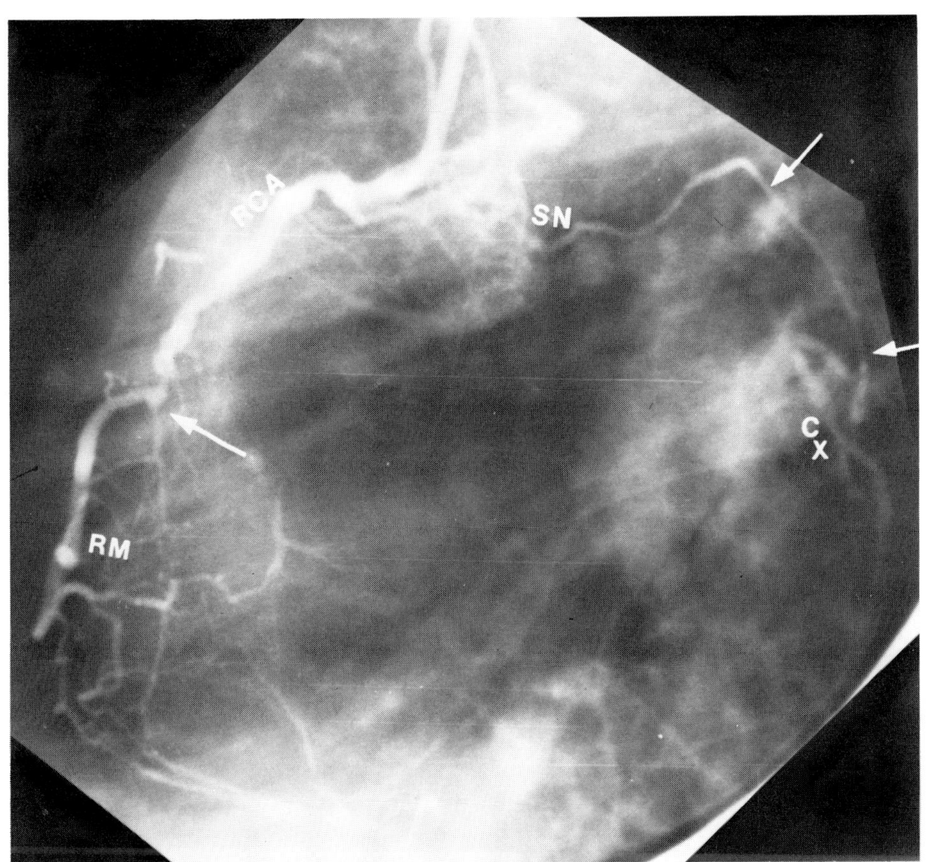

FIGURE 10.11

Figure 10.12: Right coronary arteriogram; left anterior oblique projection.

A. The right coronary artery (RCA) is occluded shortly after its origin and between the origins of the conus and first right marginal (RM) arteries. Two sources of collateral exist to the other segments of the RCA; the first over the free wall of the right ventricle to a second right marginal branch; the other through bridging intracoronary collateral branches (small markers). The posterior descending artery (PDA) is filled as a result of this collateral circulation. The sinus node (SN) artery serves as collateral circulation (between right pointers) to the left circumflex (CX).

B. Diagrammatic representation of **A**.

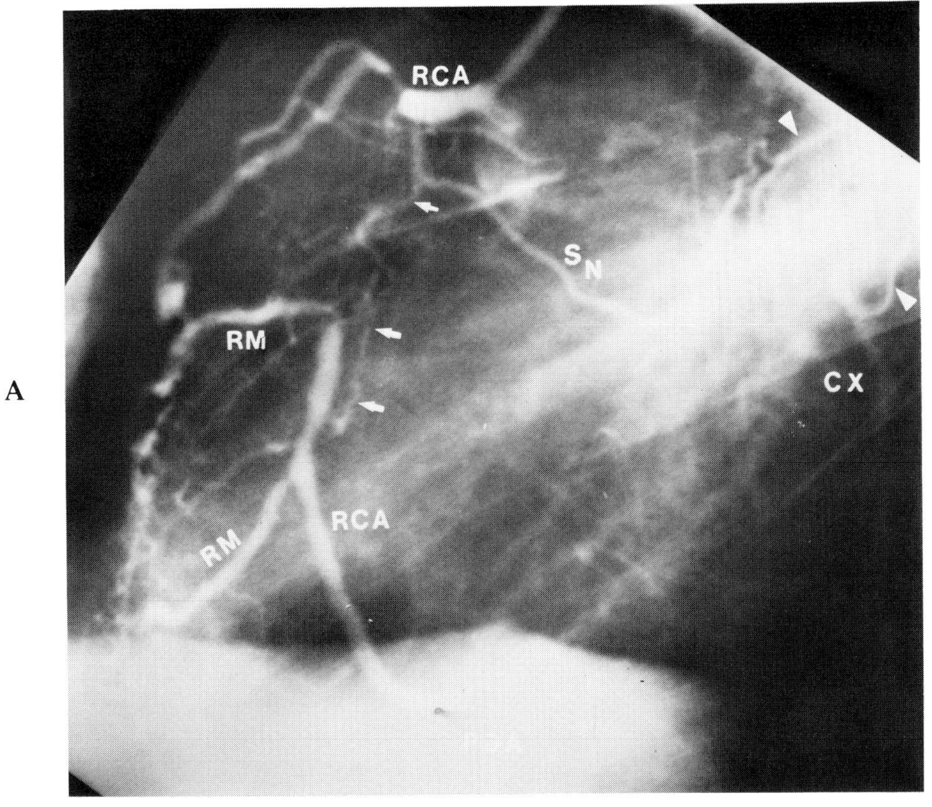

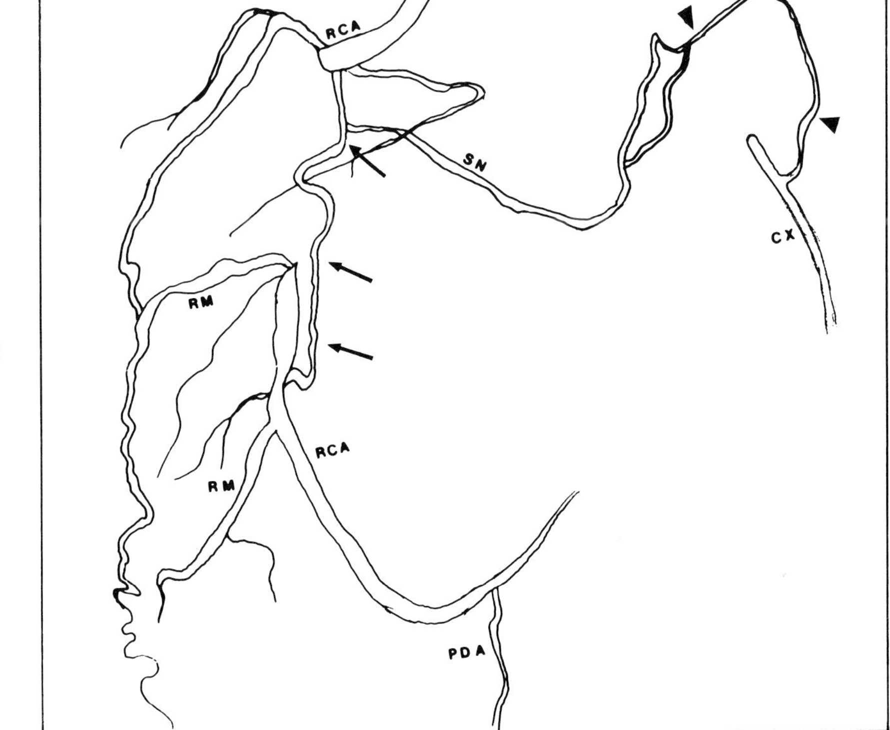

FIGURE 10.12

Figure 10.13: Left coronary arteriogram; right anterior oblique projection.

A. A branch of the left marginal artery (LM) is occluded (upper arrow). The other branch of the LM has a 70-90% stenosis. A diagonal branch (D) from the left anterior descending artery (LAD) fills the distal segment of this occluded LM branch (lower arrow). In addition collateral circulation from the left anterior descending artery also fills a left ventricular branch of the distal right coronary artery (DRCA). This is an example of the left anterior descending artery providing collaterals to both the left circumflex (CX) and distal right coronary arteries.

B. Diagrammatic representation of A.

S = septal branch of left anterior descending artery.

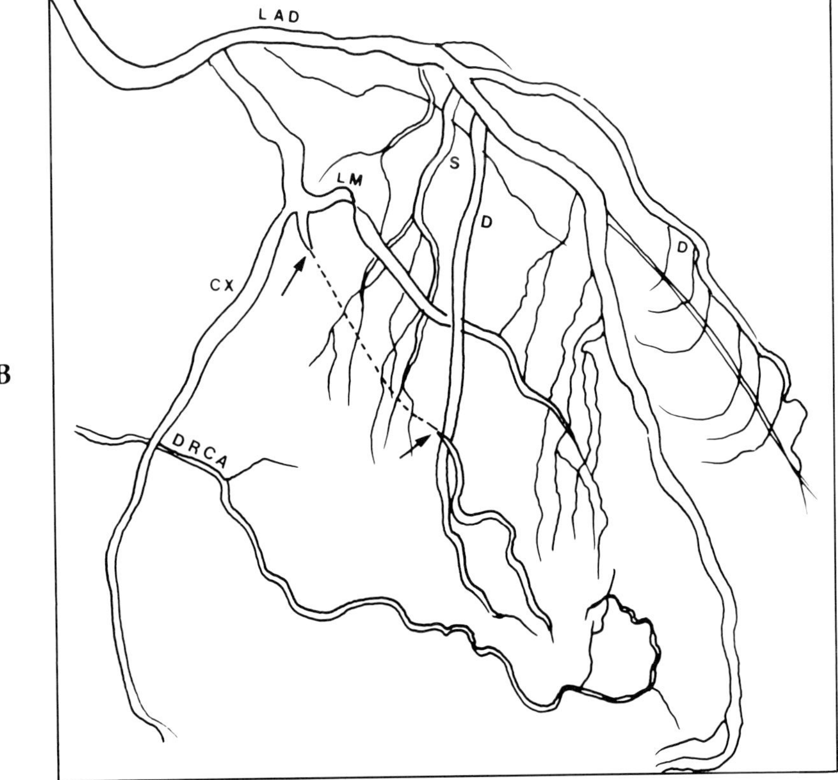

FIGURE 10.13

Figure 10.14: Left coronary arteriogram; right anterior oblique projection. The left anterior descending coronary artery is occluded (arrow) after the origin of the first diagonal vessel. The left circumflex artery is occluded after the first left marginal branch (LM). There is a 70-90% stenosis (arrow) at the origin of the left marginal artery. Collateral channels originating from the left marginal artery (LM) are seen filling the second left marginal artery (lower LM), the distal left circumflex artery, as well as adjacent segments of the left anterior descending and posterior descending (PDA) arteries.

LCA = left main coronary artery.

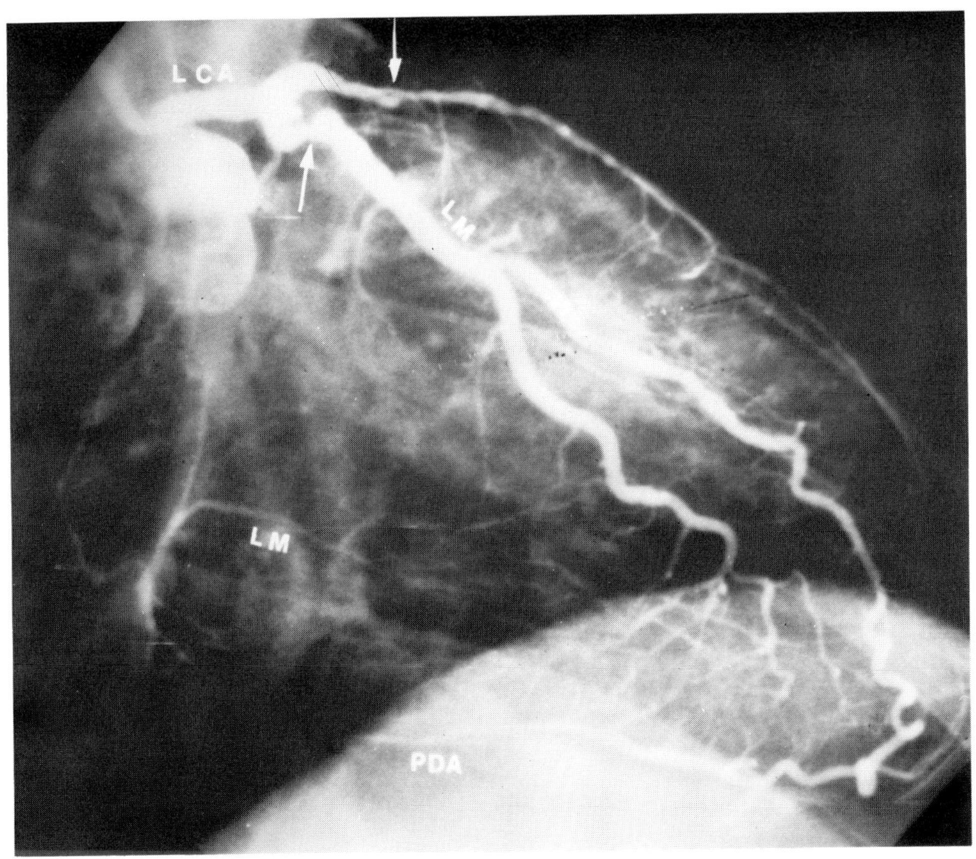

FIGURE 10.14

Figure 10.15: Left coronary arteriogram; right anterior oblique projection.

A. Total occlusion of the left circumflex artery is demonstrated. A well developed septal artery (S) from the left anterior descending (LAD) provides partial filling of the posterior descending artery (PDA) through its septal artery (lower S).

B. Later phase of same injection now demonstrates almost complete filling of the posterior descending artery (PDA) as well as filling of the distal left circumflex through its left marginal (LM) branch.

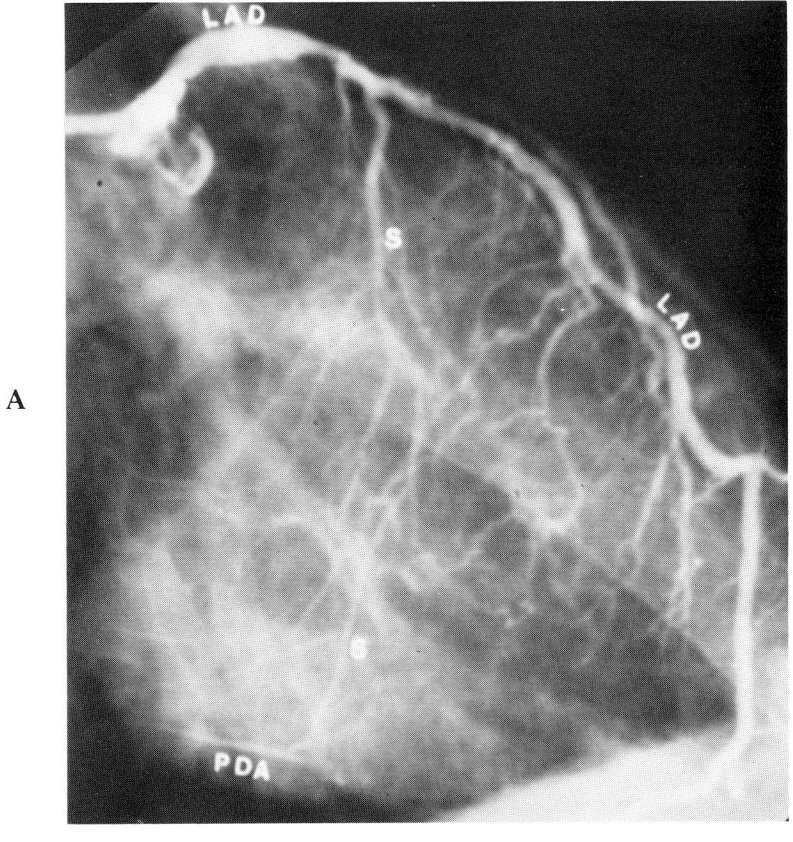

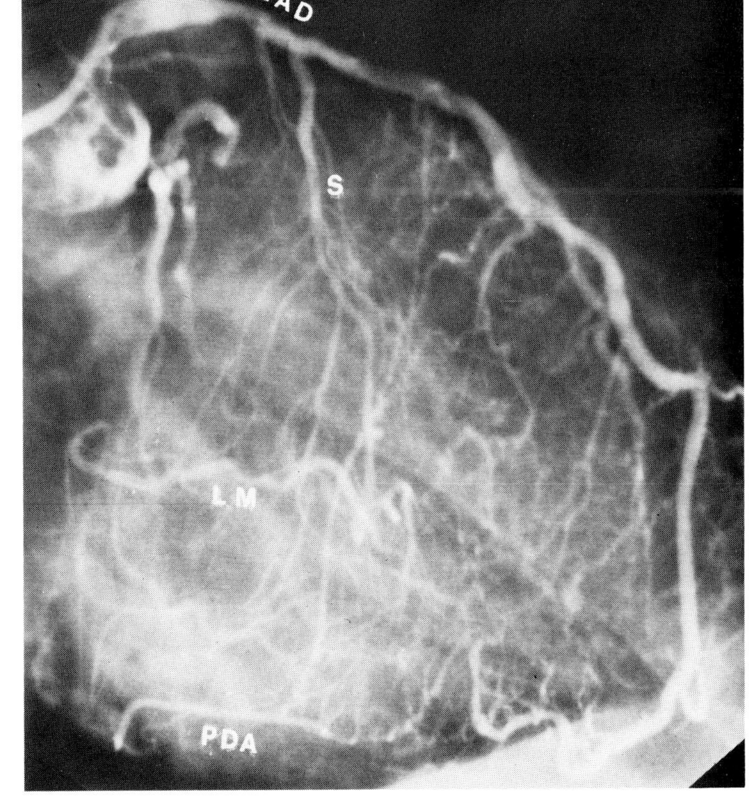

FIGURE 10.15

Figure 10.16: Left coronary arteriogram; right anterior oblique projection. Two examples of collateral channels to the right coronary artery.

A. The left circumflex artery is occluded near its origin. Intercoronary collaterals from the left circumflex artery prior to its occlusion (pointers) running over the free wall of the left atrium fill the distal right coronary artery and posterior descending artery (PDA). The left anterior descending (LAD) provides additional collateral to the posterior descending artery over the apex. The left anterior descending artery has a severe stenosis (arrow) in its proximal one-third. The septal branches (S) of the left anterior descending artery also function as collateral circulation to the PDA.

B. Again, an occluded left circumflex artery provides collaterals over the free wall of the left atrium (pointers) to the posterior descending artery (PDA). Additional collateral circulation is provided through the septal (S) vessels of the left anterior descending (LAD). This LAD also has a severe stenosis (arrow) in its proximal one-third.

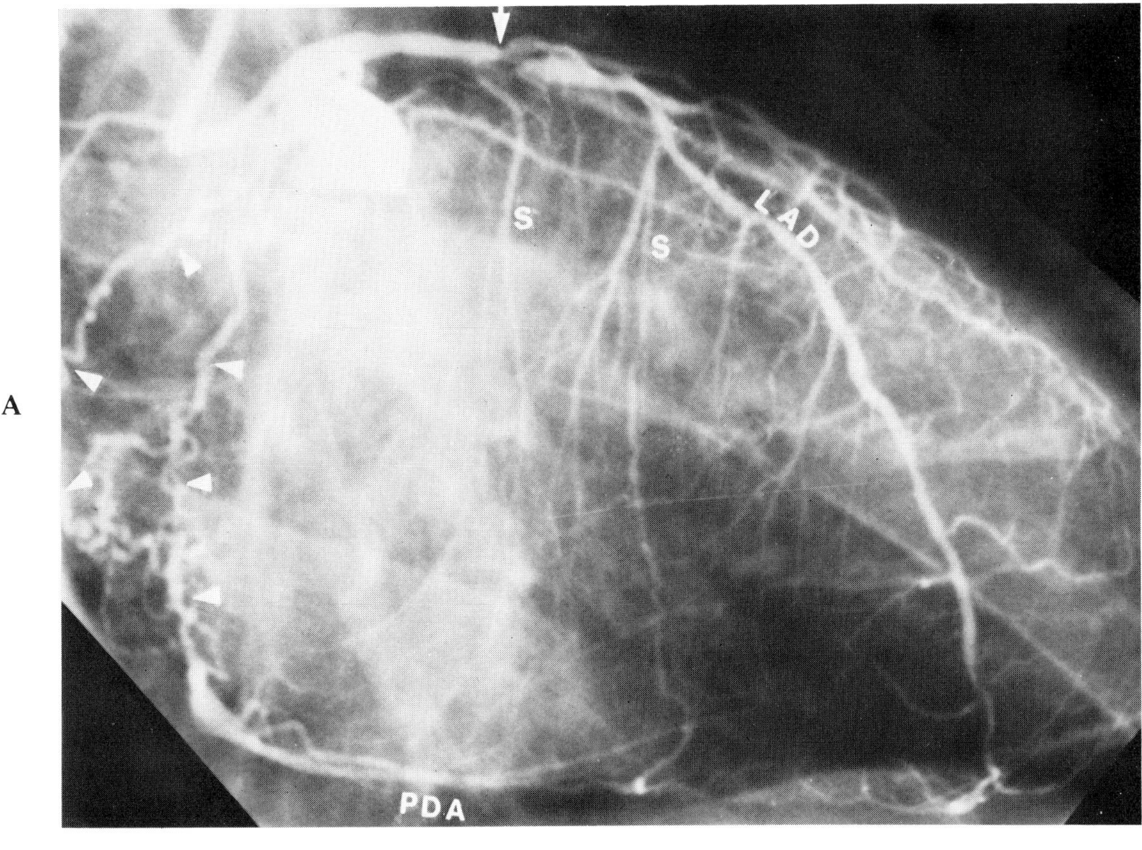

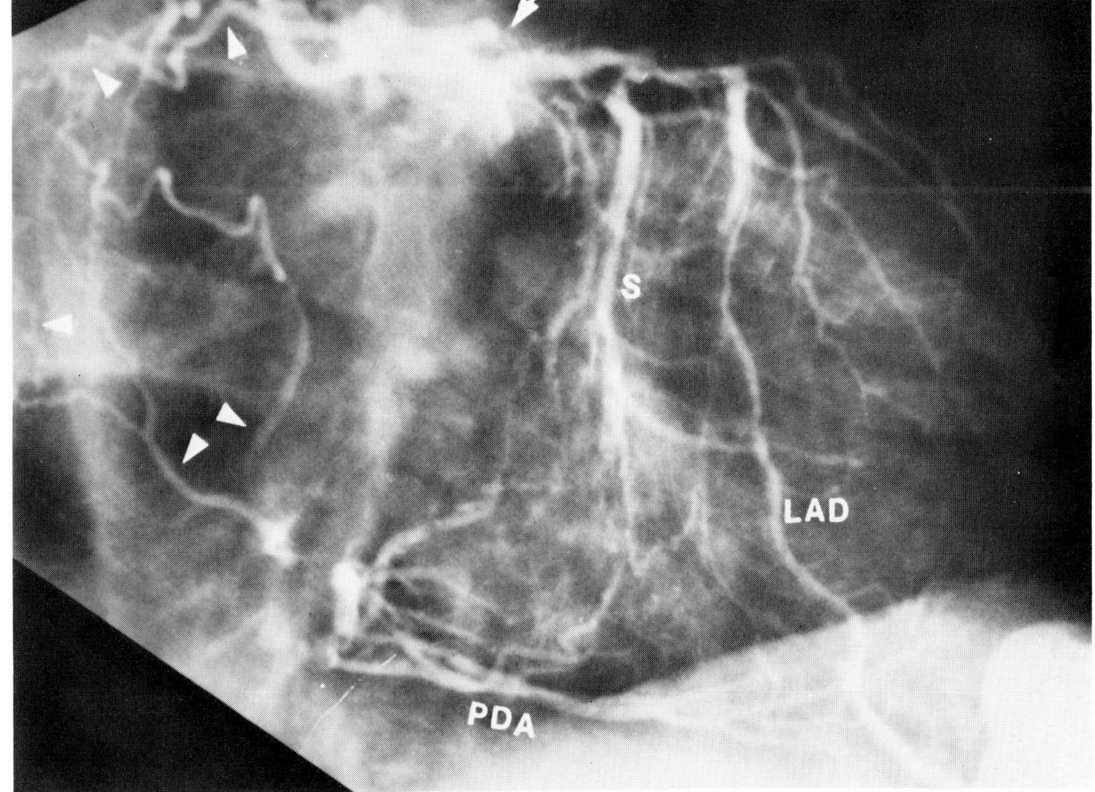

FIGURE 10.16

Figure 10.17: Left coronary arteriogram; right anterior oblique projection.

A. A short left circumflex artery (CX) gives off a large atrial collateral channel (pointers) which allows filling of the posterior descending artery (PDA) of an occluded right coronary artery. Septal branches (S) of the left anterior descending artery provide collateral circulation to the PDA also. In addition there is occlusion of the left anterior descending artery (arrow).

LM = left marginal branch of circumflex artery.

B. Diagrammatic representation of **A**.

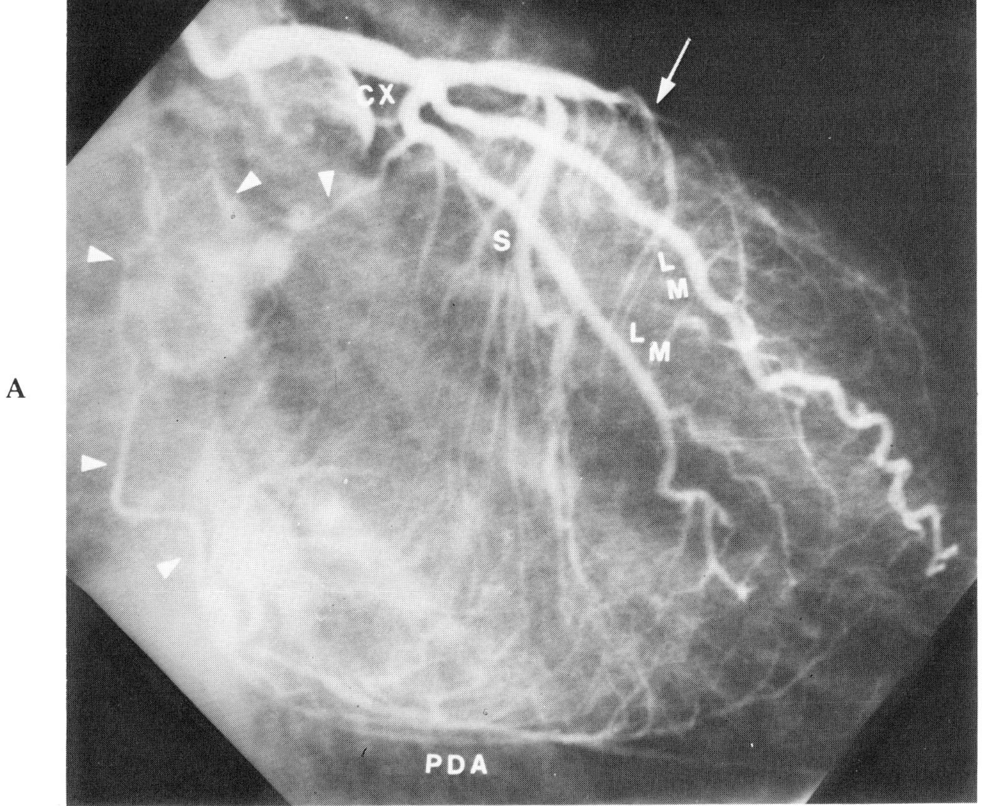

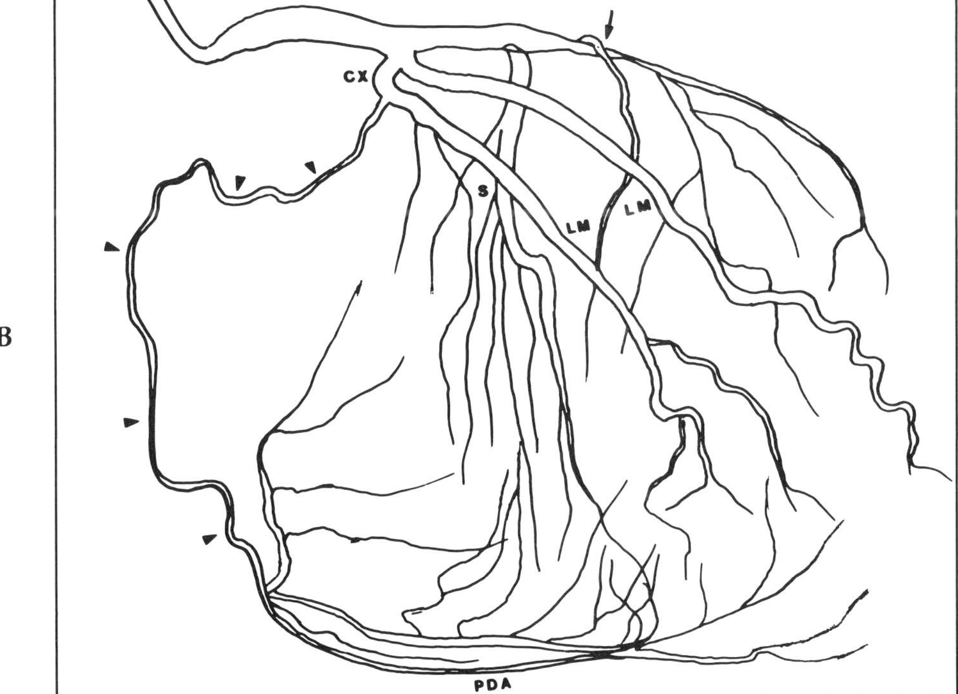

FIGURE 10.17

Figure 10.18: Left coronary arteriogram; right anterior oblique projection. An example of filling of the posterior descending artery (PDA) and left ventricular branch of the distal right coronary artery (pointers) from the left anterior descending artery (LAD) by collateral circulation over the apex of the left ventricle.

LM = left marginal branch of circumflex artery.

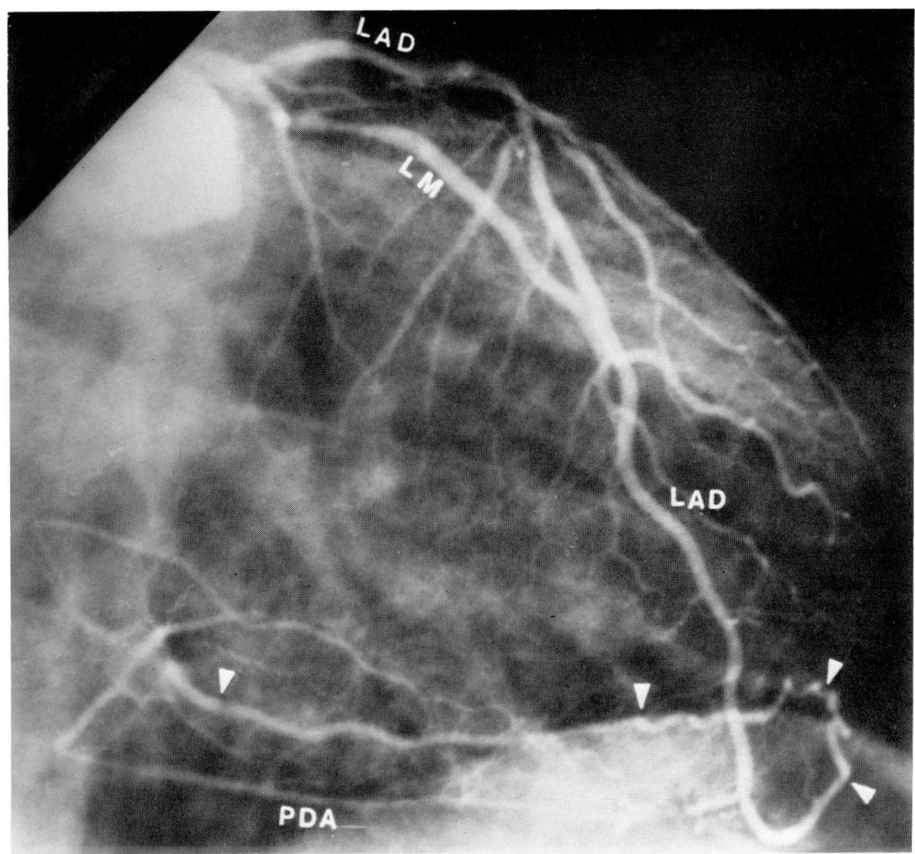

FIGURE 10.18

Figure 10.19: Left coronary arteriogram; lateral projection; same patient as in Figure 10.17. The left atrial circumflex branch (pointers) of the left circumflex artery (CX) filling the posterior descending artery (PDA) is seen projected over the posterior and inferior surface of the left atrium. The total occlusion of the LAD (arrow) is better demonstrated.

S = septal branches of the left anterior descending artery. LM = left marginal branch of circumflex artery.

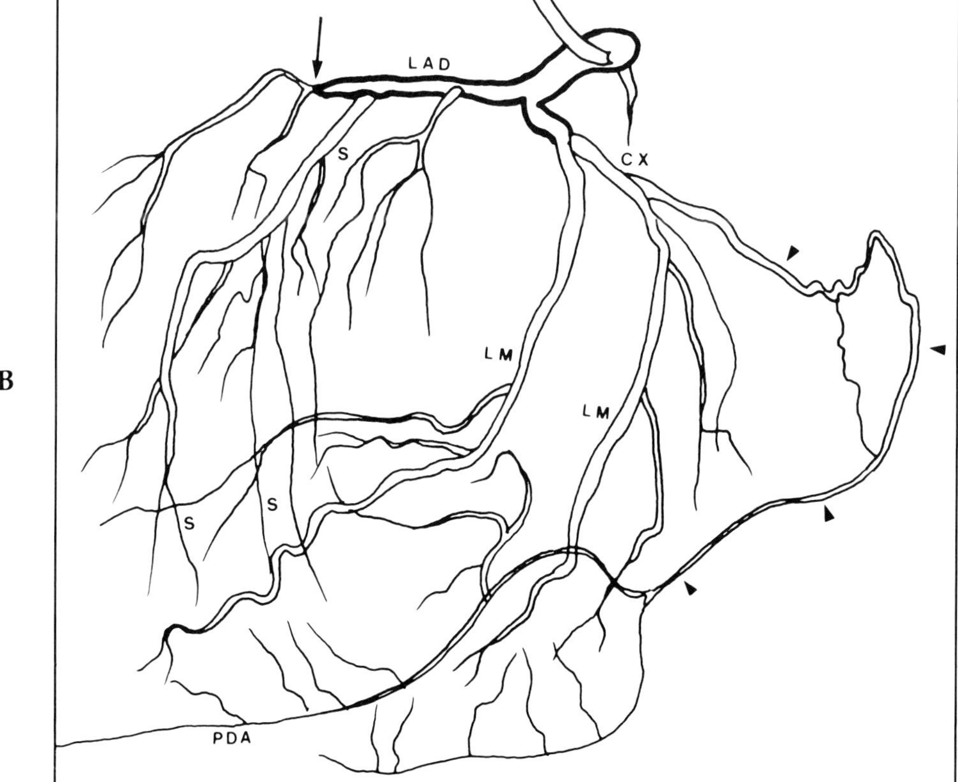

FIGURE 10.19

Figure 10.20:   Right coronary arteriogram; right anterior oblique projection.

A. There is total occlusion of the right coronary artery (RCA) after the right marginal artery (RM). Intracoronary collaterals provide filling of another right marginal branch (lower RM). There is no filling of the main channel of the RCA.

B. Diagrammatic representation of **A**.

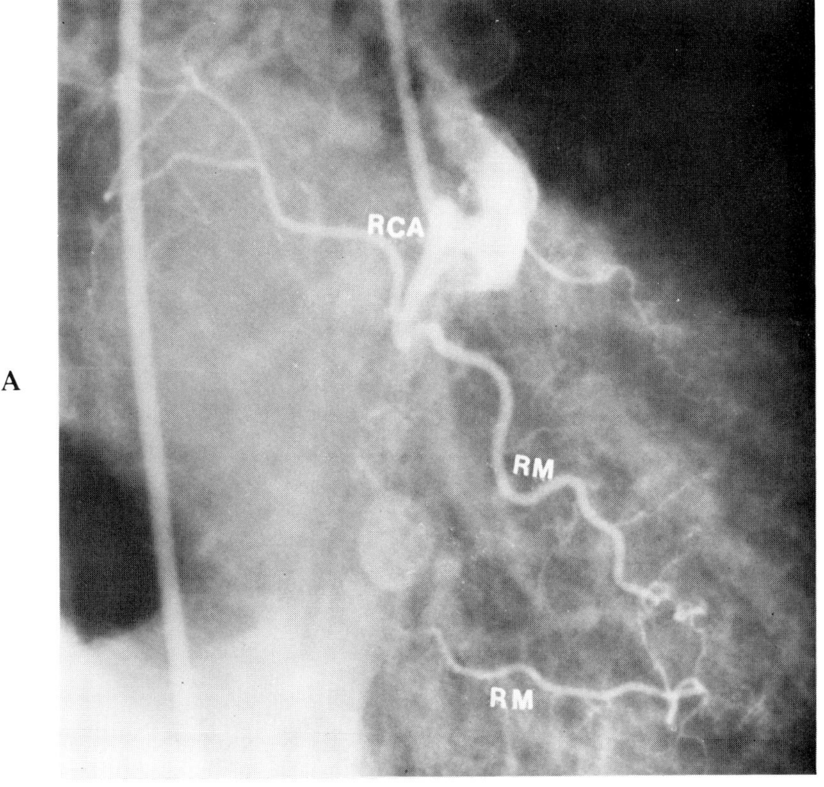

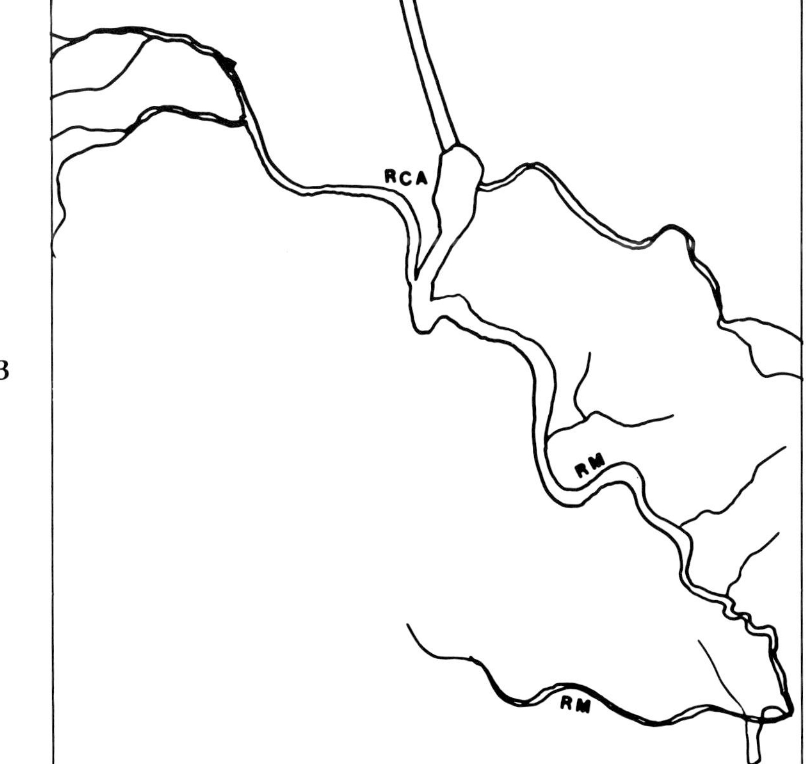

FIGURE 10.20

Figure 10.21: Right coronary arteriogram; right anterior oblique projection. **A**, **B** and **C** are sequential phases in the same artery following injection.

A. The right coronary artery is occluded in the proximal one-third (arrow) after giving rise to a large tortuous collateral channel (pointers) which courses over the right atrium.

B. The middle one-third of the right coronary artery (RCA) fills via this collateral channel. The segment of the proximal one-third of the RCA which does not fill is between the arrows. The conus (C) branch of the RCA also fills.

C. The middle one-third of the RCA, while diffusely diseased, and the right marginal (RM) are well filled as a result of this collateral.

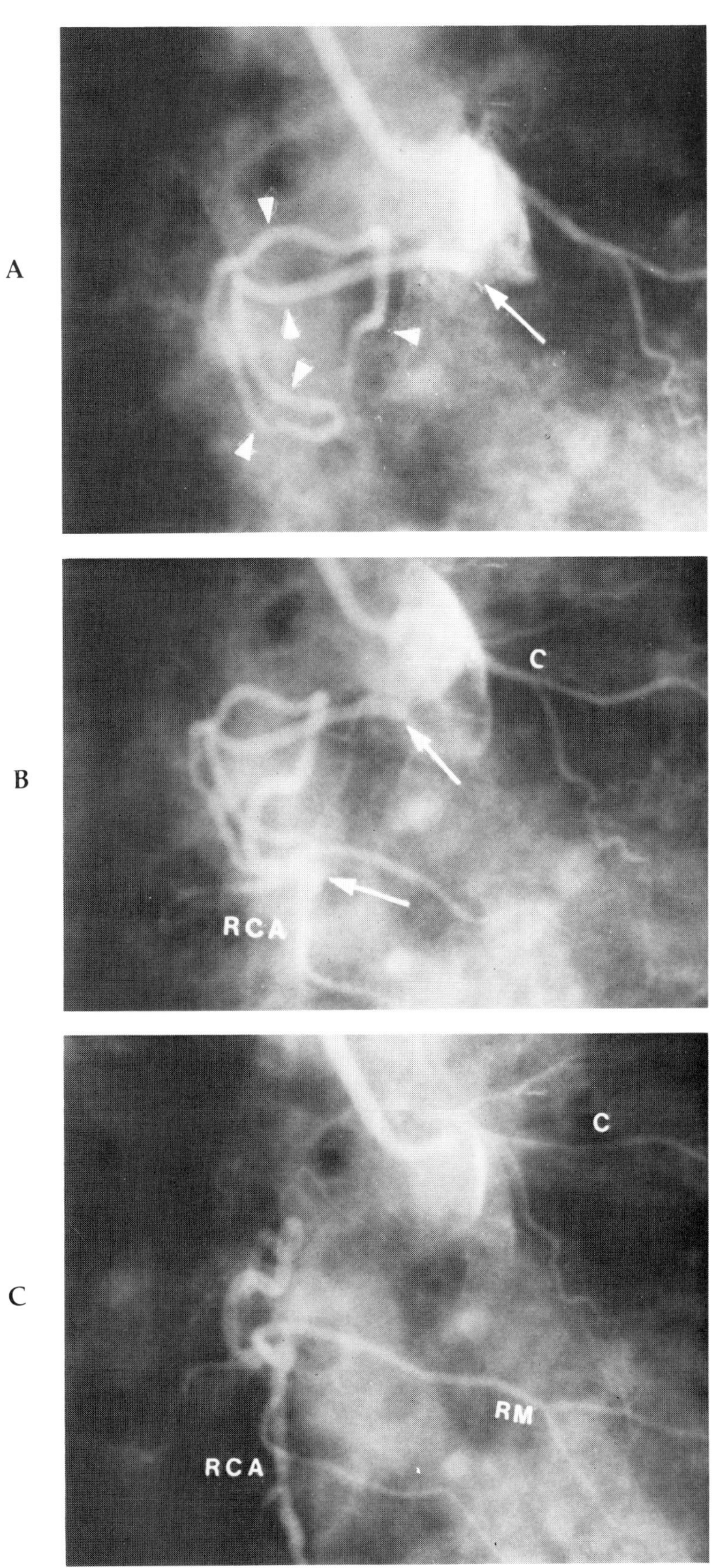

FIGURE 10.21

Figure 10.22: Right coronary arteriogram; lateral projection of same patient as in Figure 10.21. **A, B** and **C** are sequential phases following injection of contrast material.

A. The occluded right coronary artery (RCA) and the collateral vessel (pointers) are very well demonstrated.

B. The collateral channel (pointers) lying over the right atrium is now seen partially filling the middle portion of the right coronary artery (RCA). The segment between the arrows is the occluded segment of the right coronary artery.

C. The most proximal portion of the right coronary artery is no longer seen. The distal segment of the collateral channel (pointers) is still visualized and the middle portion of the right coronary artery (RCA) is very well demonstrated. The arrow indicates the native right coronary artery. This is an example of an unusually well developed intracoronary collateral channel lying over the right atrial wall.

RM = right marginal branch of the right coronary artery.

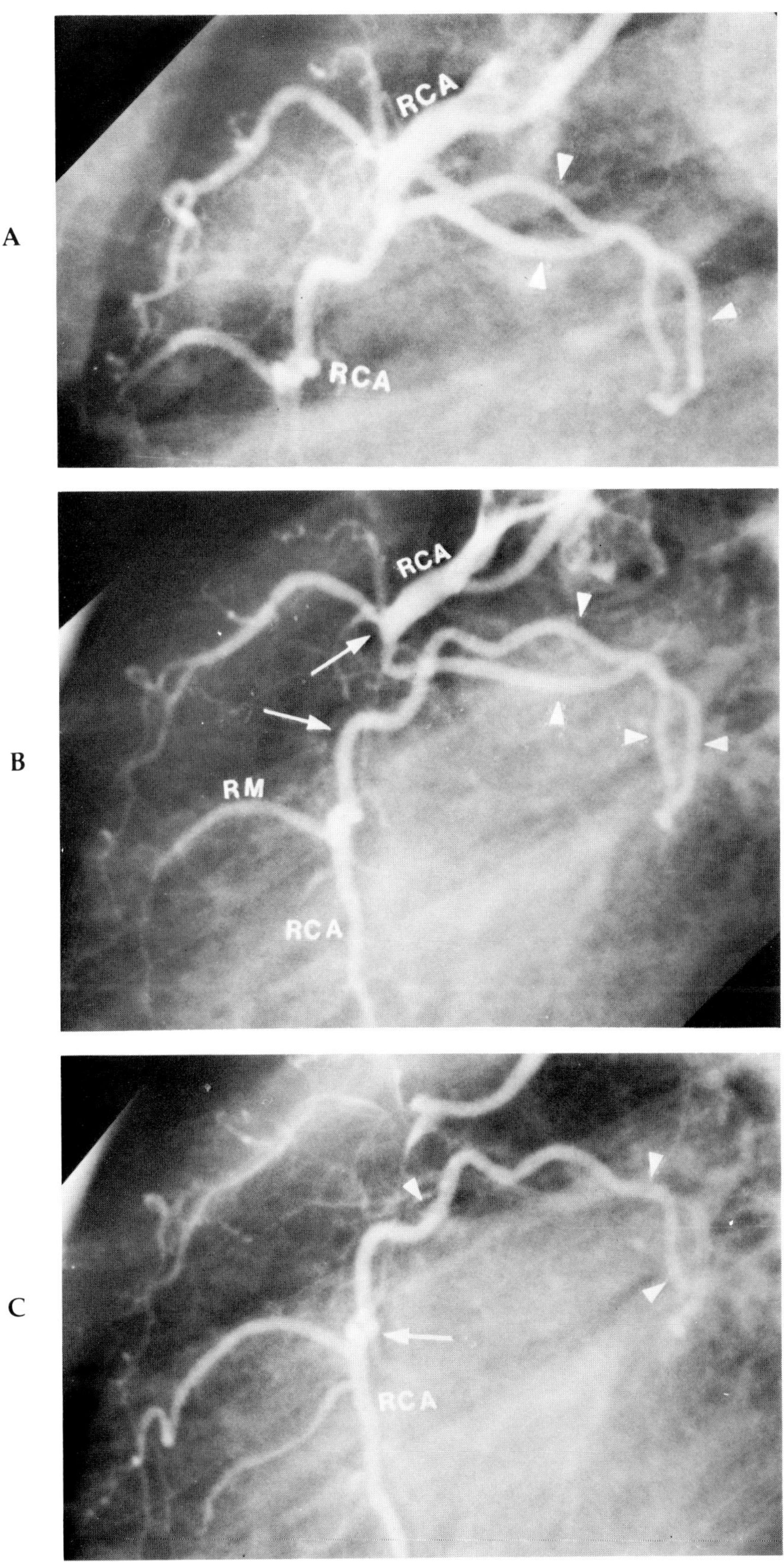

FIGURE 10.22

Figure 10.23: Right coronary arteriogram in two different patients both in left anterior oblique projection.

A. The right coronary (RCA) is totally occluded in its distal portion. The arteria anastomotica auricularis magna (AAM) Kugel's artery, (pointers) provides collateral filling of the distal right coronary artery (DRCA).

B. The right coronary artery (RCA) is occluded proximally (pointer) and intracoronary collateral circulation fills the middle and distal portions of the right coronary artery (between the arrows) up to a second obstruction. Collateral flow through the arteria anastomotica auricularis magna (AAM) (pointers) fills the distal right coronary artery (DRCA, lowermost arrow).

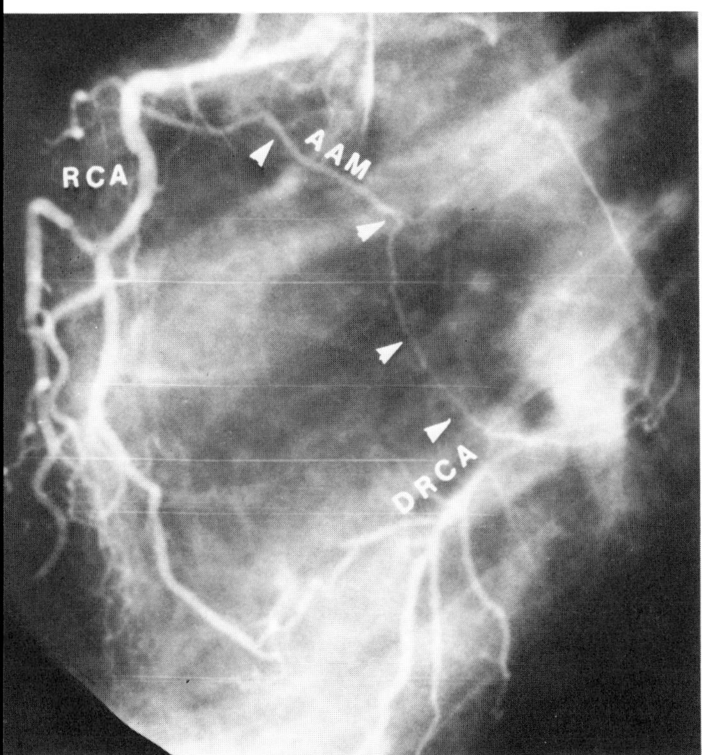

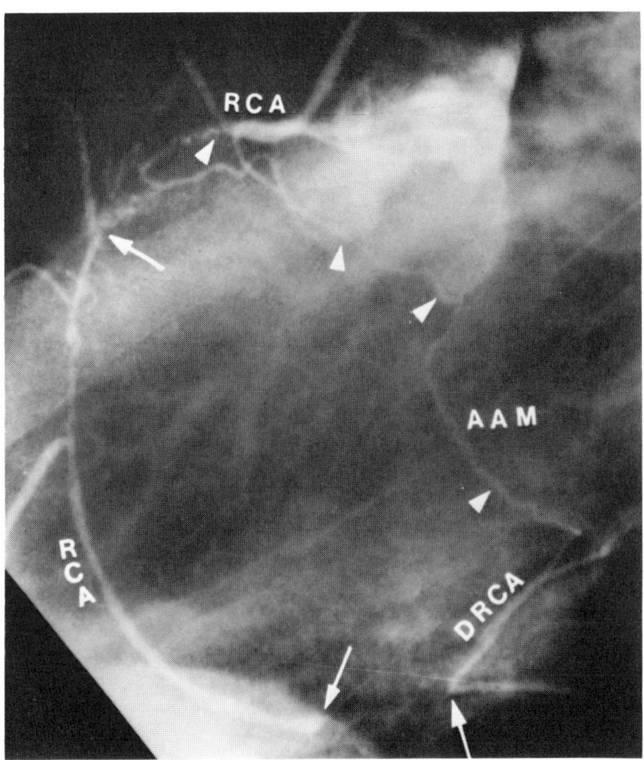

A   **FIGURE 10.23**   B

Figure 10.24: Left coronary arteriogram; **A.** Lateral projection; **B.** Left anterior oblique projection, in the same patient. In a patient with total occlusion of the right coronary artery the left anterior descending artery (LAD) provides inter-coronary collateral channels over the right ventricle to the right coronary artery (pointers). The left anterior descending has a high grade proximal stenosis after the origin of the diagonal (D) and septal (S) arteries. In **B**, there is filling of the middle and distal portions of the right coronary artery (RCA). This is an example of unusual collateralization from the left anterior descending artery over the anterior wall of the right ventricle to the right coronary artery.

DRCA = distal right coronary artery. CX = left circumflex artery. LM = left marginal branch of circumflex artery.

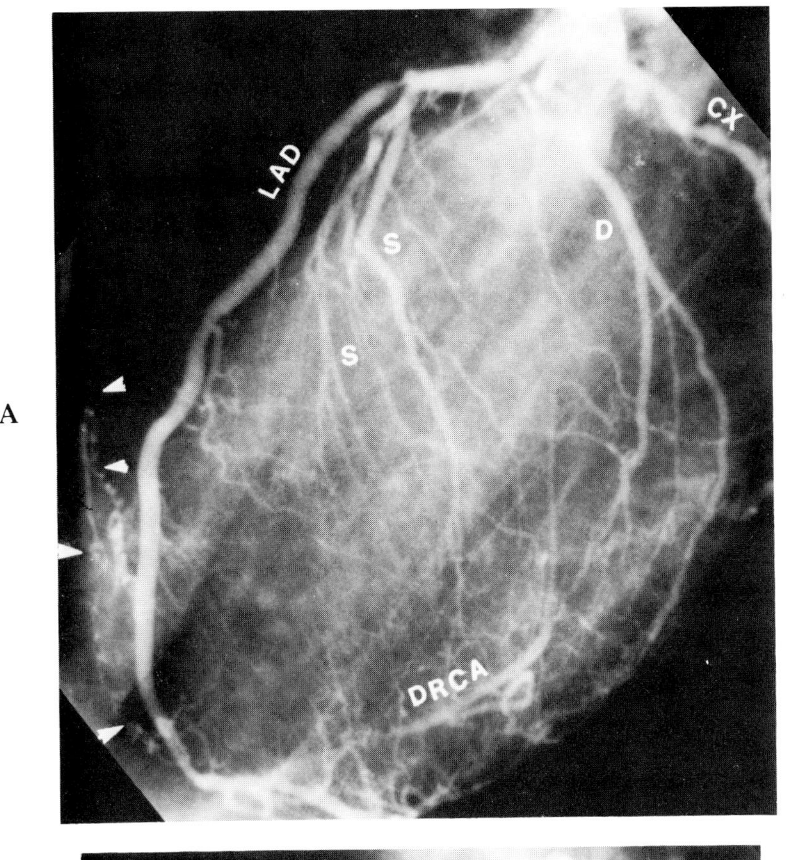

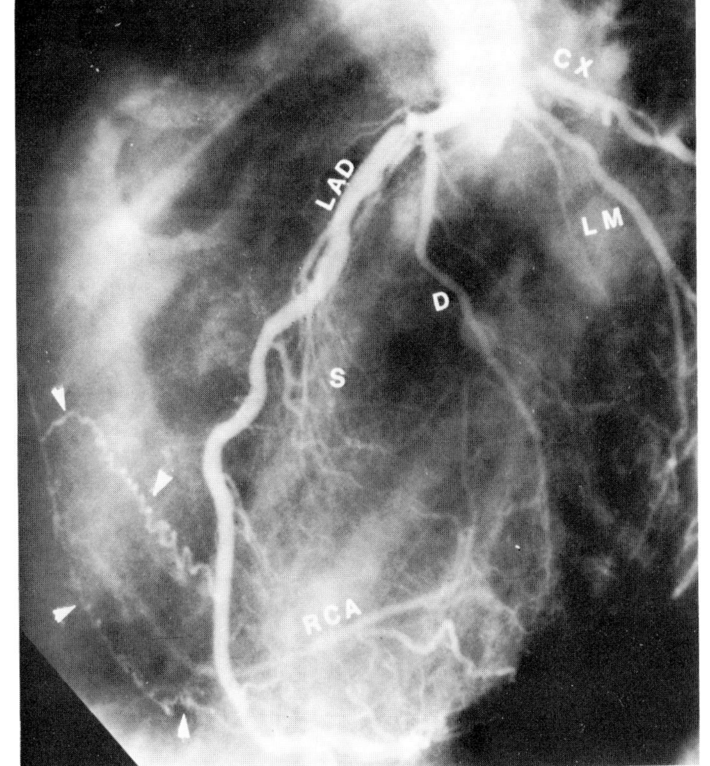

FIGURE 10.24

Chapter 11

Coronary Anatomy in Left Ventricular Aneurysm

A left ventricular aneurysm may develop following acute myocardial infarction. In a large series of hearts examined at necropsy of patients who had sustained remote or recent myocardial infarction, the incidence of left ventricular aneurysm, as defined by strict pathologic criteria, was 3.5%.[1] The majority of these aneurysms were located on the anterior and/or apical surface of the left ventricle (Figures 11.1, 11.3).

The standard chest x-ray in the posterior-anterior and lateral projections is not adequate for detecting aneurysms of the left ventricle, especially if they are inferior in location. Left ventricular angiography is most useful and the angiographic characteristics of a left ventricular aneurysm have been well defined.[2] Akinetic or dyskinetic segments (Figure 11.1) of left ventricle usually correlate best with areas of myocardium which are thinned and replaced by fibrous tissue.

Since left ventricular aneurysm is most commonly associated with coronary artery disease, arteriography is essential for complete evaluation of patients with proven or suspected aneurysm. Post-mortem and ante-mortem angiographic studies usually show severe coronary artery disease which may be extensive or confined to the artery supplying the segment of the myocardium replaced by the aneurysm. Occasionally, however, the coronary arteriograms may fail to detect any coronary disease.[3]

The anatomic distribution and the angiographic appearance of the coronary arteries frequently suggest the presence of an aneurysm. There may be a marked paucity of arteries over the site of the aneurysm (Figure 11.2); the vessels may be sharply cut-off, or end abruptly (Figure 11.2); absence or a marked decrease in angiographically detectable collateral circulation may be apparent (Figures 11.2, 1.4); the branches of the major arteries may be quite prominent, but vessels over the aneurysm and at its borders will frequently appear quite small or delicate (Figure 11.4); finally, the major vessels frequently will appear to branch at very wide angles to each other (Figure 11.4).

In this chapter two examples of left ventricular aneurysm with the associated coronary arteriograms are shown.

References

1.   Dubnow, M.H., Burchell, H.B., and Titus, J.L.: Postinfarction ventricular aneurysm: A clinicomorphologic and electrocardiographic study of 80 cases. *American Heart Journal,* **70**:753-760, 1965.
2.   Gorlin, R., Klein, M.D., and Sullivan, J.M.: Prospective correlative study of ventricular aneurysm: Mechanistic concept and clinical recognition. *American Journal of Medicine,* **42**:512-531, 1967
3.   Greenberg, H. and Dwyer, E.M. Jr.: Myocardial infarction and ventricular aneurysm in a patient with normal coronary arteries. *Chest,* **66**:306-308, 1974.

Figure 11.1:   Left ventricular angiogram, A-P projection: **A.** Diastole; **B.** Systole (different magnification). The left ventricular aneurysm in the patient whose coronary arteriograms are shown in Figure 11.2, is demonstrated by the pointers and arrows. The aneurysm is anterolateral and apical.

The oblong radioopaque marker near the center of **A** and upper middle in **B** is the central x-ray beam marker.

AO = aorta. LV = left ventricle.

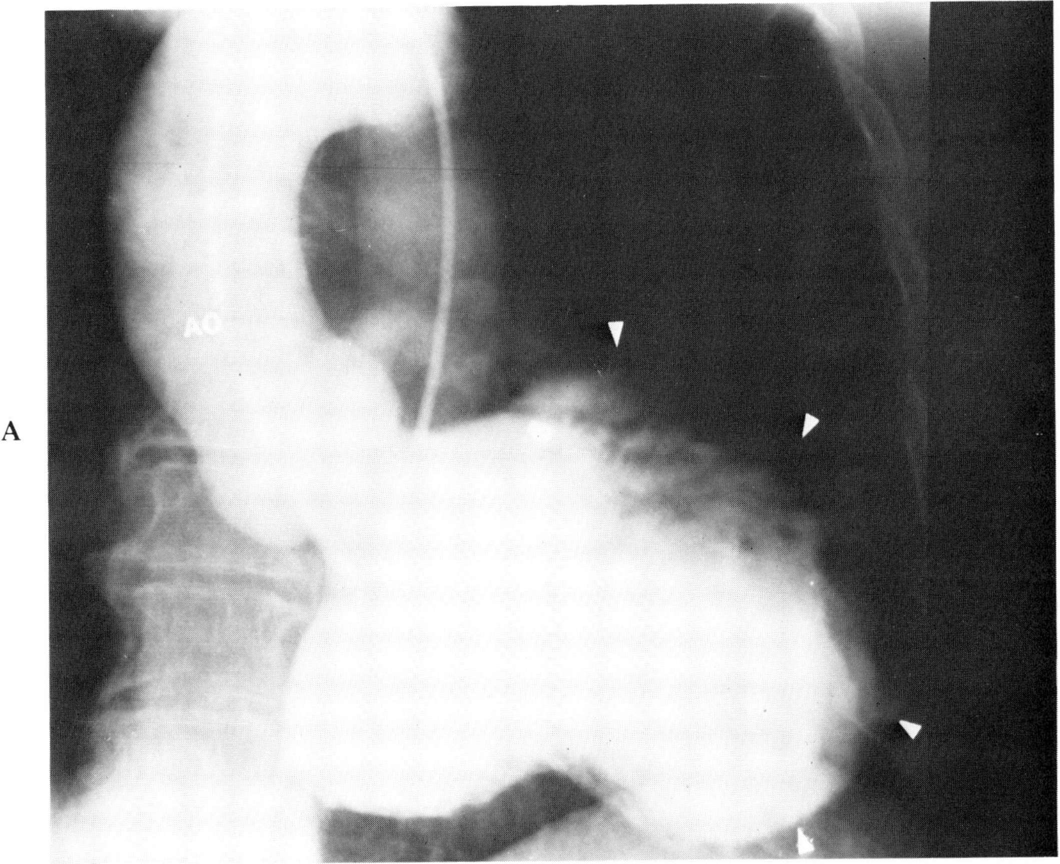

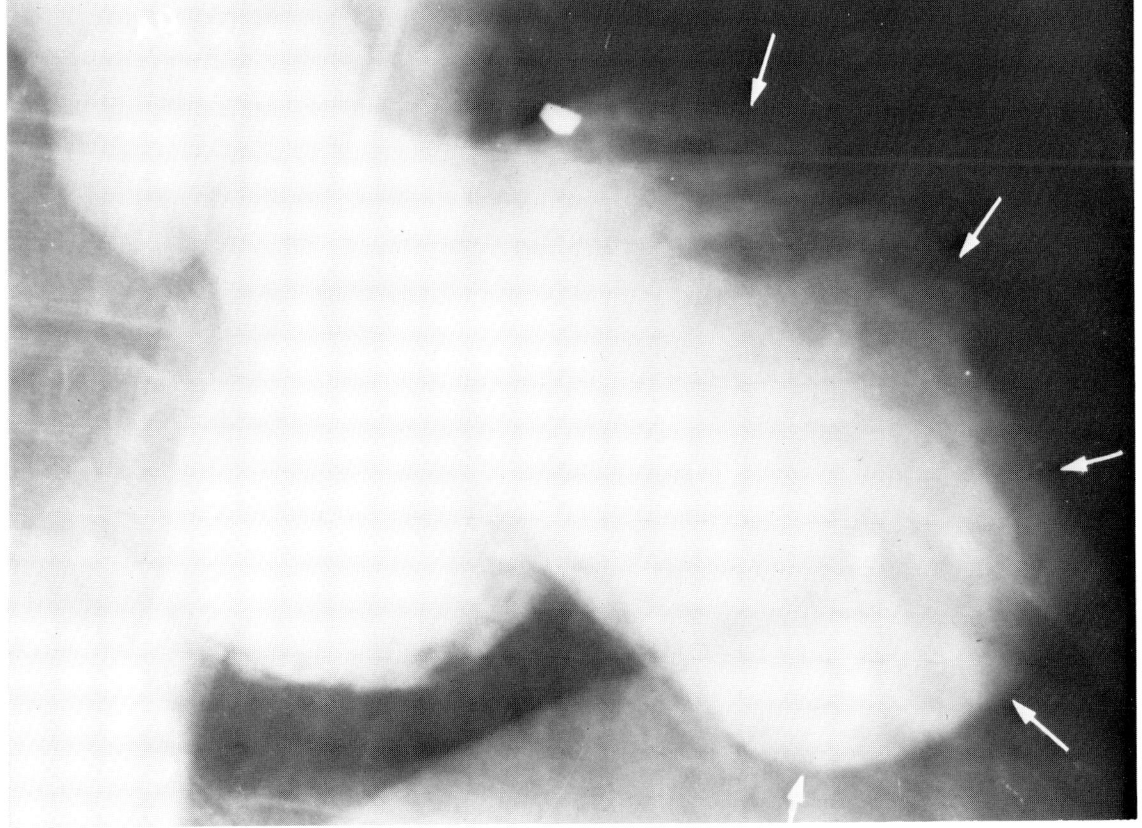

FIGURE 11.1

Figure 11.2:   Left and right coronary arteriograms in patient with left ventricular aneurysm.

A. Left coronary arteriogram; lateral projection. Complete occlusion of the left anterior descending artery (arrow). There is a network of collateral vessels from the left marginal artery (LM), but opacification of the distal left anterior descending artery is not achieved.

B. Right coronary arteriogram; lateral projection. The right coronary artery (RCA) is normal. Collateral flow from the septal (S) branches of the posterior descending artery fill branches of the left anterior descending artery (LAD). Again it is difficult to identify the main channel of the left anterior descending artery as its branches are pruned.

CX = left circumflex artery. RM = right marginal branch of right coronary artery.

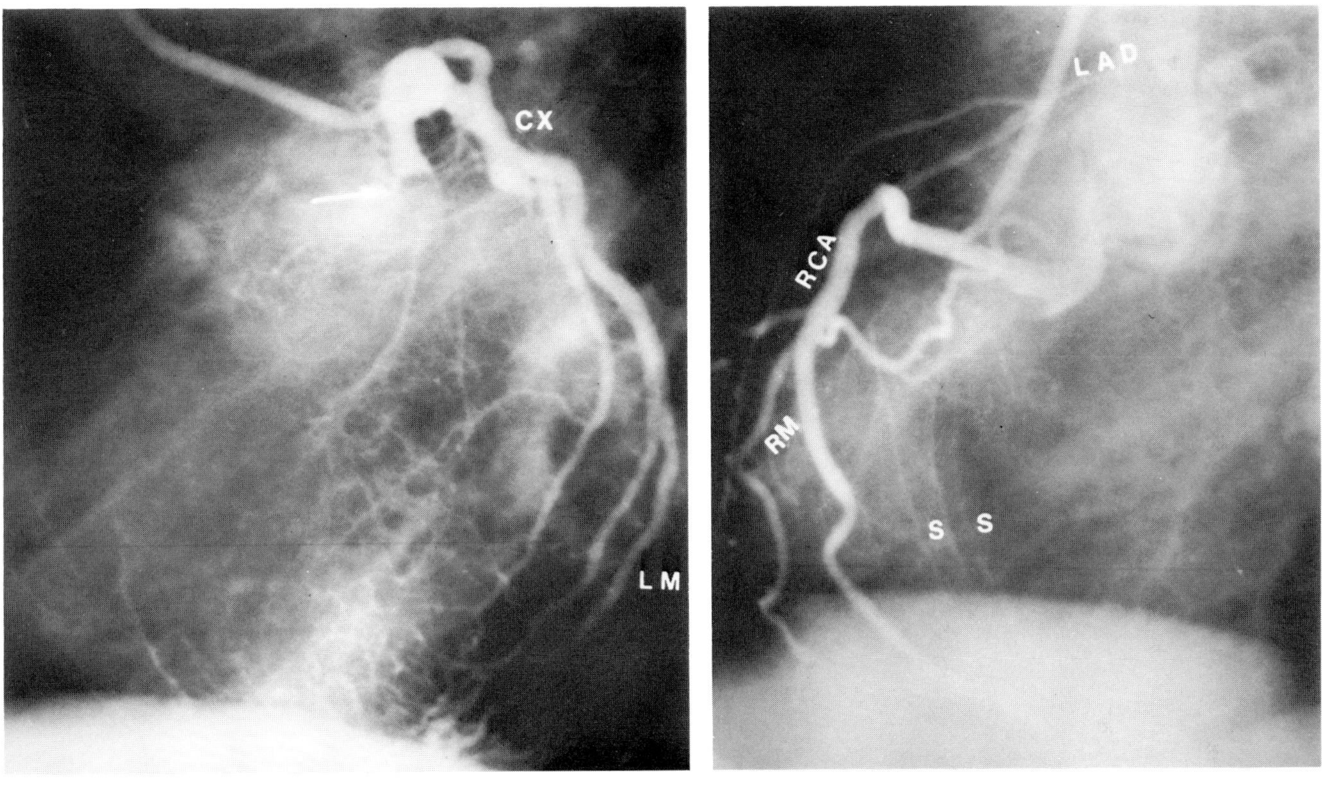

A   **FIGURE 11.2**   B

Figure 11.3:   Left ventricular angiogram, lateral projection: **A**. Diastole; **B**. Systole. This is the left ventricular aneurysm in the patient whose left coronary arteriogram is shown in Figure 11.4. The aneurysm is demonstrated by the arrows and is anterior and apical.

AO = aorta. LV = left ventricle.

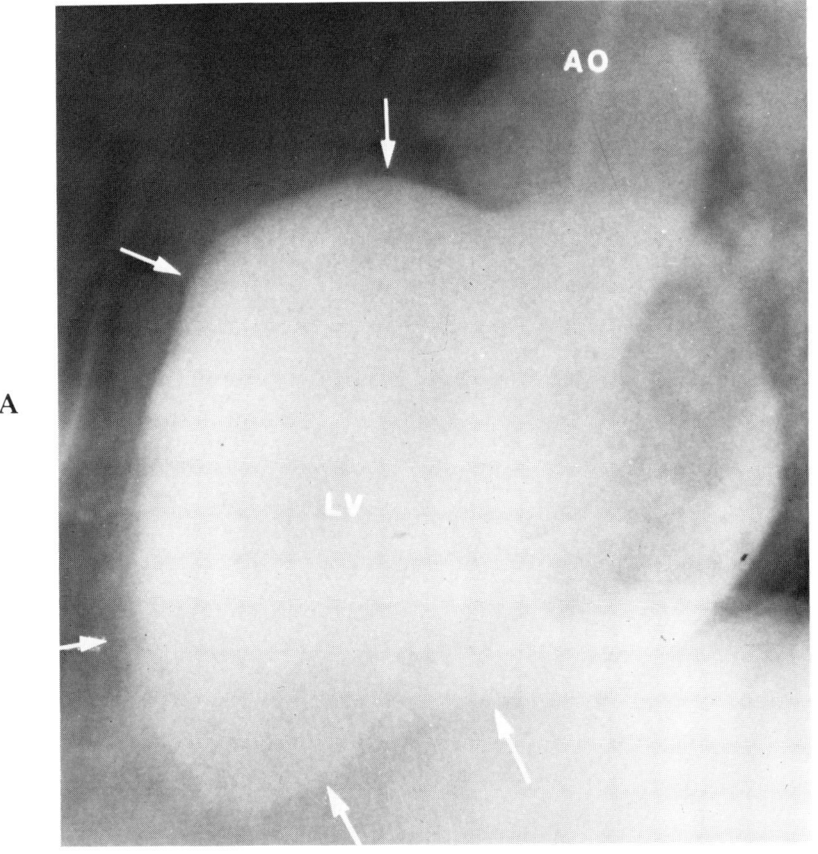

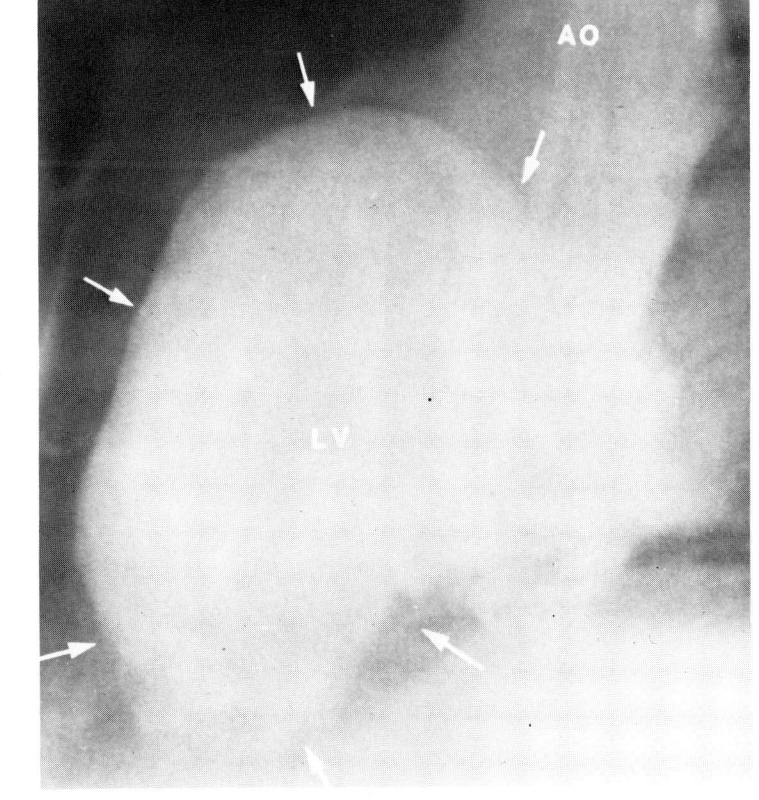

FIGURE 11.3

Figure 11.4:   Left coronary arteriogram in patient with a left ventricular aneurysm; **A**. Right anterior oblique projection; **B**. Left anterior oblique projection; **C**. Lateral projection.

A. There is a severe stenosis (70-90%) at the origin of the left anterior descending coronary artery (LAD, arrow). Distal to this stenosis there are two size "C" vessels lying on the anterior wall of the left ventricle. These vessels are elongated and appear pruned of their branches. The distal left anterior descending artery is difficult to identify. The left circumflex artery (CX) is normal and gives off three left marginal branches (LM) before giving off the posterior descending artery (PDA). The left system is dominant.

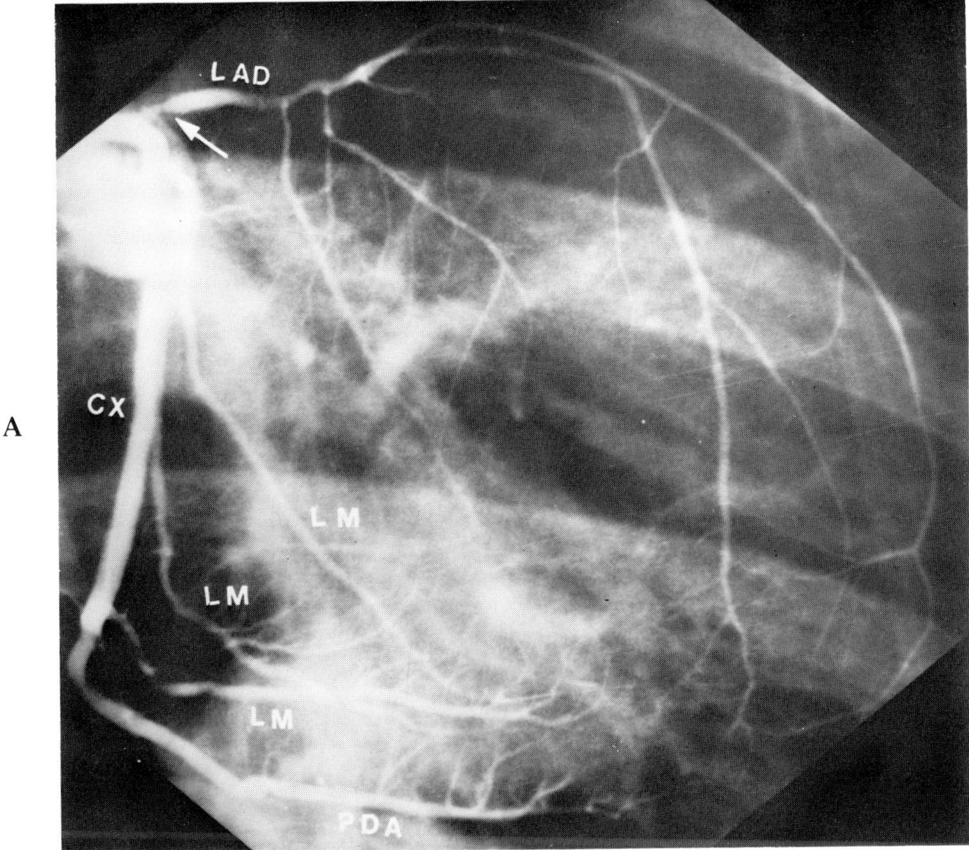

FIGURE 11.4

Figure 11.4:   **B.** In this projection the LAD appears to stretch over the aneurysm.

C. The elongated vessel lying anteriorly is assumed to be the left anterior descending artery (LAD).

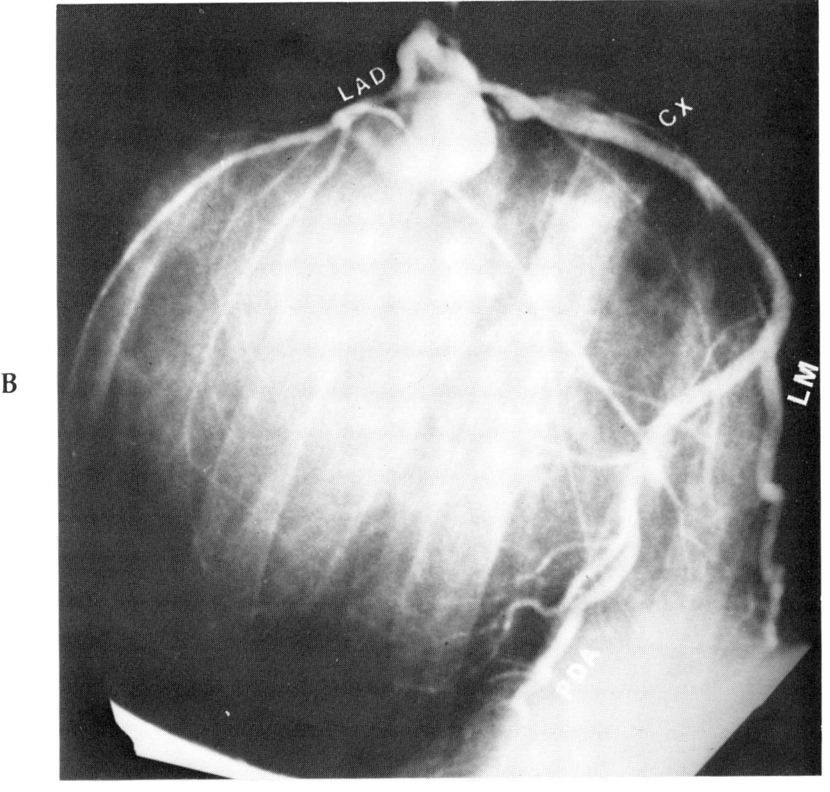

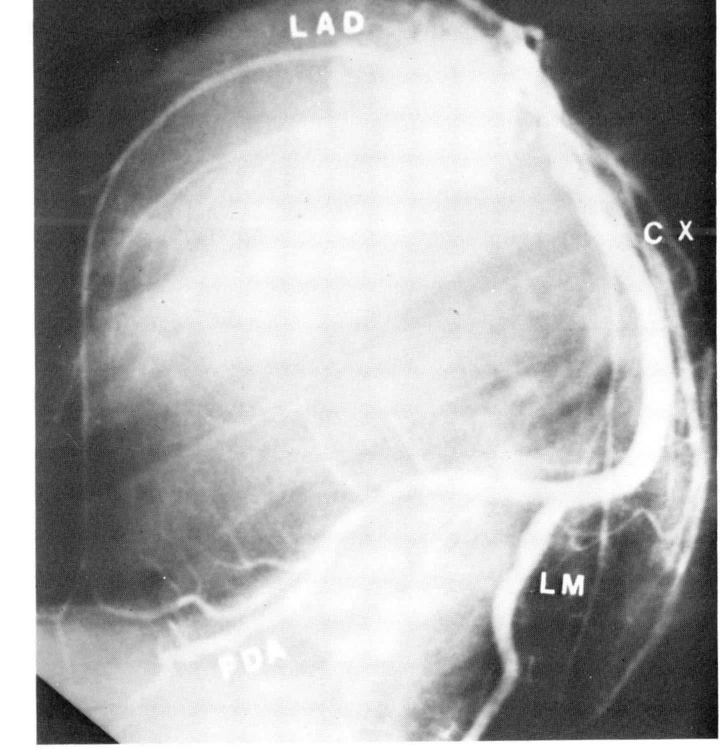

FIGURE 11.4

Chapter 12

Saphenous Vein Bypass Grafts

Post-operative evaluation of patients with coronary artery disease who have received aortocoronary saphenous vein bypass grafts frequently includes coronary arteriography and saphenous vein graft visualization. The angiographic study of such patients requires some modification in technique.[1]

The percutaneous transfemoral approach is utilized. A pigtail left ventricular catheter is introduced first and aortic and left ventricular pressures measured. Left ventricular biplane angiography is then performed at 6 frames per second for five seconds following injection of 60 ml of sodium and meglumine diatrizoates (Renografin®). The exposed film is then processed while angiography of the native coronary circulation is performed in the usual manner. The left ventriculogram provides visualization of a significant portion of the ascending aorta and provides information as to the location of the aorto-saphenous vein anastomoses and patency of the grafts (Figure 12.1). Since the film is immediately processed this information is available when coronary arteriography is completed and selected saphenous vein angiography is begun.

Visualization of the native coronary circulation is performed by selective injection of the left coronary artery first. Then following right coronary arteriography the preformed right coronary catheter is available for selective opacification of the saphenous vein grafts. This method will thus decrease the number of catheter changes required to complete the study. The preformed right coronary catheter is usually adequate for catheterizing the grafts to the left anterior descending coronary artery and the left circumflex or left circumflex marginal arteries. Catheterization of the right coronary artery may require the use of a special bypass catheter.

In our experience we have found it most useful to place the patient in the lateral position when searching for the site of the aorto-saphenous vein anastomosis. Once the catheter is at the orifice of the saphenous vein graft, the projections utilized for selective opacification of the graft are as previously described for the coronary arteries. Special care must be taken to visualize the entire graft in order to detect any abnormalities at its origin, at the site of anastomosis with the coronary artery and in its course.

Saphenous vein grafts to the left anterior descending coronary artery and the left circumflex artery usualy originate from the left side of the ascending aorta, close to the pulmonary artery. They course anteriorly almost perpendicular to the aorta, and curve around the pulmonary artery. At this point the graft to the left anterior descending coronary artery courses anteriorly and the graft to the left circumflex artery, or its marginal branch, curves posteriorly (Figure 12.1).

The graft to the left anterior descending coronary artery is anastomosed to the aorta most superiorly, followed by the anastomotic site of the left circumflex graft. The graft to the right coronary artery is anastomosed to the ascending aorta only 2−5 centimeters above the origin of the right coronary artery, and is thus in the lowest position on the ascending aorta. It runs inferiorly along the right side of the cardiac silhouette as it courses to its distal anastomosis with the right coronary or posterior descending artery.

Characteristics of properly functioning grafts have been well described.[1] The graft size should be proportional to that of the grafted vessel at the anastomotic site and the opacification of the native coronary artery should be complete (Figures 12.2-12.6). Retrograde filling of the grafted vessel to its point of obstruction (Figures 12.3-12.5, 12.7 A, 12.8 C, 12.9 B), retrograde filling of non-grafted vessels (Figures 12.8 C) and collateral filling of non-operated diseased vessels (Figures 12.2, 12.4, 12.7, 12.9 B, 12.10 B) also are findings frequently observed in patients with grafts which are functioning well.

Although found to be patent, grafts may nevertheless function poorly. The size of the graft may be too large for the lumen of the grafted vessel (Figure 12.10) and a stenosis may be present. Most commonly stenosis of a graft occurs at its distal anastomotic site. Other signs of a poorly functioning graft are persistence of contrast agent in the graft and, of course, poor distal opacification of the grafted artery. A totally occluded graft may be demonstrated by a small "dimple" at the site of the aortic anastomosis.

Study of the native circulation also provides important information concerning graft function. Frequently there is no opacification or poor opacification of the grafted vessel distal to its stenosis (Figure 12.11). This is due to predominant flow of non-opacified blood from a well functioning graft to its artery. Occasionally reflux into the graft is observed (Figures 12.8 A, 12.11, 12.12) and may signify poor flow through the graft. An unchanged pattern of flow through the coronary circulation may signify poor function or occlusion of the saphenous vein grafts. Progression of coronary artery disease (Figure 12.13) may be observed in patients with patent grafts.

Proper and complete post-operative angiographic evaluation of patients who have received saphenous vein bypass grafts includes left ventricular angiography, coronary arteriography and selective saphenous vein graft visualization.

Reference

1.   Rösch, J., Judkins, M.P., Green, G.S., and Kidd, H.: Aortocoronary venous bypass grafts: Angiographic study of 84 cases. *Radiology,* **102**:567-573, 1972.

Figure 12.1:   Biplane left ventricular angiogram in patient with three saphenous vein bypass grafts. **A**. Anterior-posterior projection. **C**. Lateral projection.

A. The graft to the left anterior descending artery (1) and the left circumflex artery (2) are demonstrated coming to the left of the ascending aorta (AO) and anterior to the main pulmonary artery.

C. All three grafts are visualized. The graft to the left anterior descending artery (1) originates in the most cephalic position. The graft to the left circumflex artery (2) originates just below the graft to the left anterior descending artery. Both of these grafts initially run parallel to the ascending aorta but then diverge, with graft to the left anterior descending artery curving anteriorly and the graft to the left circumflex artery curving posteriorly. The graft to the right coronary artery (3) originates just above the right coronary sinus of Valsalva and curves anteriorly and inferiorly.

LV = left ventricle.

B. Diagrammatic representation of **A**.

D. Diagrammatic representation of **C**.

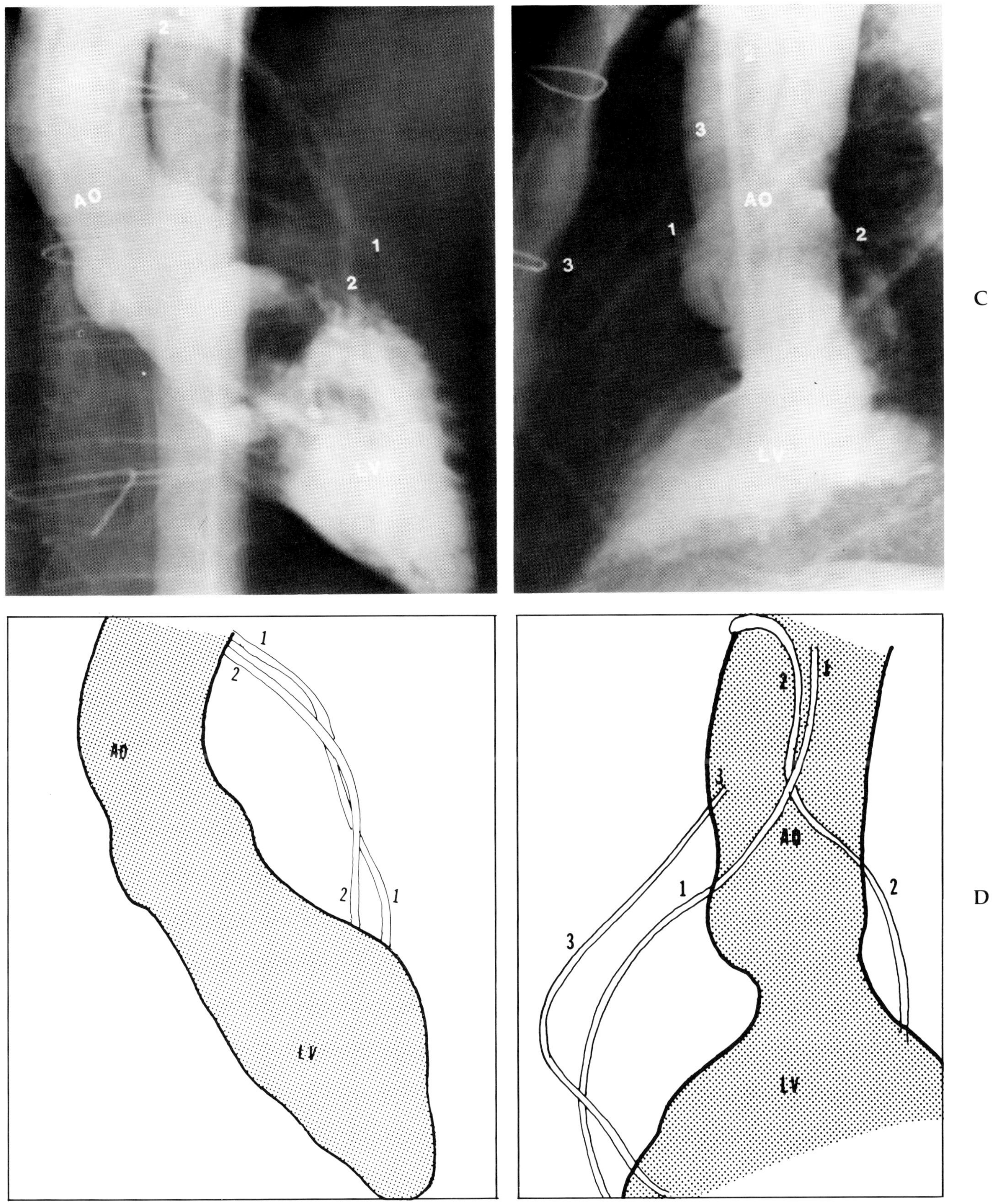

FIGURE 12.1

Figure 12.2:   Saphenous vein graft, aorta to left anterior descending coronary artery (LAD). **A**. Right anterior oblique projection and **B**. Lateral projection, in the same patient. The graft anastomoses with the middle of the LAD and there is good continuity between graft and artery (arrow). There is a well developed collateral system through the septals (S) to the posterior descending coronary artery, (PDA). There is no retrograde flow into the proximal one-third of the LAD.

G = graft.

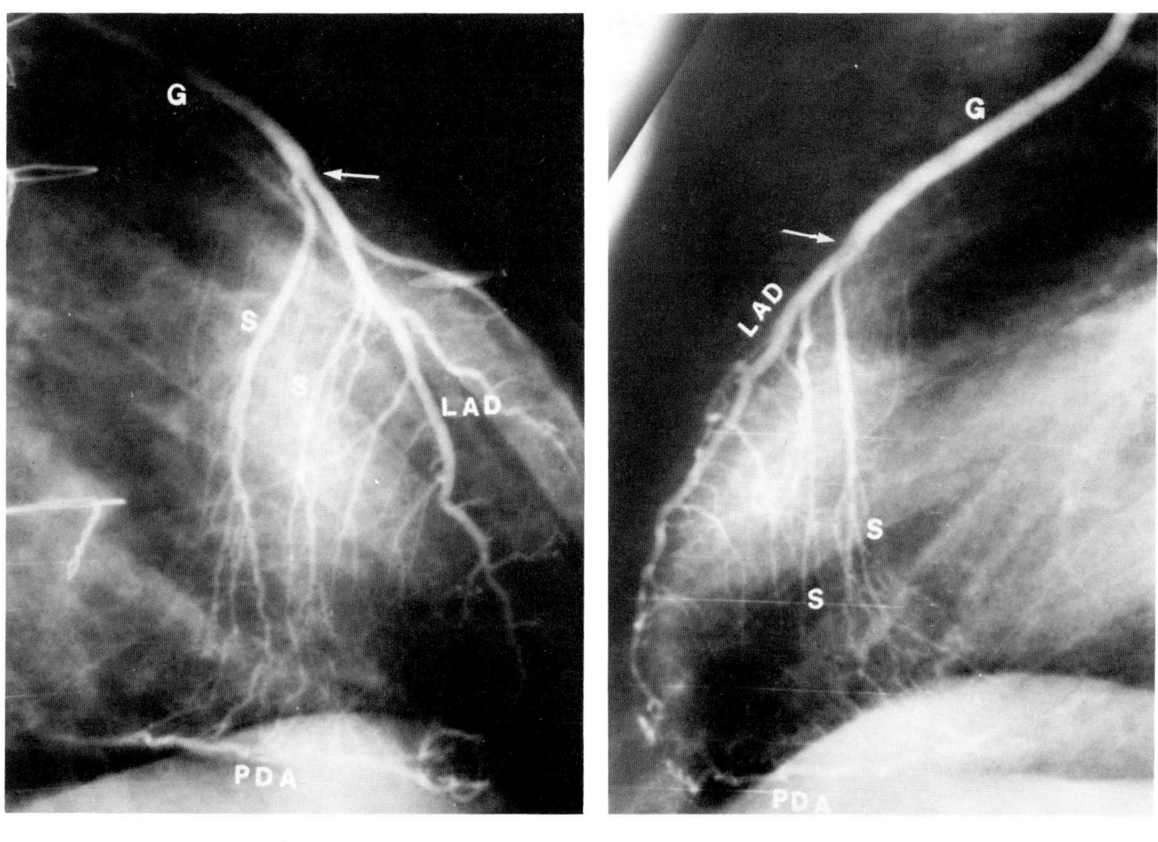

A   FIGURE 12.2   B

Figure 12.3:   Saphenous vein graft, aorta to left anterior descending coronary artery. **A.** Lateral projection and **B.** Left anterior oblique projection, in the same patient. Both projections demonstrate antegrade flow into the distal left anterior descending artery (LAD) as well as retrograde flow into the proximal LAD and its septal (S) and diagonal (D) branches. In **B** the site of anastomosis is well visualized (arrow).

G = graft.

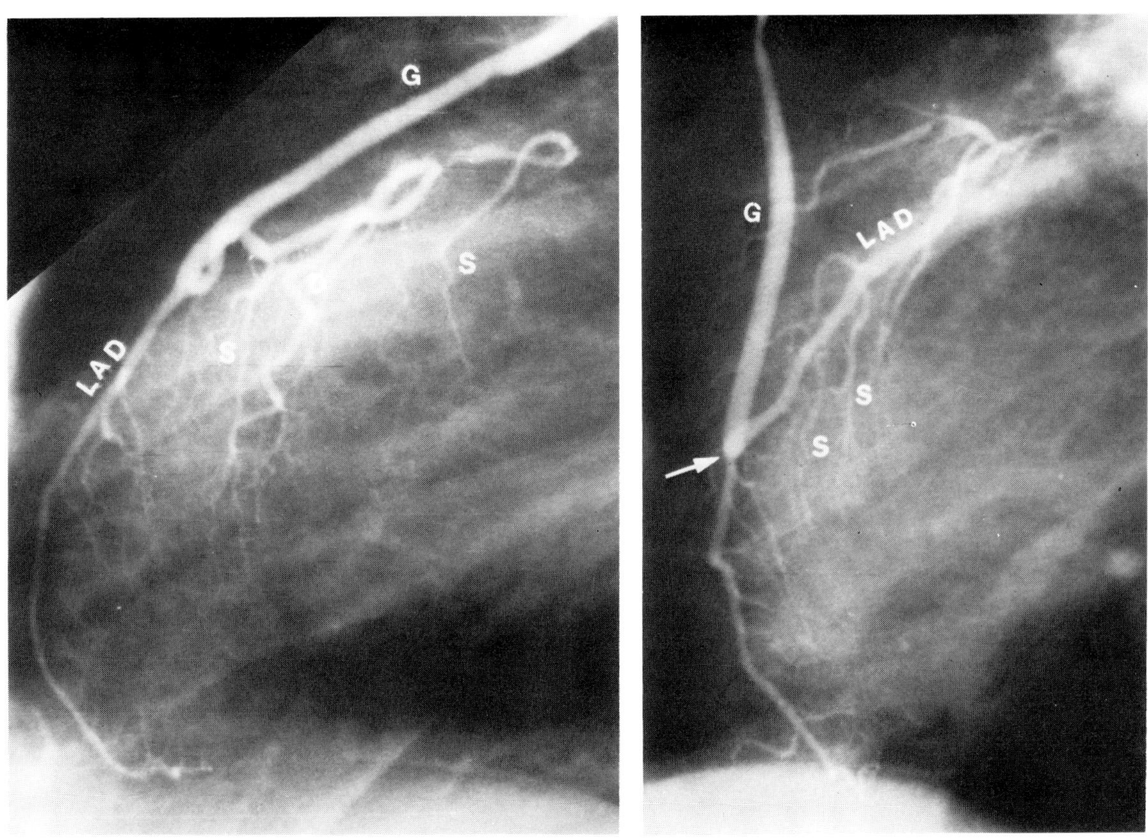

A   **FIGURE 12.3**   B

Figure 12.4:   Saphenous vein graft, aorta to right coronary in a patient with a completely occluded right coronary artery. Right anterior oblique projection. **A.** Early phase; **B.** Later phase.

A. The well opacified graft (G) fills the proximal right coronary artery (RCA) and the posterior descending artery (PDA).

B. The graft (G) is now only partially opacified but there is better visualization of the right coronary (RCA) and posterior descending (PDA) arteries. There is also visualization of the left anterior descending (LAD) and circumflex (CX) arteries indicating a well developed collateral network. This is a good example of a patent and effective graft.

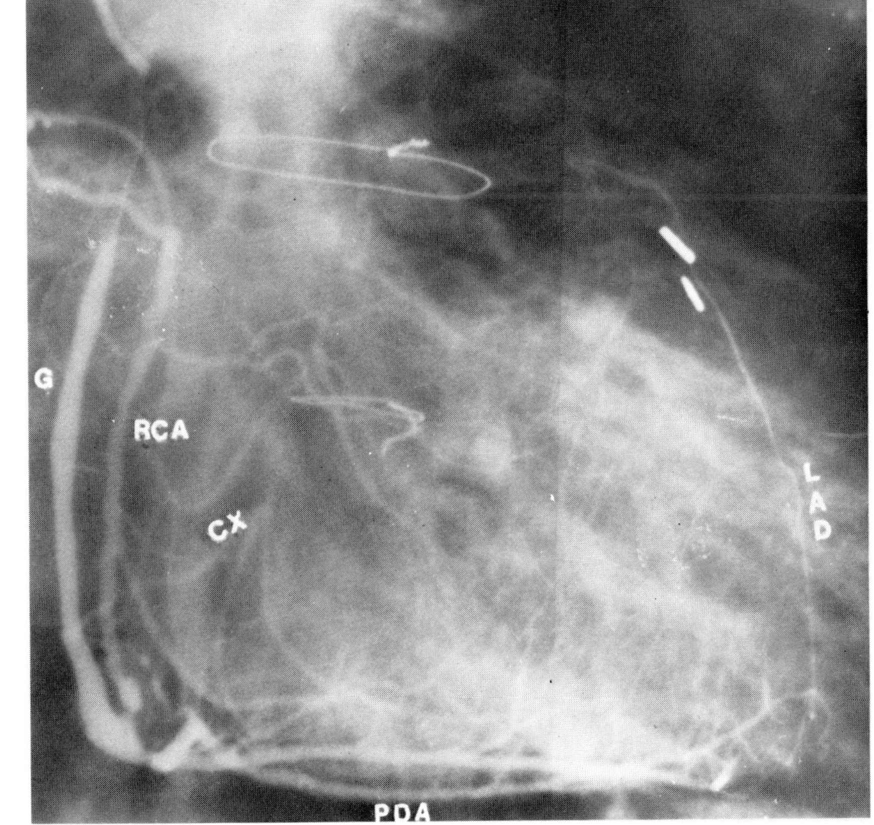

FIGURE 12.4

Figure 12.5:   Saphenous vein graft, aorta to right coronary artery.

A. Lateral projection. A patent graft (G) anastomoses to the right ventricular marginal branch. The posterior descending (PDA) and distal right coronary arteries (DRCA) fill via this anastomosis.

B. Diagrammatic representation of **A**.

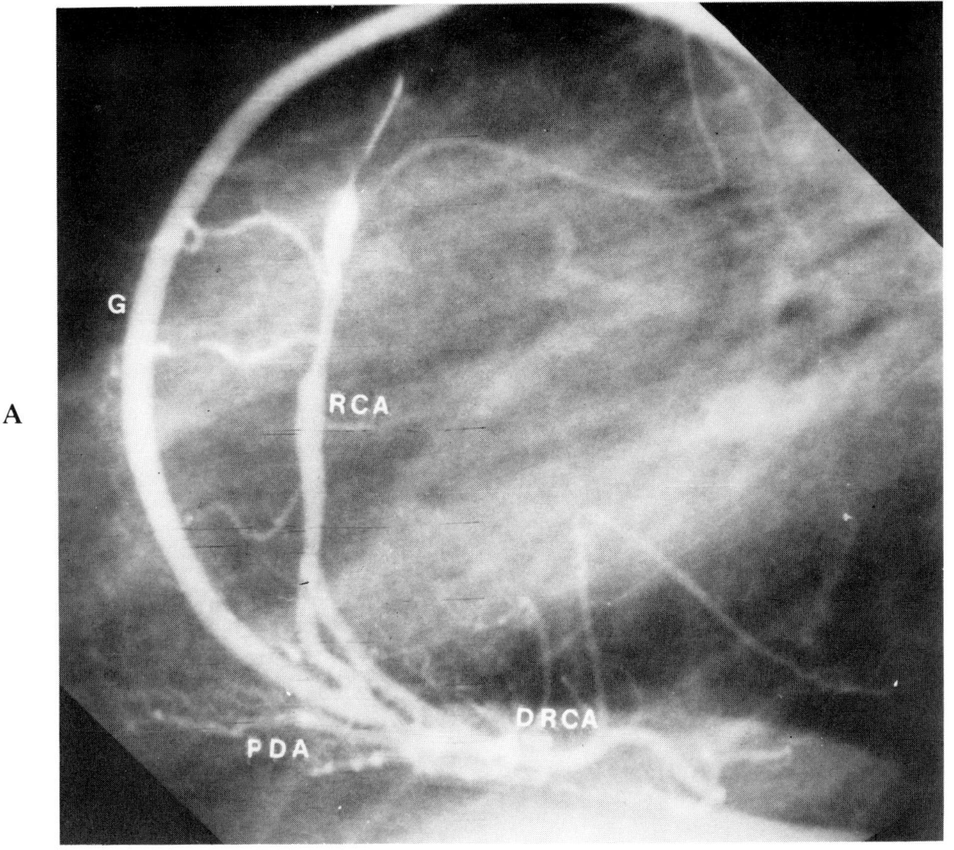

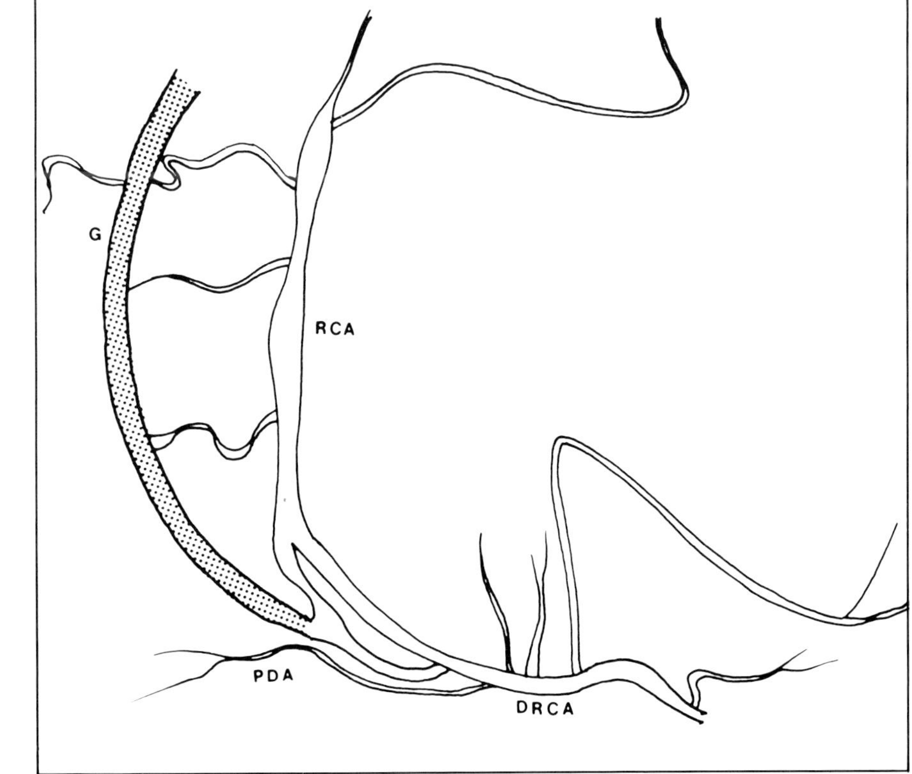

FIGURE 12.5

Figure 12.6:   Saphenous vein graft, aorta to right coronary artery in patient with a totally occluded right coronary artery. Left anterior oblique projection. The patent graft (G) which is nearly equal in size to the right coronary artery provides optimal flow to its distal branches. The distal right coronary artery (DRCA) is an unusually long vessel extending well into the left atrioventricular sulcus (arrows). Retrograde flow into the proximal right coronary artery was not demonstrated.

AV = atrioventricular node branch of right coronary artery. PDA = posterior descending branch of right coronary artery.

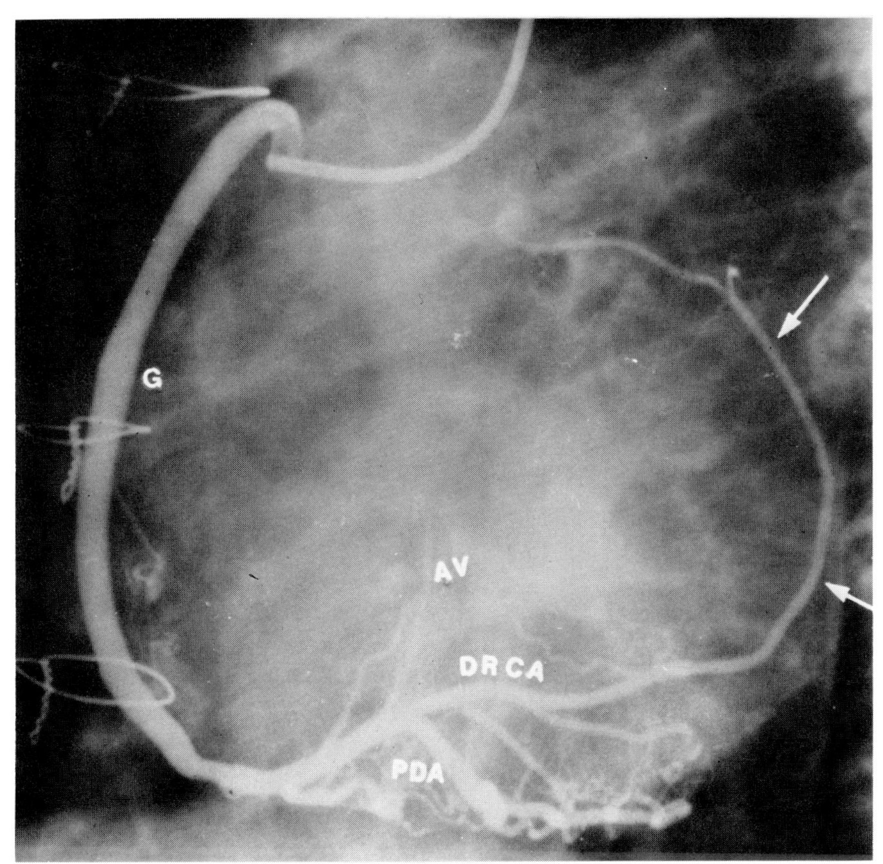

FIGURE 12.6

Figure 12.7:   Saphenous vein graft, aorta to left marginal branch of the circumflex artery. **A** and **B** in left anterior oblique projection in two patients.

A. The graft (G) supplies flow to the left marginal artery (LM) and by retrograde flow to the left circumflex artery (CX). There is a large collateral network from the circumflex artery to the distal right coronary artery (DRCA).

B. In this patient the graft (G) fills the left marginal artery (LM) only. There is no retrograde flow and collateral networks are not demonstrated.

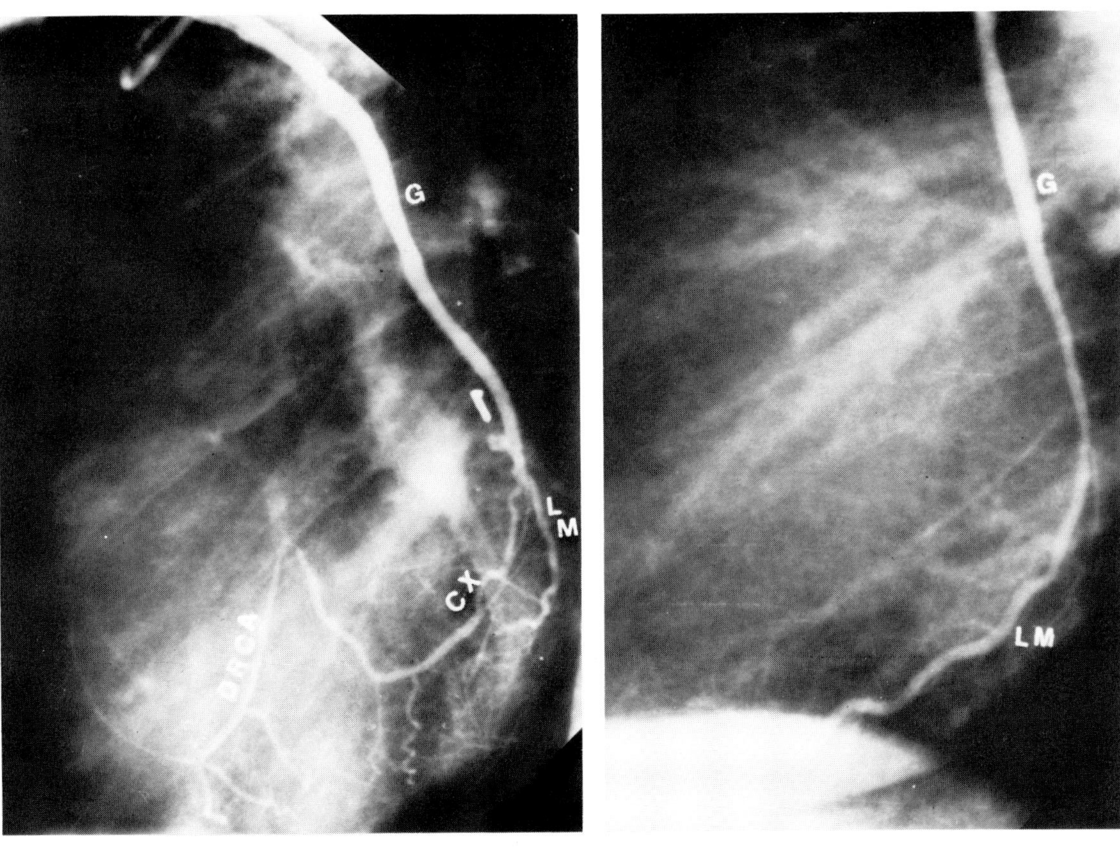

A   FIGURE 12.7   B

Figure 12.8:   **A**. Left coronary arteriogram, left anterior oblique projection; **C**. Saphenous vein graft, aorta to left marginal branch of the left circumflex artery, in the same patient.

A. Injection of contrast material into the left main coronary artery demonstrates retrograde filling of the graft (G) to the left marginal artery (LM). Well demonstrated is the significant (70-90%) stenosis (arrow) of the left main coronary artery as well as good opacification of the left anterior descending artery (LAD), its septal (S) and diagonal (D) branches and the left circumflex artery (CX).

C. Injection of contrast material into the graft (G) to the left marginal artery demonstrates antegrade filling of the left marginal artery (LM) but also marked retrograde flow to the left circumflex (CX), left main coronary artery (arrow) and left anterior descending (LAD) arteries. These angiograms demonstrate bi-directional flow of blood in the arteries and the graft.

B. Diagrammatic representation of **A**.

D. Diagrammatic representation of **C**.

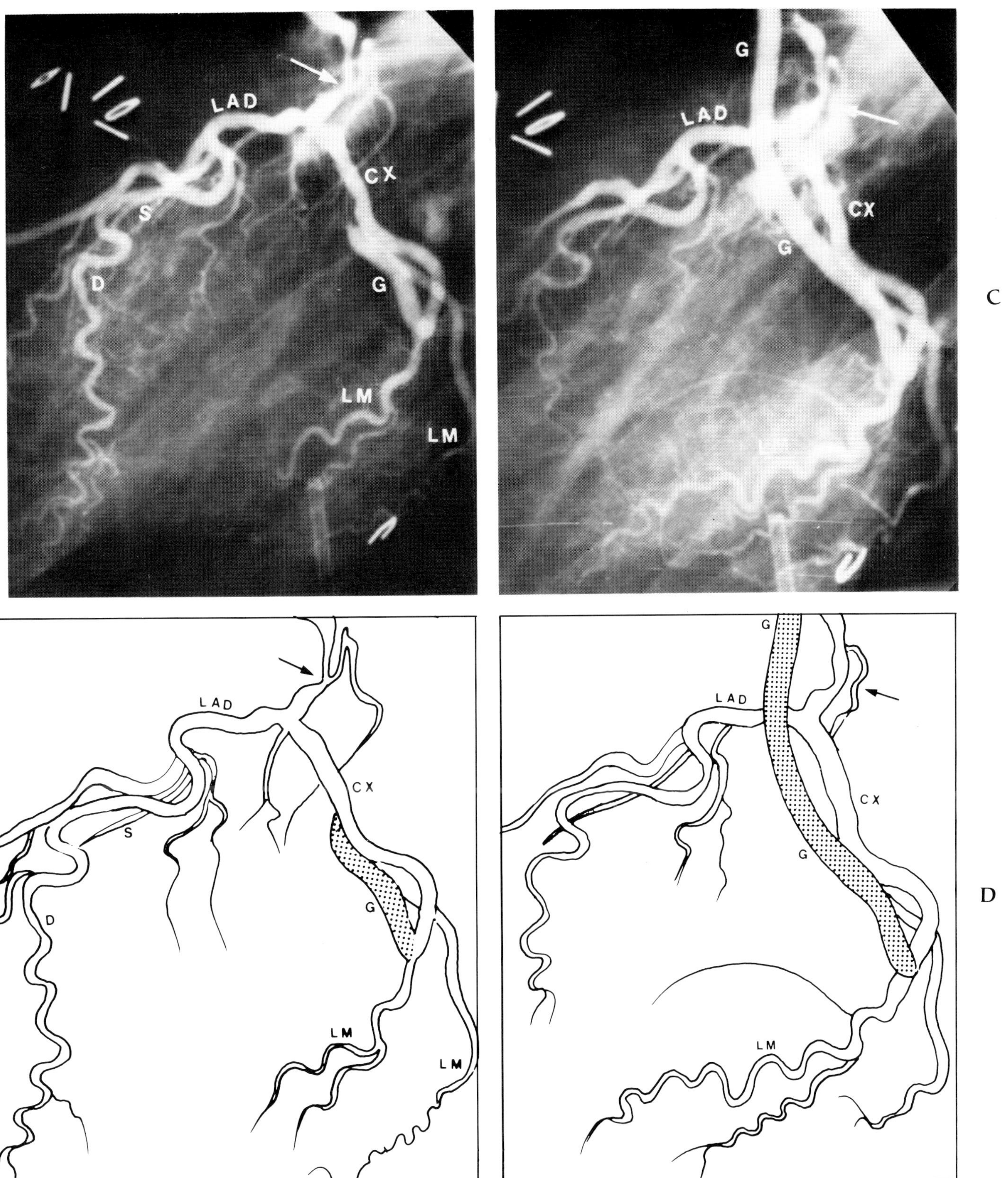

FIGURE 12.8

Figure 12.9:   Saphenous vein graft, aorta to right coronary artery in a patient with a totally occluded right coronary artery. Lateral projection. **A** and **B** shows two phases of the cardiac cycle. In **A** the patent graft (G) overlaps the proximal right coronary artery. In **B** the proximal right coronary artery (RCA), the distal right coronary artery (DRCA) and the posterior descending (PDA) arteries are well filled and easily visualized. The sinus node artery (SN) fills from the retrograde flow and the left circumflex artery (CX) fills via collaterals from the DRCA.

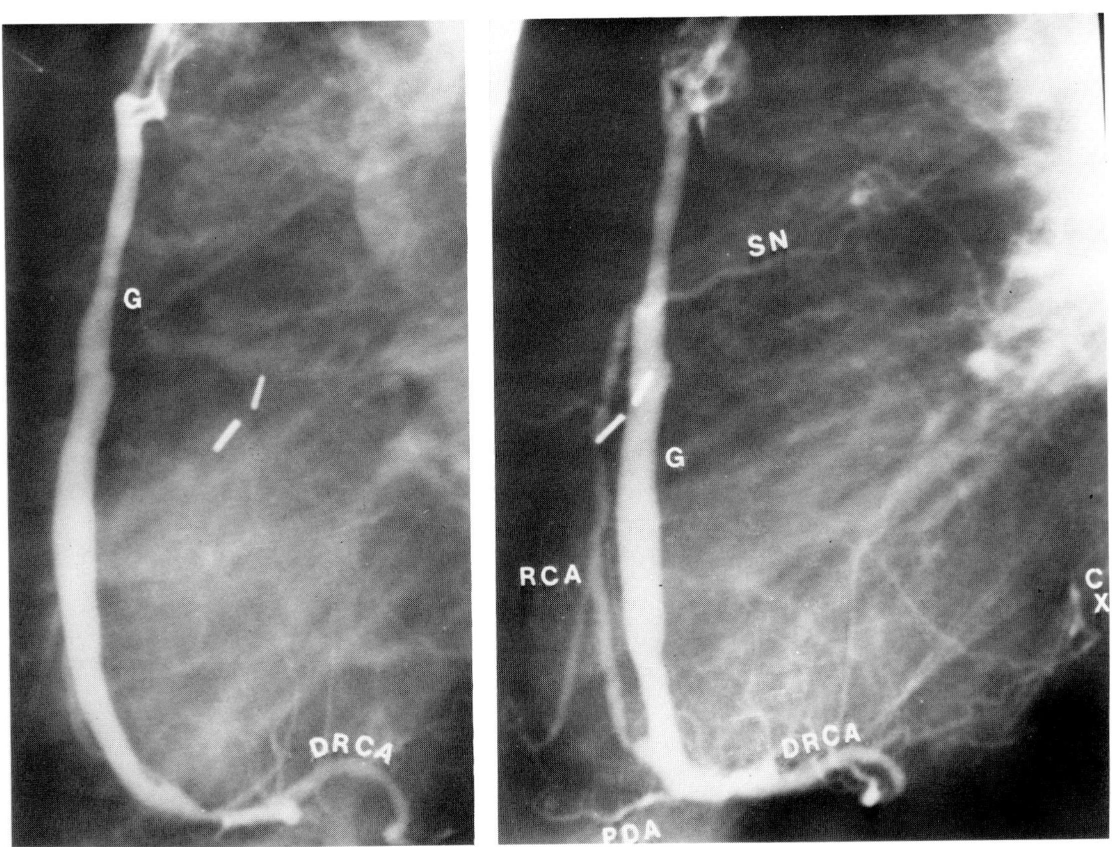

A   **FIGURE 12.9**   B

Figure 12.10:   Saphenous vein graft, aorta to left anterior descending coronary artery. **A** and **B** in lateral projections.

A. There is a marked disproportion in size between the graft (G) and the artery (LAD) with poor filling of the left anterior descending artery (LAD) in both the antegrade and retrograde directions. A diagonal branch (D) is demonstrated.

B. There is greater disproportion between the graft (G) and artery (LAD) and there is total lack of opacification of the distal left anterior descending artery. Only a short segment of the LAD is visualized proximal to the site of anastomosis. Collateral flow through the septals (S) opacifies the posterior descending coronary artery (PDA).

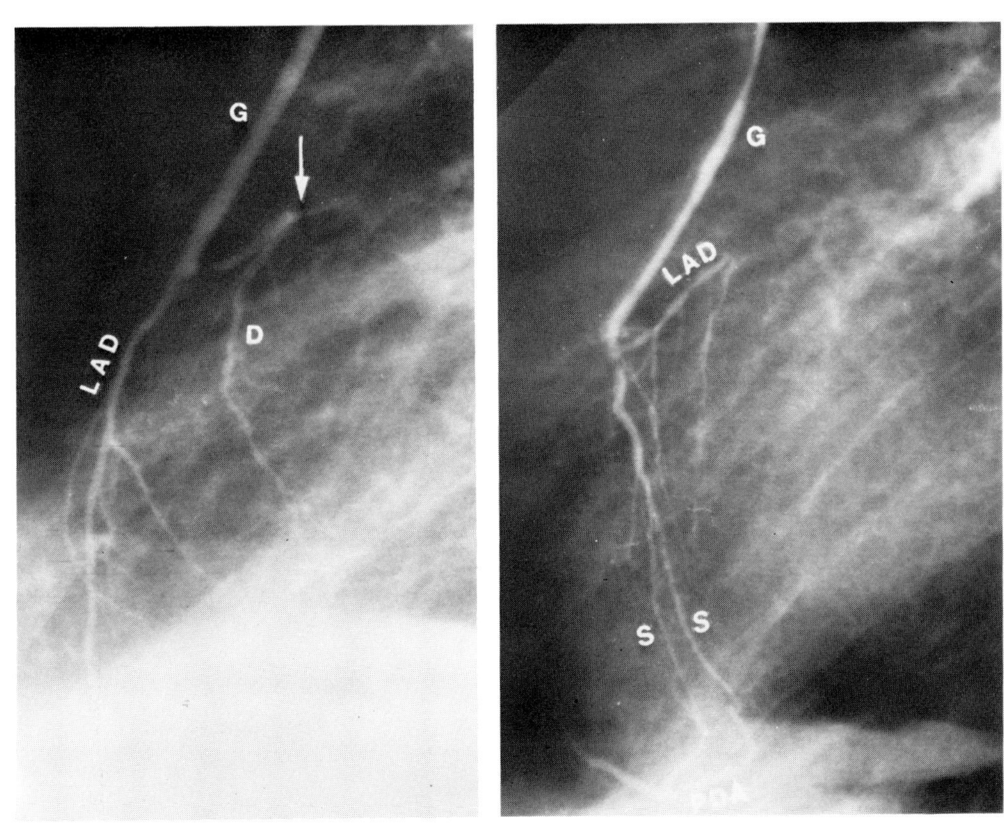

A　　　　**FIGURE 12.10**　　　　**B**

Figure 12.11: Left coronary arteriogram, lateral projection.

A. There is tenting of the left anterior descending coronary artery (LAD) at the junction of the proximal and middle thirds of the LAD at the site of anastomosis of the graft (G). There is obvious reflux into the graft. Partial opacification or layering of contrast material in the distal LAD is due to predominant flow of non-opacified blood from the graft to the LAD.

B. Diagrammatic representation of **A**.

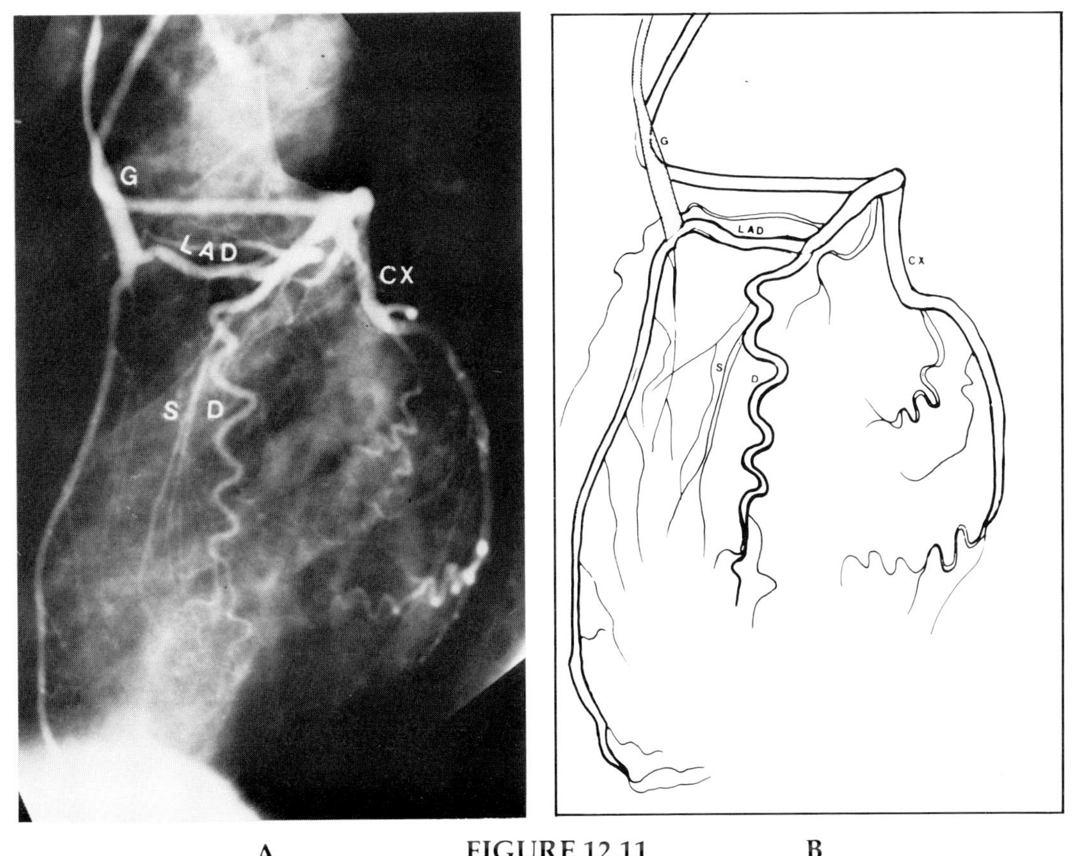

A   FIGURE 12.11   B

Figure 12.12: Left coronary arteriogram, right anterior oblique projection. **A**. Early phase; **C**. Later phase. Post-operative study of a patient with stenosis of the left main coronary artery.

A. Injection into the left coronary artery demonstrates retrograde filling of the saphenous vein graft (G) to the left marginal (LM) branch of the left circumflex artery (CX).

B. Diagrammatic representation of **A.**

A

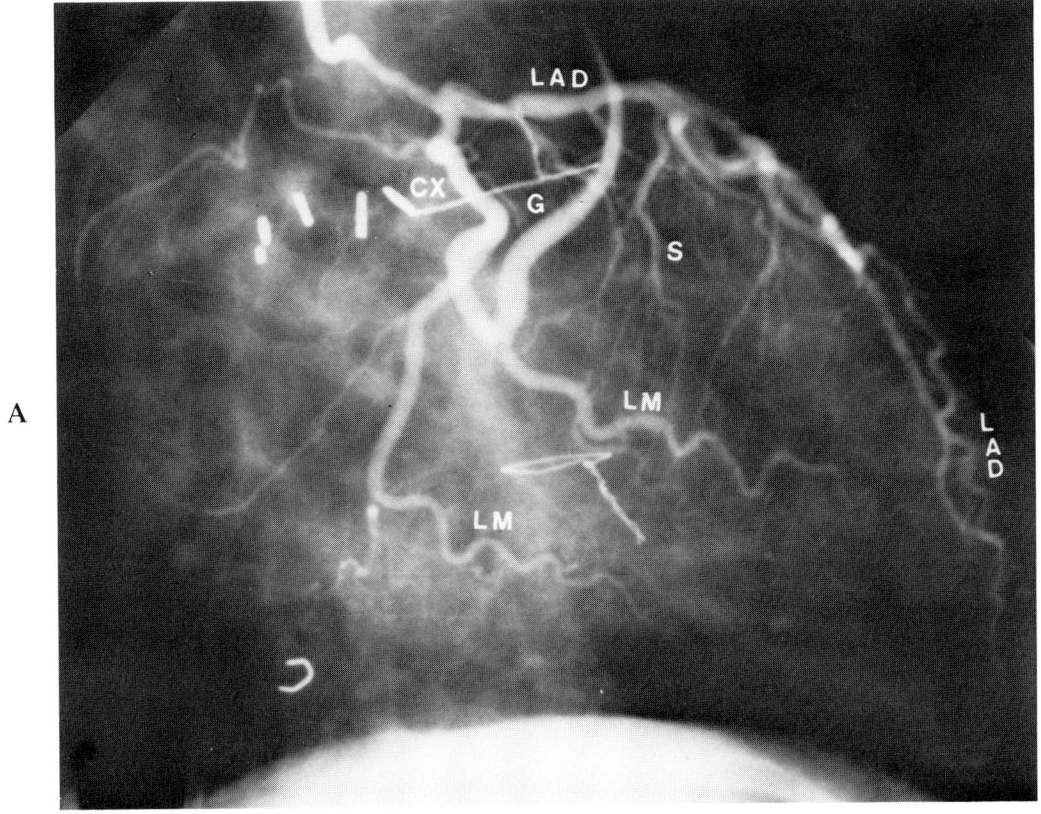

B

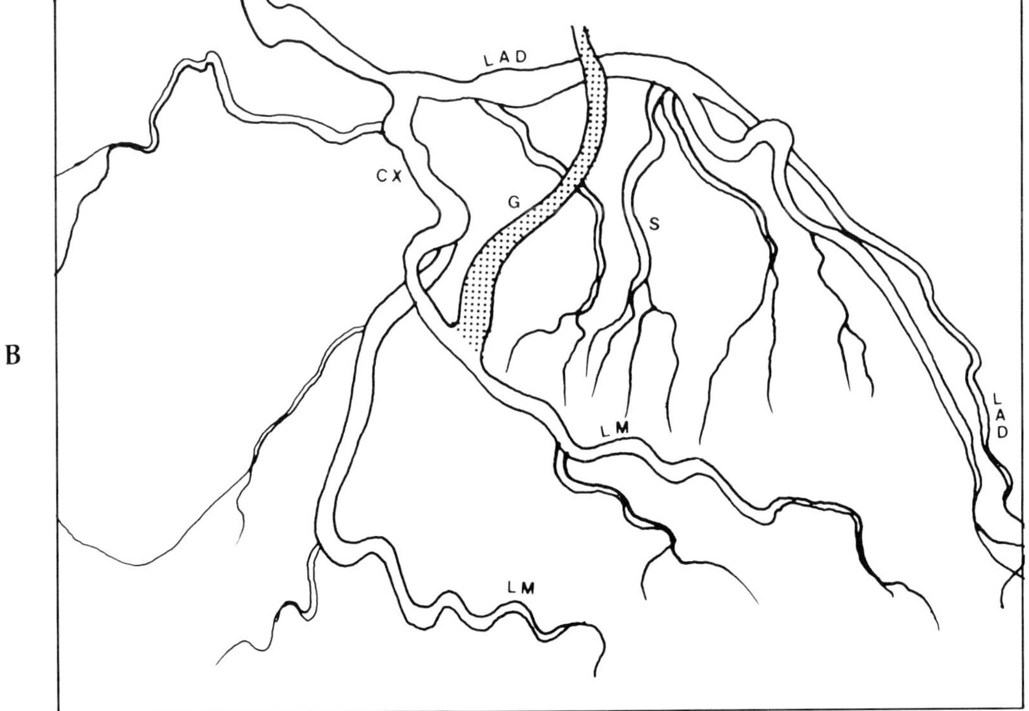

FIGURE 12.12

Figure 12.12:   C. In this later phase the graft to the left anterior descending artery (LAD) is also seen to fill in retrograde fashion (lower G and arrow).

S = septal branch of left anterior descending artery.

D. Diagrammatic representation of C.

C

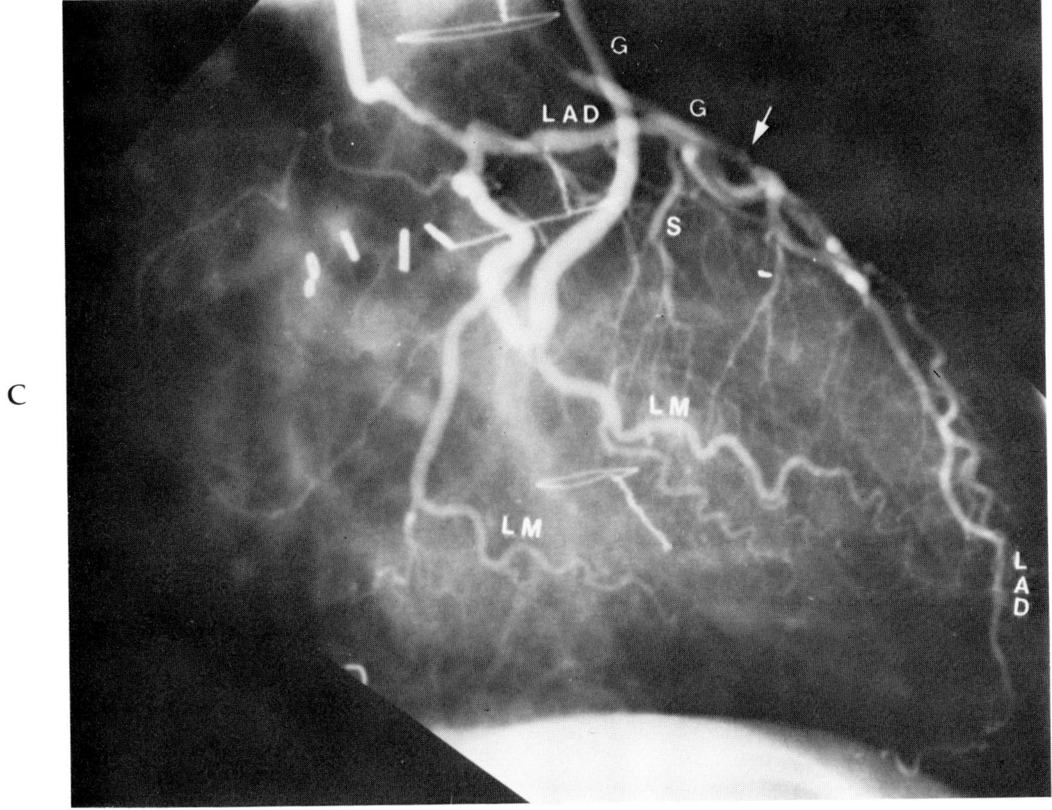

D

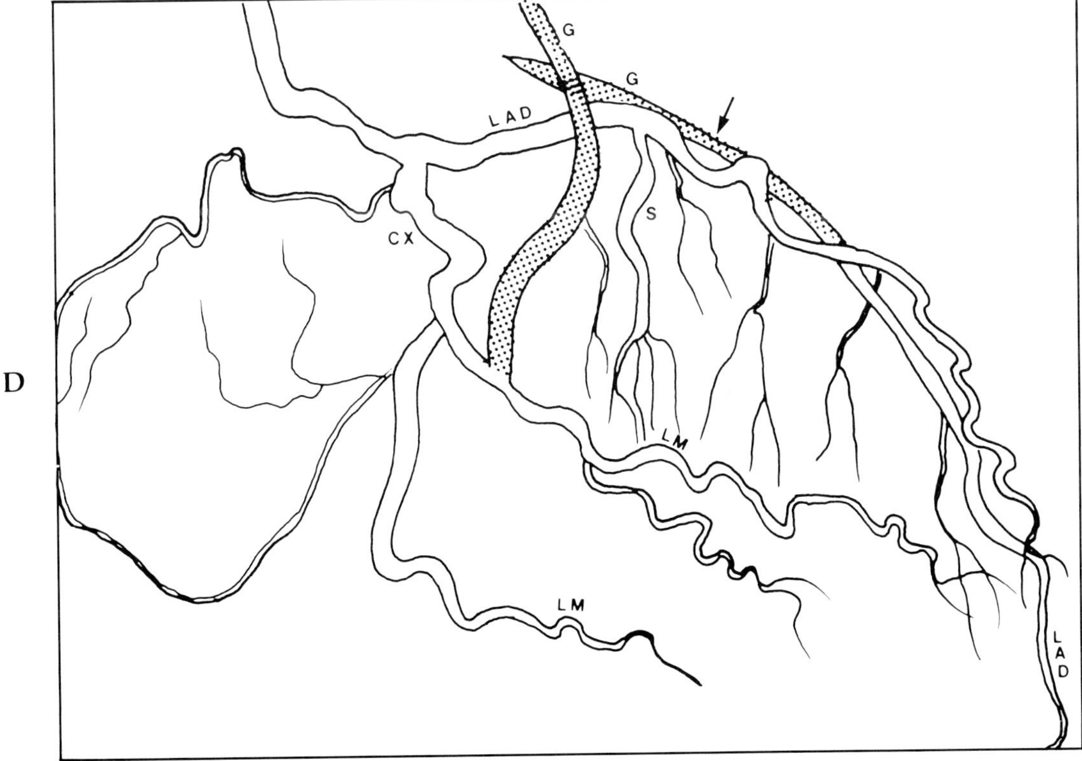

FIGURE 12.12

Figure 12.13: Left coronary arteriogram, left anterior oblique projection. **A.** Pre-operative study; **B.** Post-operative study seven months later.

A. There is a significant (70-90%) stenosis of the left main coronary artery (LCA, arrow). The left anterior descending coronary artery (LAD) and the left circumflex artery (CX) are well seen.

B. There is significant progression in the severity of the lesion in the left main coronary artery (LCA, arrows). The saphenous vein grafts from aorta to LAD and CX were demonstrated to be patent. This is an example of progression of coronary disease in grafted arteries at sites proximal to anastomosis of patent grafts.

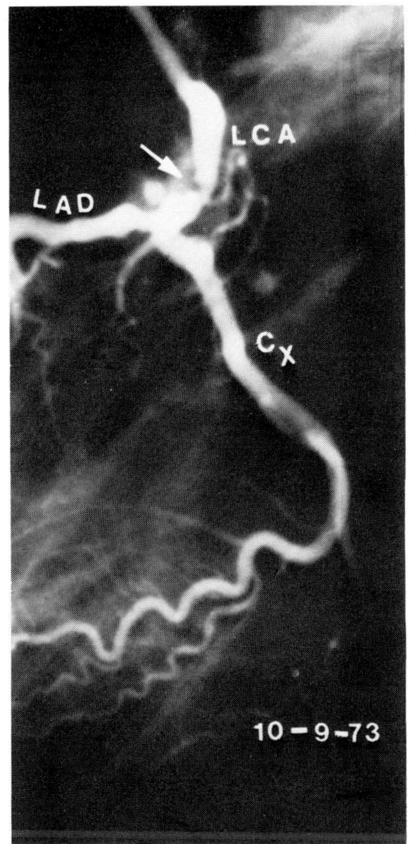

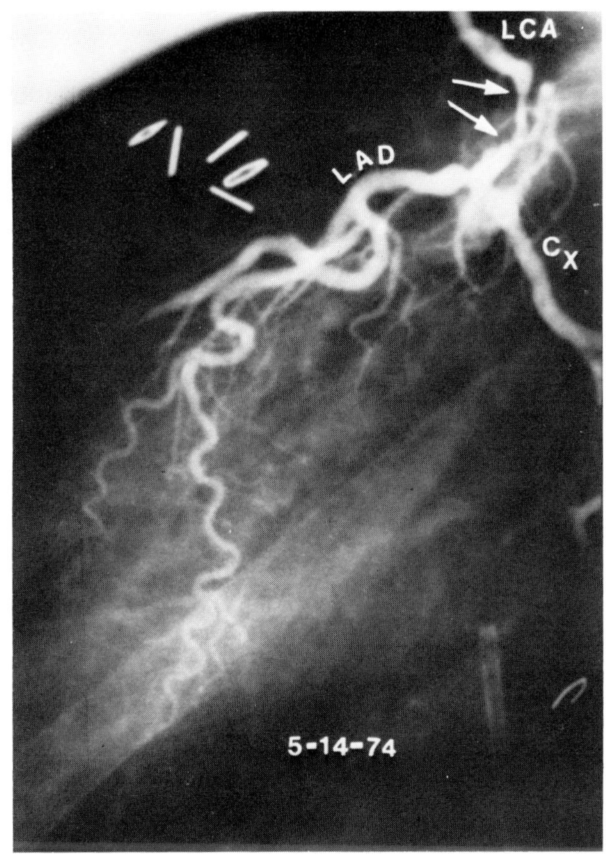

A   **FIGURE 12.13**   B